SECOND EDITION

Eat Well & *Keep Moving*

An Interdisciplinary Curriculum for Teaching Upper Elementary School Nutrition and Physical Activity

Lilian W.Y. Cheung, DSc, RD
Harvard School of Public Health

Hank Dart, MS
Health Communication Consultant

Sari Kalin, MS
Harvard School of Public Health

Steven L. Gortmaker, PhD
Harvard School of Public Health

A CD-ROM OR DVD ACCOMPANY
THIS BOOK – SEE WALLET ON
INSIDE LEFT COVER

Human Kinetics

Library of Congress Cataloging-in-Publication Data

Eat well & keep moving : an interdisciplinary curriculum for teaching upper elementary school nutrition and physical activity / Lilian W.Y. Cheung ... [et al.]. -- 2nd ed.
   p. cm.
 Previous edition has main entry under Lilian W.Y. Cheung.
 ISBN-13: 978-0-7360-6940-3 (soft cover)
 ISBN-10: 0-7360-6940-2 (soft cover)
 1. Nutrition--Study and teaching (Elementary) 2. Exercise--Study and teaching (Elementary) I. Cheung, Lilian W. Y., 1951- II. Cheung, Lilian W. Y., 1951- Eat well & keep moving. III. Title: Eat well and keep moving.
 TX364.C44 2007
 372.3'7--dc22

                    2007014820

ISBN-10: 0-7360-6940-2
ISBN-13: 978-0-7360-6940-3

The Web addresses cited in this text were current as of July 9, 2007, unless otherwise noted.

Acquisitions Editor: Bonnie Pettifor Vreeman; **Managing Editor:** Amy Stahl; **Assistant Editor:** Jackie Walker; **Copyeditor:** Jocelyn Engman; **Proofreader:** Joanna Hatzopoulos Portman; **Permission Manager:** Dalene Reeder; **Graphic Designer:** Bob Reuther; **Graphic Artist:** Denise Lowry; **Photo Manager:** Jason Allen; **Cover Designer:** Keith Blomberg; **Illustrator (cover):** Mary Anne Lloyd; **Photographer (interior):** Tom Roberts, unless otherwise noted; **Art Manager:** Kelly Hendren; **Associate Art Manager:** Alan L. Wilborn; **Illustrators:** Alan L. Wilborn, Keri Evans, Tom Roberts, Sharon Smith, and Denise Lowry; **Printer:** Sheridan Books

Printed in the United States of America   10 9 8 7 6 5 4 3 2 1

Human Kinetics
Web site: www.HumanKinetics.com

United States: Human Kinetics, P.O. Box 5076, Champaign, IL 61825-5076
800-747-4457
e-mail: humank@hkusa.com

Canada: Human Kinetics, 475 Devonshire Road Unit 100, Windsor, ON N8Y 2L5
800-465-7301 (in Canada only)
e-mail: orders@hkcanada.com

Europe: Human Kinetics, 107 Bradford Road, Stanningley, Leeds LS28 6AT, United Kingdom
+44 (0) 113 255 5665
e-mail: hk@hkeurope.com

Australia: Human Kinetics, 57A Price Avenue, Lower Mitcham, South Australia 5062
08 8372 0999
e-mail: info@hkaustralia.com

New Zealand: Human Kinetics, Division of Sports Distributors NZ Ltd., P.O. Box 300 226 Albany, North Shore City, Auckland
0064 9 448 1207
e-mail: info@humankinetics.co.nz

To all children, parents, educators,
and school food service personnel

Contents

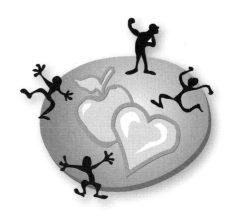

Preface

Eat Well & Keep Moving is a school-based program that equips children with the knowledge, skills, and supportive environment they need to lead more healthful lives by choosing nutritious diets and being physically active. Research shows that a good diet and physical activity can significantly reduce the risk of obesity and chronic diseases such as heart disease, high blood pressure, and type 2 diabetes, all of which can begin early in childhood. However, many children are not eating the food and getting the exercise they need to combat these chronic diseases and promote good lifelong health. Indeed, the rate of child overweight is on the rise in the United States and around the world; type 2 diabetes, once found primarily in adults, is increasingly being diagnosed in youths. It is especially disconcerting that, as children age and move into adolescence and then adulthood, they become progressively less active and choose less healthy diets. This trend makes it even more important for children to develop healthful habits early in life so that these practices can be sustained into adulthood.

The *Eat Well & Keep Moving* program was launched to provide teachers and school staff with the tools that students need to lead healthier lives. Initially designed as a joint research project between the Harvard School of Public Health and Baltimore City Public Schools, *Eat Well & Keep Moving* has evolved into a comprehensive program that can be introduced in other school systems throughout the country, including urban, suburban, and rural schools. The program received the Dannon Institute Award for Excellence in Community Nutrition in 2000. Since the publication of the first edition of *Eat Well & Keep Moving* in 2001, the program has been disseminated throughout all 50 U.S. states and across more than 20 countries.

Unlike traditional health curricula, *Eat Well & Keep Moving* is a multifaceted program encompassing all aspects of the learning environment, from the classroom, the cafeteria, and the gymnasium to school hallways, homes, and even community centers. This comprehensive approach, as recommended by the Centers for Disease Control and Prevention's coordinated school health program model, helps reinforce crucial messages about nutrition and physical activity and increases the chance that students will eat well and keep moving throughout their lives.

Numerous existing curricula address either nutrition or physical activity independently, yet few address nutrition and physical activity simultaneously. This program is a significant addition to elementary school curricula, not only because it was among the first to address both nutrition and physical activity, but also because it was among the first to address children's physical inactivity (namely television viewing and computer game playing). In this updated edition of *Eat Well & Keep Moving,* we have incorporated recommendations from the *Dietary Guidelines for Americans 2005,* and we have included two new lessons on sugar-sweetened beverage consumption, a key determinant of child overweight.

The six interlinked components of *Eat Well & Keep Moving*—classroom education, physical education, school-wide promotional campaigns, food service, staff wellness, and parent involvement—work together to create a supportive learning environment that promotes the learning of good lifelong habits. But *Eat Well & Keep Moving* does more than just work well for students. As it uses existing school resources, fits within most school curricula, contains camera-ready teaching materials, and is inexpensive to implement, teachers and schools find it easy to adopt as well. Feedback from the teachers who have taught the curriculum has been exceptionally positive. In particular, teachers have praised the integration of *Eat Well & Keep Moving* lesson plans into core subject areas, and they see that integration as fundamental to the program's success. Schools are hard-pressed to find time for "extra" subjects; with the integrated design of *Eat Well & Keep Moving*, nutrition and physical activity can be taught by classroom teachers in core subject areas (including math, language arts, and science). For information on how the lessons align with state standards in core subject areas, visit the *Eat Well & Keep Moving* Web site, www.eatwellandkeepmoving.org.

You can make the *Eat Well & Keep Moving* program as broad or as focused as you like. Choose the approach that works best for you. Focusing solely on the classroom portion of the program will provide students with excellent knowledge and skills that they can apply throughout life. The program is at its strongest, though, when it includes the entire school community: other teachers (classroom and physical education teachers), food service staff, the school food environment and policies, and parents or guardians. The power of the *Eat Well & Keep Moving* messages is enhanced even further when students are exposed to these messages in other classes, experience them in the cafeteria and school hallways, and put them into practice at home with their parents or guardians. Implementing *Eat Well & Keep Moving*—either the curriculum or the broad program—can also help schools meet new federally mandated wellness policy criteria.

The *Eat Well & Keep Moving* book and accompanying CD-ROM provide all the information you need to implement the program, whether you are introducing it into a single classroom or expanding it to an entire school community or school system. We encourage you to customize the content of the program according to your school and student population profile. For example, schools can tailor the foods, language, and customs of the lesson plans and activities to their student population.

Eat Well & Keep Moving Components

Parts I and II of the *Eat Well & Keep Moving* book contain the interdisciplinary fourth- and fifth-grade classroom lessons that provide students with in-depth exposure to the program's nutrition and physical activity themes. Through a feature unique to these lessons, students learn about nutrition and physical activity while actually being physically active in the classroom. This feature is especially valuable in schools where physical education is limited or not available.

Part III, Promotions for the Classroom, offers students and teachers fun and engaging ways to put the themes of the program into practice. These promotions include class walking clubs, a week of featuring fruits and vegetables through Get 3 At School and 5+ A Day, the Freeze My TV contest, and the Tour de Health game.

Parts IV, V, VI, and VII contain the physical education lessons, the FitChecks, the FitCheck physical education microunits, and the additional physical education microunits. The physical education lessons offer students more traditional physical education activities, many of which also integrate nutrition topics. Students learn as they move, and by doing so they begin to appreciate the importance of both eating well and being physically active. The FitCheck is a tool for self-assessment of activity and inactivity. Teachers and students are taught how to use this tool in order to evaluate how students are progressing. The FitCheck physical education microunits are designed to be used with the FitCheck materials to teach students about a variety of topics in physical activity. Likewise, the additional physical education microunits are brief 5-minute lessons that cover a wide range of physical activity topics.

Both the FitCheck microunits and the additional microunits have been formatted differently from the rest of the book. These units use many bulleted lists to provide you with an easy outline to follow while you are delivering the lessons to your students. You will notice text boxes within the microunits. These text boxes contain additional information that you can share with your students to help them learn even more about the topic at hand.

The appendixes describe stretches and strength exercises that you will use throughout the book, and they also house the Eat Well cards and the Keep Moving cards. These cards offer a quick and fun way for students to synthesize and put into practice the nutrition and physical activity information they learn through the lessons and other promotions.

The *Eat Well & Keep Moving* CD-ROM provides in-depth implementation manuals and supporting materials for each part of the program as well as information for running workshops to train fellow teachers, food service staff, and community members about nutrition and physical education. It contains a comprehensive list of Web resources on nutrition, physical activity, improving the school environment, school wellness policies, and other related topics. It also includes the classroom and physical education lessons, worksheets, and other reproducibles contained in this book.

Even more important than the scope of your school's approach to implementing the *Eat Well & Keep Moving* program is the fact that you are teaching your students how important it is to eat well and keep moving. This lesson will not only help them be healthier and happier students right now but will also give them the knowledge and skills they need for good lifelong health.

Acknowledgments

The *Eat Well & Keep Moving* program was developed over five years by a team headed by Lilian Cheung and Steven Gortmaker. The ideas for the program evolved among the faculty at the Harvard School of Public Health after the 1991 Harvard Conference on Nutrition and Physical Activity for Youth, cochaired by Lilian Cheung and Julius Richmond. In 1993, the program began in earnest with support from Christy and John Walton of the Walton Family Foundation. Christy and John Walton had long been concerned about the state of children's nutrition and the role of public schools. We want to express our sadness over John's death in 2005; his good work lives on through *Eat Well & Keep Moving*. The Waltons introduced Lilian Cheung and her colleagues to the Baltimore City Public Schools, where the pilot program for *Eat Well & Keep Moving* started in 1993. Research documenting the effectiveness of *Eat Well & Keep Moving* was published in 1999 (Gortmaker et al., 1999). The program was such a resounding success that the Baltimore City Department of Education made it available to all public elementary schools in Baltimore.

Eat Well & Keep Moving was the result of a strong collaboration among faculty members from the Departments of Nutrition, Society, Human Development, and Health, Epidemiology, and Biostatistics at the Harvard School of Public Health. The team of co-investigators included Lilian Cheung, Steven Gortmaker, Karen Peterson, Graham Colditz, and Nan Laird. *Eat Well & Keep Moving* owes its success to many dedicated individuals spanning a wide range of expertise, including educators, academic researchers, nutritionists, food service specialists, and physical education teachers. The authors wish to thank those listed in the following paragraphs for their dedication, hard work, and perseverance. *Eat Well & Keep Moving* would never have become a reality without them.

There are numerous individuals whose contributions have been invaluable to the completion of this second edition. We would like to thank Lori Marcotte for her work updating lessons and writing new materials; Juliana Weinstein for her updates to the lessons, the Eat Well cards, and the CD-ROM; and Margaret Connors for creating the nature walk activities. We also offer our thanks to Susan Carle, Kyle Miller, and Alicia Pendergast, health educators with the Boston Connects program, for their timely testing of new and revised lessons in the Boston Public Schools; thanks also to Patrice DiNatale and Maureen Kenney of Boston College for facilitating our connection with Boston Connects.

Special thanks to the authors of the *Planet Health* microunits (Carter et al., 2000, 2007), Jill Carter, Jean Wiecha, Karen Peterson, Steven Gortmaker, and Suzanne Nobrega, for adapting 11 units for use with *Eat Well & Keep Moving* and updating them for this second edition. We would like to thank the *Planet Health* team, along with Kendrin Sonneville, for developing and sharing with us the Balanced Plate for Health. Thanks are also due to Suzanne Nobrega, project coordinator for the *Planet Health* revision, for being a liaison to the *Planet Health* revision team and contributing ideas to the CD-ROM; to Jill Carter, for her ideas for new extension activities and the sugar-sweetened beverage lesson; to Dariush Mozaffarian, for his review of our background material on trans fat; to Frank Hu and David Ludwig, for sharing their insights on sugar-sweetened beverages and blood glucose response; to Laurie Torf and Patricia Gregory of Harvard University Dining Services, for contributing the Peach Salsa recipe and assisting with other recipe updates; and to Teresa Fung, for her review of the final manuscript of the second edition.

The first edition of *Eat Well & Keep Moving* would not have been realized without the help of the original Harvard team that created the program. Our sincerest thanks go to Ginny Chomitz for her leadership early on and for overseeing process evaluation; Jay Hammond Cradle, our strategic liaison between Harvard and Baltimore and the person who truly made it possible for the program to be a success; Marianne Lee for her skillful project management; Wendy Fraser, Julie Fredericksen, and Ronita Wisniewski for coordinating the project as well as playing key roles in materials development; Karen Peterson for her global vision of public health nutrition and the importance of intervention studies; Graham Colditz and Alison Field for their insights and forthright advice; Nan Laird for her guidance in statistical methods; and Kevin Morris, Shari Sprong, Shirley Hung, Kelley Wells, Darlene Ratliff, and Teresa Fung for their input into the manuals. We owe special thanks to Barbara Lind for leading retreats that inspired us all and to Jon Chomitz for his artistic inputs in the photographic essay and the design of the *Eat Well & Keep Moving* logo. We thank Helen Klipp for helping us pull together the *Eat Well & Keep Moving* grant.

We are grateful to Harvey Fineberg, former Harvard University Provost, and Barry Bloom, Dean of the Harvard School of Public Health, for endorsing *Eat Well & Keep Moving*. We thank Walter Willett, Chair of the Department of Nutrition, for his wise counsel and his unwavering support. We appreciate too the efforts of John Lichten at the Harvard School of Public Health for his skillful assistance in the contract management, and we thank Eleanor Livingston for her administrative support.

We owe a great debt of gratitude to our other colleagues in Baltimore; special thanks to Reba Bullock and Edith Fulmore of the Department of Curriculum and Instruction for working with us in development of the classroom lessons and teacher trainings, as well as assistance from their colleagues Andrea Boyer, April Lewis, and Brenda Holmes. Vivian Brake for playing a leading role in the food service programs, Jan Desper Maybin for her staff wellness work, Alanna Taylor for parental involvement components, and Ruth Bushnell for her innovative work in creating classroom-based physical activity lesson plans. Special thanks go to Former Superintendent Walter Amprey; Matthew Riley of the Baltimore City Department of Education; and Leonard Smackum, director of the Department of Food and Nutrition Services, and his colleagues Joann Bell, Shirley Kane, and Kathleen Wilson.

Eat Well & Keep Moving would never have left the drawing board without the dedication of the principals from the collaborating schools. They are truly the unsung heroines who continue to inspire and nurture their students. Thank you for their honest feedback and guidance. Specifically, we want to recognize Doris Graham of Dr. Rayner Browne Elementary School; Rosemunde Smith and Flora Johnson of Mary E. Rodman Elementary School; Shirley Johnson of Edgewood Elementary School; Ann Moore of Sarah M. Roach Elementary School; Janice Noranbrock of Mildred Monroe Elementary School; and Julia Winder of Graceland Park-O'Donnell Heights. In addition, we would like to thank the principals from participating schools: Bernice Welcher of City Springs Elementary School; Barbara Hill and Betty Ross of George Street Elementary School; Iris Harris of Collington Square Elementary School; Addie Johnson of Robert W. Coleman Elementary School; Mayess Craig of Walter P. Carter Elementary School; Dale Parker-Brown and Patricia Dennis of Montebello Elementary School; Margaret Wicks and Jean Tien of Holabird Elementary School; and Elizabeth L. Turner of Tench Tilghman Elementary School.

We would like to thank all lead teachers and teachers who assisted in the training and evaluation of the program: Verbena Redmond of Dr. Rayner Browne Elementary School; Sandra Watt of Edgewood Elementary School; Myra Smith of Graceland Park-O'Donnell Heights; Marian J. McCrea of Mary E. Rodman Elementary School; Cecelia Cooper of Mildred Monroe Elementary School; and Dorothy M. Simpson of Sarah M. Roach Elementary School. We especially appreciate the efforts of the fourth- and fifth-grade teachers in Baltimore elementary schools who taught the lessons and gave us valuable feedback. Moreover, we express our gratitude to all food service staff, students, parent liaisons, and parents in participating schools.

We acknowledge with thanks the assistance provided by volunteer organizations in Baltimore: the American Cancer Society, Maryland Cooperative Extension Services, Maryland Food Committee, National Black Women's Health Project, and Operation Frontline.

Special thanks are due to Abt Associates and especially to Mary Kay Fox (now at Mathematica Policy Research) for her leadership and competence in managing data collection and to Mary Jo Cutler for her input in food service and training. We thank Scott Wikgren, Amy Tocco, Bonnie Pettifor Vreeman, Amy Stahl, and their talented editorial staff at Human Kinetics for their help in making *Eat Well & Keep Moving* available nationally and internationally.

We are very grateful for the guidance of a distinguished advisory board: William Dietz (chair), Cheryl Achterberg, Dorothy Caldwell, Janet Collins, Dale Conoscenti, Tony Earls, John Foreyt, David Herzog, Nancy Harmon Jenkins, Sue Kimm, Katherine Merseth, Julius Richmond, Alex Roche, James Sallis, Cassandra Simmons, and Walter Willett. We thank the United States Department of Agriculture for recognizing the excellence of this program in granting *Eat Well & Keep Moving* a Promising Practice award in 1997.

We express our gratitude to the Walton Family Foundation for the generous funding that brought this project to life, and in particular we thank John and Christy Walton for years of supporting and championing this project. Finally, we thank all the children who participated in *Eat Well & Keep Moving*. Their critiques gave us invaluable insights toward developing a successful program. They continue to inspire us, and we wish them a healthy and bright future.

Lilian Cheung
Hank Dart
Sari Kalin
Steve Gortmaker
July 2007

Carter, J., J. Wiecha, K.E. Peterson, and S.L. Gortmaker. 2000. *Planet Health*. Champaign, IL: Human Kinetics. Carter, J., J. Wiecha, K.E. Peterson, S.L. Gortmaker, and S. Nobrega, S. 2007. *Planet Health: An Interdisciplinary Curriculum for Teaching Middle School Nutrition and Physical Activity*. Champaign, IL: Human Kinetics. Gortmaker, S.L., L.W.Y. Cheung, K.E. Peterson, G. Chomitz, J.H. Cradle, H. Dart, M.K. Fox, R.B. Bullock, A.M. Sobol, G. Colditz, A. Field, and N. Laird. 1999. Impact of a school-based interdisciplinary intervention on diet and physical activity among urban primary school children: Eat well and keep moving. *Archives of Pediatrics and Adolescent Medicine, 153*: 975-83.

Introduction

The *Eat Well & Keep Moving* book comprises two main sections: section 1, which contains the classroom lessons and promotions, and section 2, which contains the physical education lessons and microunits. In addition, the *Eat Well & Keep Moving* CD-ROM expands the program beyond your classroom to food services, other teachers, and students' homes.

Section 1

The classroom component (parts I–III) of *Eat Well & Keep Moving* combines nutrition and physical activity lessons, discussion cards (Eat Well cards and Keep Moving cards), and promotional activities to create a reinforcing and supportive learning environment for students.

The lessons on nutrition and physical activity are the most prominent feature of the classroom component. The 26 multidisciplinary lessons for fourth and fifth grades (13 for each grade) provide students with the knowledge and skills they need to choose healthful eating patterns and be physically active. Developed with elementary school teachers, these lessons

- are meant to be integrated into core subject areas,
- follow a format familiar to educators,
- meet educational standards,
- require minimal teacher training, and
- are simple and easy to use.

Parts I and II: Classroom Lessons on Nutrition and Physical Activity

The classroom lessons on nutrition and physical activity are the cornerstone of *Eat Well & Keep Moving.* The fourth-grade (part I) and fifth-grade (part II) lessons use multidisciplinary teaching and unique approaches to equip students with the knowledge and lifelong skills they need to choose a nutritious diet and be physically active.

Designed to fit easily into a school's curriculum, the lessons address a wide range of learning outcomes and can be taught across numerous subject areas (such as math, language arts, social studies, and visual arts). See table I.1 on page xvii for a detailed list of the competencies addressed by the classroom lessons. Depending on your school, the lessons can be taught either as part of the regular core subjects or as health education.

Lesson Messages

The *Eat Well & Keep Moving* classroom lessons focus on six simple messages for students. These messages are called the *Principles of Healthy Living*:

- Eat 5 or more servings of fruits and vegetables each day.
- Choose whole-grain foods and limit foods and beverages with added sugar.
- Choose healthy fat, limit saturated fat, and avoid trans fat.
- Eat a nutritious breakfast every morning.
- Be physically active every day for at least an hour per day.
- Limit television and other screen time to no more than 2 hours per day.

Through lessons on overall health, the five food groups, best-choice foods within the food groups, safe physical workouts, and the Balanced Plate for Health, students learn the value of these six messages and acquire the knowledge and skills to put them into practice. To help you see at a glance which of these key messages are emphasized in each lesson, icons representing each message are found on the opening page of each lesson, as well as on each transparency and worksheet.

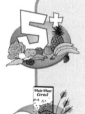

Go for 5⁺ Fruits and Veggies—More Is Better!
▶ Eat 5 or more servings of fruits and vegetables each day.

Get Whole Grains and Sack the Sugar!
▶ Choose whole-grain foods and limit foods and beverages with added sugar.

Keep the Fat Healthy!
▶ Choose healthy fat, limit saturated fat, and avoid trans fat.

Start Smart With Breakfast!
▶ Eat a nutritious breakfast every morning.

Keep Moving!
▶ Be physically active every day for at least an hour per day.

Freeze the Screen!
▶ Limit television and other screen time to no more than 2 hours per day.

▶ Icon key.

▶TABLE I.1 Eat Well & Keep Moving Education Components

Classroom activity*	Quantity	Description
PARTS I AND II—CLASSROOM LESSONS		
Part I—Fourth grade	13	Classroom lessons on wellness, the five food groups, sugar-sweetened beverages, whole grains, healthy fat, fruits and vegetables, snacking, the Balanced Plate for Health, limiting television and other screen time, and the safe workout
Part II—Fifth grade	13	Classroom lessons on wellness, the five food groups, sugar-sweetened beverages, whole grains, healthy fat, fruits and vegetables, snacking, the Balanced Plate for Health, limiting television and other screen time, and the safe workout
PART III—PROMOTIONS FOR THE CLASSROOM		
Class Walking Clubs	1	Yearlong class walking clubs
Freeze My TV	1	Weeklong activity focusing on limiting students' television and screen time
Get 3 At School and 5+ A Day	1	Weeklong activity focusing on getting at least 3 servings of fruits and vegetables while at school and at least 5 servings for the entire day
Tour de Health	1	A question-and-answer game that reinforces the six key healthy living messages of Eat Well & Keep Moving; includes the My Tour de Health booklet
Eat Well cards	18	Brief discussions focusing primarily on healthful selections in the cafeteria
Keep Moving cards	2	Brief discussion of physical activity topics addressed in the classroom and physical education lessons
PARTS IV, V, VI, VII—PHYSICAL EDUCATION ACTIVITIES		
Fourth- and fifth-grade lessons	5	Physical education lessons following the safe workout while also addressing nutrition issues
Fourth- and fifth-grade FitCheck	2	Tool for student self-assessment of activity and inactivity
Fourth- and fifth-grade FitCheck PE microunits and additional PE microunits	9	Brief 5 min. activities teaching a variety of nutrition and physical education topics; 4 are designed to be used with the FitCheck, and 5 cover other physical activity and nutrition topics

*For information on how the classroom lessons align with state standards in math, language arts, science, social studies/history, health, and physical education, visit the Eat Well & Keep Moving Web site, www.eatwellandkeepmoving.org.

Lesson Format

The Eat Well & Keep Moving lessons are clear and easy to use. Each lesson is described step by step, and each lesson begins with background information for the teacher's use. An overhead projector and copies made from the worksheet masters are two of the few materials needed that are not included with the lessons.

The lessons are designed to fit into various core disciplines (e.g., language arts, math, science, health, social studies, and art). This design not only allows the lesson to fit easily into the class schedule but also spreads the program's message across all facets of the students' school day.

Physical Activity Lessons for the Classroom

One of the many unique aspects of the *Eat Well & Keep Moving* classroom lessons is that a number of the lessons teach nutrition and physical activity issues while students are actually moving. This approach reinforces the importance of eating a nutritious diet and being physically active. Addressing both issues simultaneously helps convey this link between them to students. Also, getting students moving in the classroom can supplement a school's physical education program.

The structure of the physical activity classroom lessons is based on a five-part framework called the *safe workout.* Essentially, the safe workout teaches students the safe way to be physically active.

Each physical activity lesson leads the students through the five steps:

1. Warm-up
2. Stretch
3. Fitness activity—an active game that involves a nutrition concept
4. Cool-down
5. Cool-down stretch

After the cool-down stretch, students gather in the Stay Healthy Corner to review what they learned during the lesson. The Stay Healthy Corner can be an area of the classroom decorated with pictures or student drawings that represent the Principles of Healthy Living (e.g., healthy foods, children engaged in physical activity, and so on). Or it can be simply a time for discussion and reflection on the health messages of the lesson.

These safe workout lessons succeed in a variety of settings. While they work best in an area with open space (such as a gymnasium or a cafeteria), they have been successfully taught in the classroom itself (usually with a slight rearranging of furniture) in urban schools with class sizes of up to 30 students.

To create a large, varied collection of food pictures to use in the physical activity lessons (as well as in some of the nutrition and physical education lessons), teachers can ask students to bring in food pictures (from magazines, newspapers, and so on) or empty food packages in the weeks before the scheduled lessons. It is never too early to begin such a collection. Sets of approximately 100 food pictures may also be purchased from the National Dairy Council (800-426-8271) for around $25 U.S.

Part III: Classroom Promotions and the Eat Well Cards and Keep Moving Cards

Eat Well & Keep Moving includes four classroom promotions that build on the classroom lessons and provide students with the opportunity to put their nutrition and physical activity knowledge into practice.

Class Walking Clubs

The class walking clubs can run throughout the school year and arise directly from the lessons on fitness walking. Classes are encouraged to chart walking routes around their school and to go on walks with their teacher at least once a week. To add interest to the club, classes are encouraged to "walk" across parts of the world. Each time they walk they can accrue a certain number of miles (for example, 100 miles for every 5 minutes) and mark their progress on a map.

Freeze My TV

During the Freeze My TV week, students keep track of and try to limit the amount of their television viewing and other screen time (e.g., playing computer games, Web surfing, instant messaging). Freeze My TV ties directly to lessons 9 (fourth grade) and 21 (fifth grade). In addition to keeping track of their television and screen time, students complete graphing activities, answer questions based on their graphs, and write daily entries in the Freeze My TV Journal.

Watching television and playing video games are the main contributors to a sedentary lifestyle. Watching television also exposes children to advertisements for unhealthy foods. Getting students to limit the amount of television they watch frees up more of their time for physical activity (such as riding bikes or dancing) or working on more worthwhile projects (such as drawing or reading). One idea for supplementing Freeze My TV with art is having students create colorful posters with catchy slogans to display alternatives to watching television.

Get 3 At School and 5⁺ A Day

Students put their knowledge of healthful eating into practice during this week-long activity by trying to consume at least 3 servings of fruits and vegetables while at school. The students track their individual at-school fruit and vegetable consumption on a large class graph. In addition to getting at least 3 servings of fruits and vegetables while at school, students try to eat at least 5 servings for the entire day (more is always better). To help reach this goal, the students take home materials that reinforce this message (such as My Go for 5⁺ Tracking Chart and fruit and vegetable recipes from the Produce for Better Health Foundation Web site).

Using Eat Well cards (described later) during the Get 3 At School and 5⁺ A Day activity can further motivate students to eat their fruits and vegetables. These cards, many of which address fruits and vegetables, can be briefly discussed with students just before lunch during the week of the Get 3 At School and 5⁺ A Day activity.

Tour de Health

Tour de Health turns the *Eat Well & Keep Moving* healthy living messages into a fun and edifying game. Played in groups or as an entire class, Tour de Health can serve as a daily review for the classroom and physical education lessons as well as serve as an all-year refresher on the *Eat Well & Keep Moving* messages. The game consists of question cards covering the six healthy living messages taught throughout the *Eat Well & Keep Moving* lessons; students also get a Tour de Health scorecard (which emphasizes the healthy living messages) and an Answer Cube. When students answer the nutrition and physical activity questions on the cards correctly, they receive points. The first student or group to reach 20 points (or the student or group with the highest point total when time runs out) wins the game.

This game also includes an optional extension—the My Tour de Health booklet—that further reinforces the Principles of Healthy Living and offers an opportunity for parent involvement.

Eat Well Cards and Keep Moving Cards

Eat Well cards and Keep Moving cards reinforce key messages and link the classroom and the food service and physical education components of the program. Each card is 5.5 × 8.5 inches (14 × 22 centimeters) and contains a mixture of text and graphics. The cards present intriguing information to pique the interest of students and can be reviewed with students in as little as 3 minutes. Although brief, the Eat Well cards and Keep Moving cards play a vital role in helping students synthesize and put into practice the nutrition and physical activity information they learn through *Eat Well & Keep Moving.* These cards can also be reprinted in the school's parent newsletter, providing a valuable link between home and school.

Eat Well Cards

Eat Well cards reinforce the nutrition messages of the classroom lessons and excite students about healthful choices on the cafeteria lunch menus. With their direct relationship to the cafeteria, Eat Well cards play an integral part of the Get 3 At School and 5+ A Day activity in the classroom as well as support *Eat Well & Keep Moving* food service promotions.

For the *Eat Well & Keep Moving* Promotional Days (described in detail in the Food Service manual on the CD-ROM), a healthful food dish is highlighted each week in both the cafeteria and the classroom. Throughout the week, the dish is promoted to students in the cafeteria through table tents and posters. On the day the dish is prepared, teachers present the appropriate Eat Well card just before students go to lunch. This dual promotion helps motivate students to try the healthful dish.

Eat Well cards also remind students to eat their fruits and vegetables during the Get 3 At School and 5+ A Day promotion, when teachers are encouraged to review with students the Eat Well cards that address fruits and vegetables.

Eat Well & Keep Moving includes several ideas for using Eat Well cards in the classroom:

- Review cards with students just before lunch on an appropriate day.
- Quiz students about the information contained in the card.
- Post the Eat Well cards on a bulletin board.
- Have a group of students review a card and present the information to the entire class.
- Have the cafeteria manager present a card to the class and talk about how food is prepared in the cafeteria.

Keep Moving Cards

Keep Moving cards are similar to Eat Well cards, but they discuss physical activity issues rather than nutrition issues. Topics covered by Keep Moving cards include stretching, warming up, and physical activity recommendations. Like Eat Well cards, Keep Moving cards bolster the messages students receive outside of the classroom, in this case in the physical education class.

Eat Well & Keep Moving includes several ideas for using Keep Moving cards in the classroom:

- Review cards with students just before physical education class.
- Quiz students about the information contained in the card.
- Post the Keep Moving cards on a bulletin board.
- Have the physical education teacher come to class to present a card to the students.
- Have a group of students review a card and present the information to the entire class.

Section 2

The *Eat Well & Keep Moving* program has five physical education lessons, two versions of the FitCheck (one for the teacher and another for students), and nine microunits that complement a school's existing physical education curriculum. These lessons and microunits help students develop a lifetime habit of physical activity. They not only provide students with the skills for a safe workout but also emphasize the importance of combining good nutrition and physical activity—a concept taught throughout the program's classroom lessons.

Although similar in format to the physical activity classroom lessons, the physical education lessons and microunits are intended to be taught by the school's physical education teacher.

Lesson Format

In addition to describing the activity step by step, the physical education lessons address safety concerns and, where appropriate, include a line drawing.

The structure of the physical education lessons is based on the five-part framework of the safe workout described in section 1, although step 3 now focuses on an endurance fitness activity. If the endurance activity game laid out in the lessons is less vigorous than your students are used to, they can begin each endurance fitness activity with a jog or walk, based on this schedule:

- Lessons 31 and 32: Begin with a 4-minute jog or fast walk.
- Lessons 33 and 34: Begin with a 5-minute jog or fast walk.
- Lesson 35: Begin with a 6-minute jog or fast walk.

Because each *Eat Well & Keep Moving* physical education lesson addresses a nutrition topic, the physical education teacher may want to begin a collection of food pictures, packages, and labels. Students can help with this process by bringing in items from home. Having access to such a collection will help make the endurance fitness activities more engaging to students. Physical education teachers and classroom teachers may wish to pool their collections.

Physical educators, in addition to receiving copies of the physical education lessons, should also have access to and become familiar with the program's fourth- and fifth-grade classroom lessons. This will help teachers directly link physical education and the classroom. In addition, familiarity with the classroom lessons will allow physical educators to be a resource for classroom teachers who may have questions about some of the physical activity issues discussed in the classroom modules.

FitCheck and Microunits

The FitCheck is a tool for self-assessment of activity and inactivity, one that teachers and students can use to evaluate how students are progressing. The nine microunits (four that are designed to be used with the FitCheck materials, and five that relate to other physical education topics) are brief 5-minute lessons that cover a wide range of physical activity and nutrition topics. On days when no full-length *Eat Well & Keep Moving* physical education lesson is being taught, a microunit can be presented at the beginning of class.

CD-ROM

You can use the material on the *Eat Well & Keep Moving* CD-ROM to make nutrition and physical activity a school-wide and community-wide priority. The classroom activities and physical education lessons are powerful teaching tools in their own right, but when the *Eat Well & Keep Moving* messages are expanded to the wider school community—as suggested by the Centers for Disease Control and Promotion —their effect on students becomes even greater.

Food Service

Outside of physical education, there is no clearer tie-in to *Eat Well & Keep Moving* than the school food service. Every school day, students eat at least one meal at school, and this meal provides an excellent opportunity to reinforce the messages of *Eat Well & Keep Moving.* Reinforcement can be as simple as getting a cafeteria menu in advance and integrating it into classroom lessons or as involved as teachers working with the principal and food service manager to make permanent healthful changes to the school breakfast and lunch menus.

The CD-ROM provides detailed information for food service managers interested in making healthful changes to their school menus, including recipes, preparation tips, promotional materials, classroom tie-ins, and staff training. When implemented to its fullest, the food service component works very closely with the classroom component, as explained in the food service promotions section of the Education Guide (Manual 2) on the CD-ROM.

The link between the classroom and food service components of *Eat Well & Keep Moving* can be strengthened if teachers and the cafeteria manager openly discuss promoting the messages of the program. Teachers can invite the food service manager to give presentations in the classroom (such as an Eat Well card), and the cafeteria manager can provide teachers with regular updates on scheduled lunch menus and display on the serving line various Eat Well cards complementing the lunch items served.

Parent Involvement

Parent involvement in *Eat Well & Keep Moving* greatly bolsters the program's effectiveness. Encourage parents and family members to become involved in activities that complement the program messages students learn in school. This reinforcement increases the probability that the dietary and lifestyle changes students make will become a regular part of family and daily life.

Teachers can volunteer some of their time to organize parent activities around *Eat Well & Keep Moving* messages or can locate a parent volunteer or other teacher to spearhead such activities. The CD-ROM details different approaches to getting parents and family members involved in *Eat Well & Keep Moving*. As with all the other components of the program, your level of involvement can be as little or as great as you like. The separate components of *Eat Well & Keep Moving* stand alone very well but become even stronger when brought together.

When implemented to its full extent, the parent involvement takes a unique approach: identifying community-based health organizations to offer nutrition, physical activity, and wellness programs to parents. Additional *Eat Well & Keep Moving* activities for parent involvement include publishing nutrition and physical activity information in school newsletters and hosting program-related family activities, such as Parent Fun Nights, that allow families to see exactly what their children are learning through the *Eat Well & Keep Moving* program.

Through these *Eat Well & Keep Moving* activities, we hope that parents and guardians will become models for their children and encourage and support healthy eating practices and active lifestyles for the entire family.

Other CD-ROM Material

In addition to the food service and parent involvement material, the CD-ROM also provides

- nutrition, physical activity, and wellness workshops for teachers, and teacher training on the curriculum itself;
- the complete fourth- and fifth-grade classroom and physical education lessons;
- information for school administrators interested in *Eat Well & Keep Moving;*
- parent fact sheets and information for parent newsletters; and
- a comprehensive list of Web resources related to nutrition, physical activity, school wellness policy, improving the school environment, parental outreach, and other such topics.

Putting It All Together

All the components of the *Eat Well & Keep Moving* program complement each other. Although each component can be used independently, the power of *Eat Well & Keep Moving* is the integration of the various components into a whole-school approach.

The tables on pages xxv-xxviii offer a guide to integrating the various fourth- and fifth-grade education components. Remember that they are only a guide—the best way to integrate the program may differ from school to school, depending on each school's situation.

We encourage schools to implement as many lessons as possible, to maximize the impact of *Eat Well & Keep Moving*. If there is not enough time in the school year to implement all 13 lessons in each grade, we recommend teaching at least 7 key lessons, which cover each of the Principles of Healthy Living. These key lessons are listed in table I.4 on page xxix.

▶TABLE I.2 Fourth-Grade Implementation Grid

Classroom lessons	Promotions	Eat Well cards and Keep Moving cards	Physical education lessons*	Cafeteria activities	Parent involvement
1. Healthy Living	**31.** Tour de Health		**32.** Five Foods Countdown		
2. Carb Smart		The Power of Whole Grains	**33.** Musical Fare		• Reprint the Eat Well card in the parent newsletter. • Send home the "Eat More Whole Grains" parent fact sheet.**
3. The Safe Workout: An Introduction		Be Wise . . . Warm Up for 5 Before You Exercise			• Reprint the Keep Moving card in the parent newsletter. • Send home the "Activate Your Family!" parent fact sheet.**
4. Balancing Act					
5. Fast-Food Frenzy					• Send home the "Dietary Fats" parent fact sheet.**
6. Snack Attack			**34.** Bowling for Snacks		• Reprint the "Super Snacks" article in the parent newsletter.
7. Sugar Water: Think About Your Drink					• Reprint the "Be Sugar Smart" article in the parent newsletter. • Optional: If the lesson will be taught during warm weather, include the "Stay Cool" article in the parent newsletter.
8. The Safe Workout: Snacking's Just Fine, If You Choose the Right Kind			**31.** Three Kinds of Fitness Fun: Endurance, Strength, and Flexibility		• Reprint the Keep Moving cards in the parent newsletter.

(continued)

Classroom lessons	Promotions	Eat Well cards and Keep Moving cards	Physical education lessons*	Cafeteria activities	Parent involvement
9. Prime-Time Smartness	**27.** Freeze My TV	A Piece of the Pie?			• Reprint the Keep Moving card in the parent newsletter. • Reprint the "Tune out the TV" article in the parent newsletter. • Send home the "Take Control of TV" parent fact sheet.**
10. Chain Five	**28.** Get 3 At School and 5⁺ A Day	• To Nourish Your Body as Well as Your Soul. . . At Least 5 A Day Should Be Your Goal! • Punch Out Fruit Punch— Pick Whole Fruit • Have You Ever Heard of Pineapple Oranges? • Oranges for Each Day's Journey	**35.** Fruits and Vegetables		• Reprint the Eat Well cards in parent newsletter.
11. Alphabet Fruit (and Vegetables)					• Reprint the "Fruits and Veggies" article in the parent newsletter.
12. Brilliant Breakfast	**30.** Tour de Health (repeat)				• Reprint the "Grains" article in the parent newsletter.
13. Fitness Walking	**29.** Class Walking Clubs				• Reprint the "Keep Moving" article in the parent newsletter.

*Teaching the FitCheck, the FitCheck Microunits, and the Additional Physical Education Microunits: Use the FitCheck student self-assessment tool if it matches your students' abilities and fits into your curriculum. If you do decide to use it, we recommend scheduling FitChecks two or three times during the school year (try to make one time close to the end of the school year). The FitCheck introduction (lesson 37) and the four FitCheck Microunits (lessons 38-41) build upon one another and are best taught sequentially as a set. The Additional Physical Education Microunits (lessons 42-26) are also designed to build upon one another and are best taught sequentially as a set. However, the microunits can also be used intermittently such as on days when no full-length *Eat Well & Keep Moving* physical education lesson is being taught as long as the units are taught in the correct order.

**The parent fact sheet is also available in Spanish.

▶ TABLE I.3 Fifth-Grade Implementation Grid

Classroom lessons	Promotions	Eat Well cards and Keep moving cards	Physical education lessons*	Cafeteria activities	Parent involvement
14. Healthy Living, Healthy Eating	**31.** Tour de Health	The Power of Whole Grains	**32.** Five Foods Countdown		• Reprint the Eat Well card in the parent newslettter. • Reprint the "Grains" article in the parent newsletter.
15. Keeping the Balance					
16. The Safe Workout: A Review		Be Wise . . . Warm Up for 5 Before You Exercise			• Reprint the Keep Moving card or the "Keep Moving" article in the parent newsletter. • Send home the "Activate Your Family" parent fact sheet.**
17. Hunting for Hidden Fat					• Send home the "Dietary Fats" parent fact sheet.**
18. Beverage Buzz: Sack the Sugar					• Reprint the "Be Sugar Smart" article in the parent newsletter. • Optional: If the lesson will be taught during warm weather, include the "Stay Cool" article in the parent newsletter.
19. Snack Decisions			**33.** Musical Fare		• Reprint the "Super Snacks" article in the parent newsletter.
20. Snacking and Inactivity		A Piece of the Pie?	**34.** Bowling for Snacks		• Reprint the Keep Moving card in the parent newsletter.

(continued)

Classroom lessons	Promotions	Eat Well cards and Keep moving cards	Physical education lessons*	Cafeteria activities	Parent involvement
21. Freeze My TV	**27.** Freeze My TV				• Reprint the excerpt from the Freeze My TV Journal in the parent newsletter. • Reprint the "Tune Out the TV" article in the parent newsletter. • Send home the "Take Control of TV" parent fact sheet.**
22. Menu Monitoring					
23. Veggiemania	**28.** Get 3 At School and 5⁺ A Day	• To Nourish Your Body as Well as Your Soul . . . At Least 5 A Day Should Be Your Goal! • Punch Out Fruit Punch—Pick Whole Fruit • Have You Ever Heard of Pineapple Oranges? • Oranges for Each Day's Journey	**35.** Fruits and Vegetables		• Reprint the Eat Well card in the parent newsletter. • Reprint the Eat Well cards in the parent newsletter. • Reprint the "Fruits and Veggies" article in the parent newsletter. • Send home the "Fruits and Vegetables" parent fact sheet.**
24. Breakfast Bonanza					
25. Foods From Around the World: Italy, China, Mexico, and Ethiopia	**31.** Tour de Health (repeat)				
26. Fitness Walking	**29.** Class Walking Clubs		**31.** Three Kinds of Fitness Fun: Endurance, Strength, and Flexibility		• Reprint the "Keep Moving" article in the parent newsletter.

*Teaching the FitCheck, the FitCheck Microunits, and the Additional Physical Education Microunits: Use FitCheck student self-assessment tool if it matches your students' abilities and fits into your curriculum. If you do decide to use it, we recommend scheduling FitChecks two or three times during the school year (try to make one time close to the end of the school year). The FitCheck introduction (lesson 37) and the four FitCheck Microunits (lessons 38-41) build upon one another and are best taught sequentially as a set. The Additional Physical Education Microunits (lessons 42-26) are also designed to build upon one another and are best taught sequentially as a set. However, the microunits can also be used intermittently such as on days when no full-length *Eat Well & Keep Moving* physical education lesson is being taught as long as the units are taught in the correct order.

**The parent fact sheet is also available in Spanish.

►TABLE I.4   Key Lessons

Key messages	Fourth-grade lessons	Fifth-grade lessons	Physical education
Principles of Healthy Living (introduction to all 6 messages and to the Balanced Plate for Health)	**1.** Healthy Living	**14.** Healthy Living and Healthy Eating	**32.** Five Foods Countdown
Eat 5 or more servings of fruits and vegetables each day.	**10.** Chain Five	**22.** Menu Monitoring	**35.** Fruits and Vegetables
Choose whole-grain foods and limit foods and beverages with added sugar.	**7.** Sugar Water	**18.** Beverage Buzz	**34.** Bowling for Snacks
Choose healthy fat, limit saturated fat, and avoid trans fat.	**5.** Fast-Food Frenzy	**17.** Hunting for Hidden Fat	**43.** Be Active Now for a Healthy Heart Later (microunit)
Eat a nutritious breakfast every morning.	**12.** Brilliant Breakfast	**24.** Breakfast Bonanza	**33.** Musical Fare
Be physically active every day for at least an hour per day.	**3.** The Safe Workout: An Introduction	**15.** The Safe Workout: A Review	**31.** Three Kinds of Fitness Fun
Limit television and other screen time to no more than 2 hours per day.	**9.** Prime-Time Smartness	**21.** Freeze My TV	**39.** What Could You Do Instead of Watching TV? (microunit)

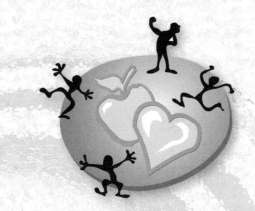

Nutrition and Physical Activity Classroom Lessons and Promotions

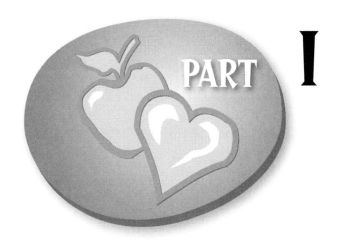

Classroom Lessons for Fourth Graders

The classroom lessons on nutrition and physical activity are the cornerstone of *Eat Well & Keep Moving.* Using a multidisciplinary teaching approach, the lessons contained in part I equip students with the knowledge and skills they need to choose a nutritious diet and be physically active both now and throughout their lives. Though effective on their own, these classroom lessons also serve as a springboard for all the other activities of *Eat Well & Keep Moving*—the promotions (part III), the physical education lessons (part IV), the FitCheck guide (part V) and FitCheck physical education microunits (part VI), the additional physical education microunits (part VII), and the cafeteria, school environment, and parent involvement components described in the CD-ROM.

Part I includes the fourth-grade lessons, in which students learn to

- eat 5 or more servings of fruits and vegetables each day;
- choose whole-grain foods and limit foods and beverages with added sugar;
- choose healthy fat, limit saturated fat, and avoid trans fat;
- eat a nutritious breakfast every morning;
- be physically active every day for at least an hour per day; and
- limit television and other screen time to no more than 2 hours per day.

Using subject areas ranging from language arts to mathematics, these lessons address, among other topics, overall health, the five food groups, smart snacking, and safe physical workouts.

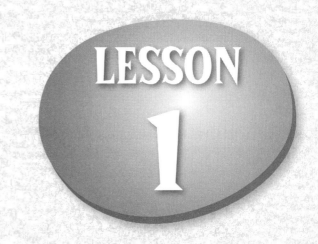

Healthy Living

BACKGROUND

Healthy living involves making lifestyle choices that maximize our physical and mental well-being. Healthy living encompasses more than just eating a nutritious and balanced diet. It also involves getting the exercise and rest our bodies need to stay healthy, as well as engaging in activities that we enjoy and that enhance our mental well-being.

It is important to recognize that our physical health and our mental health are interrelated. For example, exercising and eating a nutritious and balanced diet can help maintain physical health, boost mental health by increasing energy levels, and improve the ability to cope with stress. Spending time with friends can provide support for the many challenges we face in life as well as provide companions for physical activity. The key to healthy living is a balance of all aspects of life, including the physical, intellectual, social, and emotional.

Eating a nutritious and balanced diet and getting regular physical activity are the cornerstones of a healthy lifestyle. Eating the right foods provides us with the energy and nutrients our bodies need to stay healthy and helps fight and prevent some infections and diseases. Similarly, regular physical activity helps prevent heart disease, diabetes, cancer, osteoporosis, and a host of other diseases. What we eat and how much activity we get not only affect how our bodies perform and feel today but also affect our health for the next 10, 20, and 30 years and beyond.

BUILDING A HEALTHY FOUNDATION

The following guidelines can help you eat well and can keep you moving toward a lifetime of healthy living.

Principles of Healthy Living

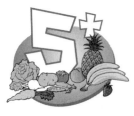

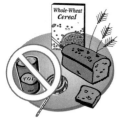

- **Eat 5 or more servings of fruits and vegetables each day.** Fruits and vegetables are packed with vitamins, minerals, antioxidants, and fiber. They also provide healthy carbohydrate that gives us energy. Choose fruits and vegetables in a rainbow of colors (especially dark-green and orange vegetables). For more on fruits and vegetables, refer to lessons 10 and 11 and to the school-wide promotion, Get 3 At School and 5⁺ A Day (lesson 28).

- **Choose whole-grain foods and limit foods and beverages with added sugar.** Minimally processed whole grains make better choices than refined grains do. Whole grains contain fiber, vitamins, and minerals, and the refining process strips away many of these beneficial nutrients. Even though some refined grains are fortified with vitamins and minerals, fortification does not replace all of the lost nutrients. In addition, refined grains get absorbed very quickly, which can cause sugar levels in the blood to spike. In response, the body quickly takes up sugar from the blood to bring sugar levels down to normal. But it may overshoot things a bit, making the blood sugar levels a bit low, and this can cause feelings of false hunger even after a big meal. Choose whole grains whenever possible, making sure that at least half of the grain servings you eat each day are made with whole grains. For more on whole grains and healthy carbohydrate, refer to lessons 2 and 12.

In addition to selecting whole-grain foods, limit your intake of sugary beverages such as soft drinks and limit foods with added sugar. Sweetened drinks are said to be filled with empty calories because they provide many calories but few of the nutrients the body needs to stay healthy and grow strong. A growing body of research suggests that consuming sugar-sweetened beverages is associated with excess weight gain in children and adults. For more on sugar-sweetened beverages, refer to lesson 7.

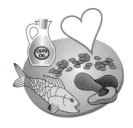

- **Choose healthy fat, limit saturated fat, and avoid trans fat.** Plant-based foods, including plant oils (such as olive, canola, soybean, corn, sunflower, and peanut oils), nuts, and seeds, are natural sources of healthy fat, as are fish and shellfish. Healthy fat can help lower the risk of heart disease, stroke, and possibly diabetes. Unhealthy fat—namely, saturated fat and trans fat—increases the risk of heart disease, stroke, and possibly diabetes. Much of the fat that comes from animals is saturated, including dairy fat, the fat in meat or poultry skin, and lard. Saturated fat should make up no more than 10% of your total calorie intake. Trans fat is formed when healthy vegetable oils are partially hydrogenated (a process that makes the oil solid or semisolid and makes the fat more stable for use in packaged foods). This is the worst type of fat because it raises the risk of heart disease in a number of different ways, and it may raise the risk of diabetes. For more on choosing healthy fat, refer to lessons 5 and 6.

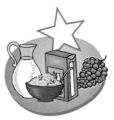

- **Eat a nutritious breakfast every morning.** Breakfast is a critical meal since it gives the body the energy it needs to perform at school, work, or home. Studies have shown that breakfast can improve learning, and it helps boost overall nutrition. Many common breakfast foods are rich in whole grains; breakfast is also a great time to get started toward the daily goal of consuming 5 or more servings of fruits and vegetables. For more on eating breakfast, refer to lesson 12.

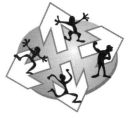

- **Be physically active every day for at least an hour per day.** Regular physical activity not only improves our physical health (by preventing several chronic diseases) but also benefits our emotional well-being. Children should get at least 60 minutes of physical activity every day. This should include moderate- and vigorous-intensity activities, and it can be accumulated throughout the day in sessions of 15 minutes or longer. For more on physical activity, refer to lessons 3, 8, and 13 as well as to the physical education lessons and microunits in parts IV through VII.

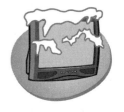

- **Limit TV and other screen time to no more than 2 hours per day.** The more television you watch, the less time you have to engage in physical activity or other healthy pursuits; the same goes for surfing the Web, instant messaging (or text messaging), and playing video games. Watching more television means watching more ads for unhealthy foods, and evidence suggests that this leads to eating extra calories. Such sedentary behavior combined with poor diet can lead to excess weight gain. Children should watch no more than 2 hours of quality television or videos each day; watching less is better. Children should limit total screen time, including watching television, playing computer games, watching DVDs, and Web surfing, to no more than 2 hours each day. For more on reducing TV viewing and screen time, refer to lesson 9 or to the school-wide promotion, Freeze My TV (lesson 27).

FOOD GROUPS AT A GLANCE

There are five basic food groups (see table 1.1): grains; vegetables; fruits; meat, fish, and beans (meat, poultry, fish, dry beans, eggs, nuts, and meat alternatives); and milk. Each food group provides nutritional benefits, so foods from each group should be consumed each day. The key to a balanced diet is to recognize that grains (especially whole grains), vegetables, and fruits are needed in greater proportion than are the foods from the meat, fish, and beans and milk groups. This concept is illustrated by the Balanced Plate for Health (see figure 1.1). A healthy and balanced diet also contains a variety of foods from within each food group, since each food offers different macronutrients (the energy-providing nutrients, namely carbohydrate, protein, and fat) and micronutrients (vitamins and minerals). Eating a variety of foods also keeps our meals interesting and flavorful. Note that the Balanced Plate for Health does not contain sweets, foods that are high in saturated or trans fats, or foods that are low in nutrients. These are "sometimes" foods, not everyday foods. "Sometimes" foods should be eaten in moderation, and they are depicted on a small side plate. For more information on food groups and the serving sizes of foods in each food group, visit the MyPyramid website, www.mypyramid.gov.

▶TABLE 1.1 Food Items From Each Food Group

Food group	Food items	Best choices*
Grains	Whole grains (barley, brown rice, buckwheat, bulgur, millet, quinoa, wheat), breads (whole wheat or rye bread, whole-grain rolls, stone-ground corn or whole wheat tortillas, whole wheat pitas), cereals (oatmeal, seven-grain hot cereal, ready-to-eat cereals made with whole oats, whole wheat, or other whole grains), pasta (whole wheat noodles, soba noodles), crackers (whole wheat crackers, whole rye crispbread), pancakes (whole wheat or buckwheat)	• Whole grains or foods made with minimally processed whole grains • Choose foods that list a whole grain as the first ingredient.
Vegetables	Collard greens, mustard greens, spinach, kale, chard, bok choy, green cabbage, red cabbage, winter squash, summer squash, zucchini, sweet potatoes, broccoli, carrots, tomatoes, corn, turnips, string beans, lettuce, onions, okra, beets, cauliflower, brussels sprouts, dry beans and peas (kidney beans, black beans, soybeans, chickpeas, lentils, black-eyed peas)	• Choose a rainbow of colors, especially dark green and orange. • Choose dry beans and peas.**
Fruits	Peaches, nectarines, cantaloupe, watermelon, grapefruit, raisins, apples, pears, oranges, bananas, strawberries, tangerines, grapes, pineapple, mangoes, blueberries, cherries, figs, kiwi fruits, avocados	• Choose a rainbow of colors. • Choose whole fruits or sliced fruits (rather than fruit juices; limit 100% fruit juice to no more than 8 ounces a day).
Meat, fish, and beans	Fish (salmon, trout, cod, shrimp, crab, scallops, light tuna, sardines), nuts (almonds, hazelnuts, walnuts), nut butters (peanut butter, almond butter), seeds (sunflower, pumpkin), dry beans and peas (kidney beans, black beans, soybeans, chickpeas, lentils, black-eyed peas), chicken, turkey, meat (beef, pork, ham), eggs, tofu and other high-protein vegetarian alternatives (tempeh, falafel, veggie burgers)	• Choose dry beans and peas,** fish, poultry, nuts, and high-protein vegetarian alternatives more often than meat. • When eating meat, choose lean cuts.
Milk	Plain milk (nonfat or 1%), low-fat flavored milk, string cheese (reduced-fat mozzarella sticks), low-fat or nonfat cottage cheese, low-fat cheddar cheese, plain low-fat or nonfat yogurt, low-fat or nonfat frozen yogurt	• Choose plain low-fat (1%) or nonfat milk, yogurt, and other dairy foods.***

*Best-choice foods contain the most nutrients and contribute to overall health.

**Dry beans and peas can also be considered part of the vegetable group.

***Students who cannot drink milk can choose lactose-free milk or calcium-fortified nondairy drinks such as unflavored and unsweetened rice milk or soy milk.

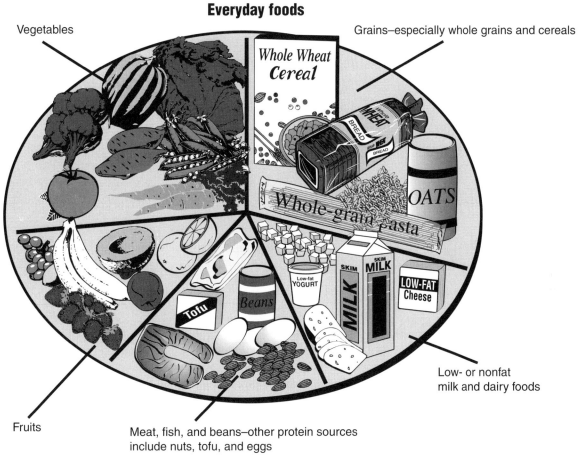

Everyday foods

Vegetables

Grains—especially whole grains and cereals

Whole Wheat Cereal

Whole-grain pasta

Fruits

Meat, fish, and beans—other protein sources include nuts, tofu, and eggs

Low- or nonfat milk and dairy foods

The key to a balanced diet is to recognize that grains (especially whole grains),vegetables, and fruits are needed in greater proportion than are the foods from the meat, fish, and beans and milk groups.

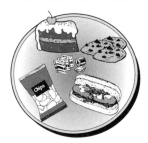

"Sometimes" foods

▶ Figure 1.1   The Balanced Plate for Health.

ESTIMATED TEACHING TIME AND RELATED SUBJECT AREA

Estimated teaching time: 1 hour, 10 minutes

Related subject area: social studies

OBJECTIVES

1. Students will understand the concept of healthy living.
2. Students will learn about the food groups and why eating a variety of foods contributes to a healthy diet.
3. Students will recognize what they can do to lead a healthier life.

MATERIALS

1. Worksheet 1, Building Block for Healthy Living (tip: copy onto card stock)
2. Worksheet 2, Help! You're the Doctor
3. Worksheet 3, The Doctor Says
4. Solutions to worksheet 2
5. Solutions to worksheet 3
6. Student Handout 1, Best-Choice Foods in Each Food Group
7. Transparency 1, Principles of Healthy Living
8. Transparency 2, The Balanced Plate for Health (display and make copies for students)

PROCEDURE

You may choose instead to ask the students to consider the lifestyles of other types of workers such as a construction worker, a cafeteria worker, or a retail employee; you may also change the setting from city to suburban or rural.

1. Discuss experiences in the everyday life of a person who lives in a city—buses, trains, cars, restaurants, busy streets, supermarkets, high-rise buildings, noise pollution. Ask students how the lifestyle of an office worker in the city can vary (and thus be healthy or unhealthy) depending on his choices. Have the students discuss the similarities and differences of these lifestyles. Record their answers on the board.

   Table 1.2 provides examples of the possible differences between a healthy and an unhealthy lifestyle.

2. Discuss with the students how people's lifestyles greatly vary and how lifestyle can affect a person's health. With the help of the students, list on the board all the things we do to stay healthy, such as exercise, rest, sleep, eat right, bathe, clean our living and work environments, visit the doctor and dentist for checkups, try to be safe, and so on.

3. Distribute worksheet 1, Building Block for Healthy Living, to each student and have students assemble the cube. Use transparency 1 to discuss the healthy living concept and the key messages for building a foundation of health.

4. Explain that foods from three food groups—grains, fruits, and vegetables—are featured in the Building Block for Healthy Living. Display and distribute transparency 2, The Balanced Plate for Health, and discuss which foods fall within each food group. We need to eat foods from all of the food groups every day. But we do not need the same amount of food from each group. Grains (especially whole grains), vegetables, and fruits are needed in greater proportion than foods from the meat, fish, and beans and milk groups.

5. Explain that physical activity is a vital component of a healthy lifestyle. Discuss the different types of physical activities that the students enjoy, and remind them that all activities (whether a team sport, something done just for fun, or a day-to-day activity like walking to school or helping around the house) help build their fitness levels and overall health.

6. Reiterate that healthy living involves a balanced and varied lifestyle. Tell students that it is important to eat a balanced and varied diet and to engage

▶TABLE 1.2　Healthy and Unhealthy Lifestyle Choices

	Active and healthy	Inactive and unhealthy
Getting to work	Walks to work (at least part of the way) or rides bike to work	Drives or takes bus to work
Taking breaks during work	Goes for a short walk during work breaks	Surfs the Web during work breaks
Eating snacks and lunch	Brings healthy snacks and lunch from home	Eats fast food at lunch or grabs snack from vending machine
Having fun after work	Walks with friends or plays sports during free time	Watches TV or surfs the Web during free time
Eating dinner	Cooks healthy meals at home	Eats out all the time, usually fast food
Shopping for food	Buys healthy, fresh food	Buys packaged, processed food

in a variety of activities in all aspects of life, including social, intellectual, physical, and emotional. For example, activities such as spending time with friends, reading, talking with family members, walking, dancing, running, playing sports, and even spending some quiet time alone add to personal well-being. Have students illustrate activities they can choose to do that will ensure that their lifestyles are varied and balanced.

7. Distribute worksheet 2, Help! You're the Doctor. Have students read about the people with health concerns and answer the questions in the spaces provided on the worksheet. Discuss the answers with the class.

8. Distribute worksheet 3, The Doctor Says. Have students consider the Building Block for Healthy Living, the Balanced Plate for Health, and the recommendation to eat a variety of foods from each food group and then suggest foods that the people discussed in worksheet 2 should consider including in their diets. (You may assign this activity to small groups who will then present their recommendations to the class.) Remind students of the five food groups and the healthy choices in each group (student handout 1, Best-Choice Foods in Each Food Group). Remind them that the Building Block for Healthy Living also gives them ideas of good food choices (whole grains, fruits, vegetables, and healthy fat but not soft drinks and foods with added sugar).

EXTENSION ACTIVITIES

1. Gather the students into small groups. Have the students take turns rolling the Building Block for Healthy Living and discussing the healthy living message that lands faceup. Ask students to discuss how they can apply the message to their own lifestyles and what changes they could make.

2. Have each student roll the Building Block for Healthy Living and create a poster illustrating the healthy living message that lands faceup. Ask the students to write letters to the cafeteria manager requesting permission to display the posters in the cafeteria.

Name _____

Building Block
for Healthy Living

Directions

1. Using scissors, cut out the entire cube on page 13 by cutting along the outside lines. Be sure to cut around the round tabs.

2. Fold the paper so that it forms the cube and tape the round tabs on the inside of the cube to hold it together.

From L.W.Y. Cheung, H. Dart, S. Kalin, and S.L. Gortmaker, 2007, *Eat Well & Keep Moving,* 2nd ed. (Champaign, IL: Human Kinetics).

(continued)

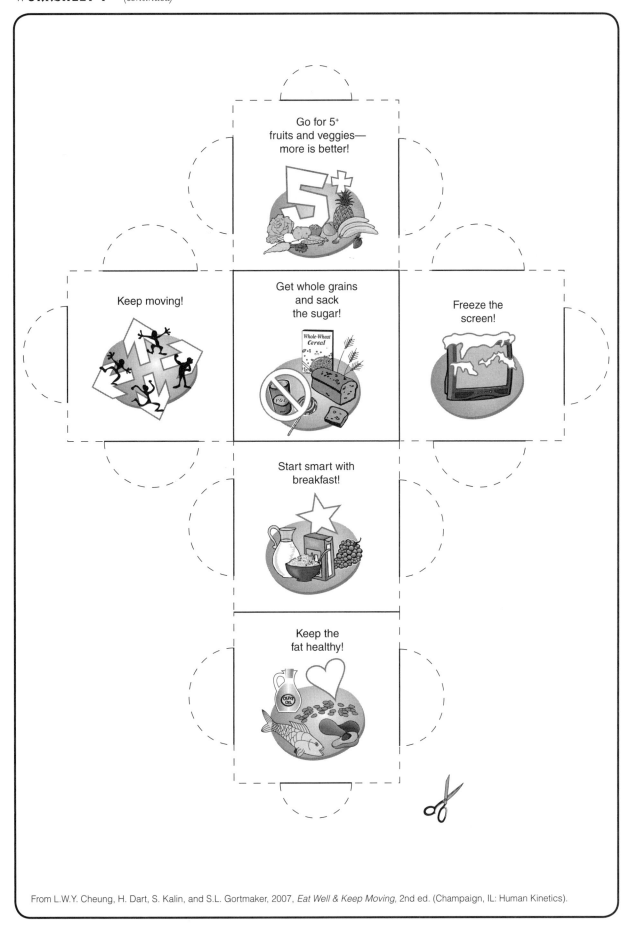

2

Name _____

Help! You're the Doctor

Directions

Read the following paragraphs and solve the problems that follow. Use the Building Block for Healthy Living.

Mr. Lee lives in the city with his wife, son, and two daughters. He works at a local bank that is 2 miles away from his house and catches the bus to the office at 8:00 each morning. He does not eat breakfast. He usually eats lunch at one of the five fast-food restaurants that are on the same street as the bank. He gets a sandwich on white bread or some pepperoni pizza, and he drinks soft drinks or lemonade with his meal. After work, he catches the bus home and then watches television after dinner in the evenings. His family is concerned because he does not have much energy to enjoy weekend outdoor activities.

Roll the Building Block for Healthy Living three times. After each roll, write down the healthy living message that lands faceup. If a message appears twice, roll again. At the end of three rolls, there should be three separate healthy living messages. For each message, write down one tip that will help Mr. Lee improve his health and feel more energetic.

1. Healthy living message: _____

_____

Tip for Mr. Lee: _____

_____

2. Healthy living message: _____

_____

Tip for Mr. Lee: _____

_____

3. Healthy living message: _____

_____

Tip for Mr. Lee: _____

_____

From L.W.Y. Cheung, H. Dart, S. Kalin, and S.L. Gortmaker, 2007, *Eat Well & Keep Moving,* 2nd ed. (Champaign, IL: Human Kinetics).

(continued)

Susan is a fourth grader who enjoyed playing basketball last season for the school team. This year she has decided not to play because she spends all her free time after school on the computer. She snacks on candy while she sits. She's becoming less active, and her bedroom is a real mess. She watches TV at night when her homework is done. Her friends are getting annoyed with her because they never see her anymore.

Explain why it is important for Susan to think about her current lifestyle. Give four suggestions that will help Susan change her current lifestyle. (Hint: Use the Building Block for Healthy Living for ideas.)

_____

_____

_____

_____

_____

_____

Michael is 14 years old. On Saturday mornings he enjoys cycling with his friends on a bike trail. He never eats breakfast, however, and he brings only unhealthy snacks (like potato chips) and no water on the ride. After just 10 minutes of cycling, he's usually exhausted. In contrast, his friends eat a healthy breakfast, drink water, and eat nutritious snacks like raisins, wheat crackers, and nuts during the ride. By the end of the morning, they are much less tired than Michael is.

Why do you think Michael's energy level is low? What are the two ways Michael can increase his energy level? (Hint: Use the Building Block for Healthy Living for ideas.)

_____

_____

_____

_____

_____

_____

From L.W.Y. Cheung, H. Dart, S. Kalin, and S.L. Gortmaker, 2007, *Eat Well & Keep Moving*, 2nd ed. (Champaign, IL: Human Kinetics).

Name _____

The Doctor Says

Just as you need a variety of activities in your life, you also need a variety of foods from each of the five food groups to stay healthy. Keep in mind the tips offered on the Building Block for Healthy Living and the Balanced Plate for Health when you plan meals and snacks for our friends.

Directions

Help Mr. Lee, Susan, and Keshawn learn about foods that will benefit their health by completing the exercises below.

1. Plan a lunch menu for Mr. Lee for the next work week that includes a variety of healthy foods from each of the food groups. You can decide if he takes his lunch from home or buys it at a store or restaurant.

    Monday: _____

    _____

    Tuesday: _____

    _____

    Wednesday: _____

    _____

    Thursday: _____

    _____

    Friday: _____

    _____

2. Choose five snacks from table 1.3 that Susan could eat that would be better for her than candy is:

From L.W.Y. Cheung, H. Dart, S. Kalin, and S.L. Gortmaker, 2007, *Eat Well & Keep Moving*, 2nd ed. (Champaign, IL: Human Kinetics).

(continued)

▶TABLE 1.3   Susan's Snack Choices

Doughnut	Doritos	Apple
Sparkling water with a splash of 100% fruit juice	Whole wheat bagel	Grapes
Chocolate chip cookies	Gatorade	Whole-grain fig bars
Soft drinks	Unsalted nuts	Plain low-fat yogurt
Peach	Banana	Low-fat cheese
Twinkies	Kool-Aid	Peanut butter
Whole wheat cereal	Carrot sticks	Raisins

3. List some healthy food choices Michael should consider for his weekend breakfast.

4. Now that you know about the foundations of healthy living, what are two things that you can do to be healthier?

From L.W.Y. Cheung, H. Dart, S. Kalin, and S.L. Gortmaker, 2007, *Eat Well & Keep Moving,* 2nd ed. (Champaign, IL: Human Kinetics).

SOLUTIONS

Help! You're the Doctor

1. There are many things Mr. Lee could do to improve his health and feel more energetic, including the following:

- *Keep moving!*

  Mr. Lee could walk the 2 miles to and from work instead of taking the bus.

  He could get off the bus a few stops early and walk the rest of the way to work.

  He could go for a walk at lunch.

  He could walk to a restaurant that is farther away than the nearby fast-food places.

- *Go for 5⁺ fruits and veggies—more is better!*

  Mr. Lee could eat less frequently at the fast-food restaurants and bring a nutritious lunch from home that includes fruits and vegetables, such as a salad with sliced chicken and a piece of fruit.

  When he does go to fast-food restaurants he could choose foods that have vegetables, such as bean soup with salad or pizza with vegetable toppings, and skip fried foods with high amounts of trans fat.

- *Freeze the screen!*

  Instead of watching television over the entire evening, Mr. Lee could also do something more physically active, such as play a sport, join a gym, play with his children, take walks with his family, do household chores, and even garden.

- *Get whole grains and sack the sugar!*

  Mr. Lee could drink water with his lunch instead of soft drinks or lemonade.

  He could bring or buy lunches that include whole grains, such as a sandwich on whole wheat bread or tabbouleh from the local deli.

- *Keep the fat healthy!*

  Mr. Lee could have a grilled chicken sandwich or some other lunch item that is low in saturated fat.

  He could choose a lunch item from a restaurant that is a good source of healthy fat, such as a salad with olive oil dressing.

  He could bring a lunch from home that features healthy fat, such as a peanut butter sandwich.

From L.W.Y. Cheung, H. Dart, S. Kalin, and S.L. Gortmaker, 2007, *Eat Well & Keep Moving*, 2nd ed. (Champaign, IL: Human Kinetics).

(continued)

- *Start smart with breakfast!*

  Mr. Lee could eat breakfast at home or at work.

2. Susan should be concerned about her new lifestyle for a number of reasons:

   She is very inactive because she stopped playing basketball and she now spends more than 2 hours on the computer and watching TV at night. While she sits, she snacks on sugary candy that probably contains unhealthy fat, many calories, and no healthy nutrients. Susan is not getting the balanced and varied diet that is very important for energy, growth, and health. On top of this, all those sweets will also greatly increase her chances of cavities. Her lifestyle is also affecting other aspects of her life: She sees her friends less frequently and is not even cleaning her room.

   There are several things that Susan can do to capture a healthy balance:

   Susan can rejoin the basketball team or try another team sport or after-school activity. This will give her the opportunity to be active as well as the opportunity to be with friends and learn about teamwork.

   By getting involved in an after-school activity other than spending time at the computer, she will be less likely to snack on candy. She can pack an extra piece of fruit or a box of raisins to munch on, or she could get a healthy snack at the after-school program.

   Susan should pay attention to how much time she spends on the computer and watching TV at night and make sure she is not getting more than 2 hours a day.

   She can also skip the computer time after school or TV at night in order to find more time to spend with friends or clean her room.

3. Michael's energy levels are low because he skips breakfast and eats unhealthy snacks. To increase his energy levels, Michael should be sure to eat a healthy breakfast that contains a balance of nutrients—ideally a meal that includes whole grains and some protein (such as a whole-grain cereal or oatmeal with nonfat or low-fat (1%) milk or whole wheat toast with peanut butter or eggs) and is low in saturated fat, trans fat, and added sugar. Also, packing nutritious snacks (like bananas, raisins, or nuts) to eat during the ride and drinking plenty of water like his friends will give him more energy as the morning of cycling wears on.

From L.W.Y. Cheung, H. Dart, S. Kalin, and S.L. Gortmaker, 2007, *Eat Well & Keep Moving*, 2nd ed. (Champaign, IL: Human Kinetics).

The Doctor Says

1. Sample lunch menus for Mr. Lee include the following:

   Monday: roast turkey sandwich with lettuce, tomatoes, and mustard on whole wheat bread; red and green pepper slices with hummus dip; a trail mix of raisins, dried papaya, whole wheat mini-pretzels, almonds, and soy nuts (with lunch or for snack); and low-fat milk (from the convenience store)

   Tuesday: whole wheat pasta tossed with vegetables, olive oil, and parmesan cheese; mixed tossed salad with an olive oil vinaigrette; a whole wheat roll; and ice water (at a local restaurant), plus an apple and grapes (packed from home to eat after lunch or for a snack)

   Wednesday: veggie burger on a whole wheat bun with lettuce and tomato, vegetable soup (in a thermos), half a cantaloupe, and low-fat yogurt (with lunch or for a snack)

   Thursday: lentil soup; a side salad with romaine lettuce or a spinach salad topped with tabbouleh, walnuts, and an olive oil vinaigrette; and bottled water (at a local deli), plus strawberries (packed from home)

   Friday: tuna salad (made with a small amount of mayonnaise or plain low-fat yogurt) on a whole wheat roll with lettuce and tomatoes, a low-fat mozzarella cheese stick, celery and carrot sticks, a pear (with lunch or for a snack), and water

2. Good snack choices include grapes, banana, apple, peach, sparkling water with a splash of 100% fruit juice, low-fat yogurt, whole wheat bagel, unsalted nuts, whole-grain fig bars, whole wheat cereal, peanut butter, carrot sticks, raisins, and low-fat cheese.

   Less healthful snack choices include Doritos, doughnut, chocolate chip cookies, soft drinks, Gatorade, Kool-Aid, and Twinkies. (For more information on why Gatorade and other sugary sports drinks are not the best snack choices for children, see the background information for lesson 7, Sugar Water, page 110.)

3. Sample healthy breakfast choices for Keshawn include the following:

   Bowl of mixed fruit and whole-grain toast

   Whole wheat pancakes with strawberries

   Hot oatmeal with fruit and 1% or skim milk

   Melon or cantaloupe with yogurt and granola (made with healthy fat and nuts; look for granola that has little added sugar)

From L.W.Y. Cheung, H. Dart, S. Kalin, and S.L. Gortmaker, 2007, *Eat Well & Keep Moving,* 2nd ed. (Champaign, IL: Human Kinetics).

(continued)

Whole-grain cereal with 1% or nonfat milk

Whole wheat English muffin with peanut butter

Hard-boiled egg with whole wheat toast

Other healthy food choices include fruit, such as bananas, peaches, or oranges; 1% or nonfat milk; 100% tomato juice (a small glass); 100% orange or grapefruit juice (a small glass; limit 100% fruit juice to no more than 8 ounces per day); nuts or nut spreads (including peanut butter); whole-grain breads or cereals; low-fat yogurt; a slice of turkey and cheese; and leftover whole wheat pasta or soba noodles.

From L.W.Y. Cheung, H. Dart, S. Kalin, and S.L. Gortmaker, 2007, *Eat Well & Keep Moving,* 2nd ed. (Champaign, IL: Human Kinetics).

Best-Choice Foods in Each Food Group

▶ **TABLE 1.4** Food Items From Each Food Group

Food group	Food items	Best choices*
Grains	Whole grains (barley, brown rice, buckwheat, bulgur, millet, quinoa, wheat), breads (whole wheat or rye bread, whole-grain rolls, stone-ground corn or whole wheat tortillas, whole wheat pitas), cereals (oatmeal, seven-grain hot cereal, ready-to-eat cereals made with whole oats, whole wheat, or other whole grains), pasta (whole wheat noodles, soba noodles), crackers or dry biscuits (whole wheat crackers, whole rye crispbread), pancakes (whole wheat or buckwheat)	• Whole grains or foods made with minimally processed whole grains • Choose foods that list a whole grain as the first ingredient.
Vegetables	Collard greens, mustard greens, spinach, kale, chard, bok choy, green cabbage, red cabbage, winter squash, summer squash, zucchini, sweet potatoes, broccoli, carrots, tomatoes, corn, turnips, string beans, lettuce, onions, okra, beets, cauliflower, brussels sprouts, dry beans and peas (kidney beans, black beans, soybeans, chickpeas, lentils, black-eyed peas)	• Choose a rainbow of colors, especially dark green and orange. • Choose dry beans and peas.**
Fruits	Peaches, nectarines, cantaloupe, watermelon, grapefruit, raisins, apples, pears, oranges, bananas, strawberries, tangerines, grapes, pineapple, mangoes, blueberries, cherries, figs, kiwi fruits, avocados	• Choose a rainbow of colors. • Choose whole fruits or sliced fruits (rather than fruit juices; limit 100% fruit juice to no more than 8 ounces per day).
Meat, fish, and beans	Fish (salmon, trout, cod, shrimp, crab, scallops, light tuna, sardines), nuts (almonds, hazelnuts, walnuts), nut butters (peanut butter, almond butter), seeds (sunflower, pumpkin), dry beans and peas (kidney beans, black beans, soybeans, chickpeas, lentils, black-eyed peas), chicken, turkey, meat (beef, pork, ham), eggs, tofu and other high-protein vegetarian alternatives (tempeh, falafel, veggie burgers)	• Choose dry beans and peas,** fish, poultry, nuts, and high-protein vegetarian alternatives more often than meat. • When eating meat, choose lean cuts.
Milk	Plain milk (nonfat or 1%), low-fat flavored milk, string cheese (reduced-fat mozzarella sticks), low-fat or nonfat cottage cheese, low-fat cheddar cheese, plain low-fat or nonfat yogurt, low-fat or nonfat frozen yogurt	• Choose plain low-fat (1%) or nonfat milk, yogurt, and other dairy foods.***

*Best-choice foods contain the most nutrients and contribute to overall health.

**Dry beans and peas can also be considered part of the vegetable group.

***Students who cannot drink milk can choose lactose-free milk or calcium-fortified nondairy drinks such as unflavored and unsweetened rice milk or soy milk.

From L.W.Y. Cheung, H. Dart, S. Kalin, and S.L. Gortmaker, 2007, *Eat Well & Keep Moving,* 2nd ed. (Champaign, IL: Human Kinetics).

Principles of Healthy Living

Go for 5 Fruits and Veggies—More Is Better!

Eat 5 or more servings of fruits and vegetables each day! Eat a variety of colors—try red, orange, yellow, green, blue, and purple.

Get Whole Grains and Sack the Sugar!

Choose healthy whole grains for flavor, fiber, and vitamins. Limit sweets. Candy, soft drinks, and other sugary drinks have almost nothing in them that is good for you. They contain just sugar.

Keep the Fat Healthy!

We need fat in our diets, but not all types of fat are good for us. Our bodies like the healthy fat that tends to come from plants and is liquid at room temperature. Examples are olive oil, canola oil, vegetable oil, and peanut oil. Our bodies do not like unhealthy fat, which is solid at room temperature. Examples include saturated fat (usually found in animal products such as meat and whole milk) and trans fat (found in fast-food fries and store-bought cookies). Of the unhealthy fat, trans fat is the worst and should rarely, if ever, be eaten.

Start Smart With Breakfast!

Eating breakfast helps you focus on schoolwork and gives you energy to play. Breakfast is a great meal for adding whole grains, fruit, and low-fat or nonfat milk to your day!

Keep Moving!

Being active is a very important part of healthy living. Do what you like most, and keep your body moving for at least an hour a day!

Freeze the Screen!

Watching TV, playing video games, or playing on the computer keeps your body still. Keep screen time as low as it can go, and never let it add up to more than 2 hours per day.

From L.W.Y. Cheung, H. Dart, S. Kalin, and S.L. Gortmaker, 2007, *Eat Well & Keep Moving*, 2nd ed. (Champaign, IL: Human Kinetics).

The Balanced Plate for Health

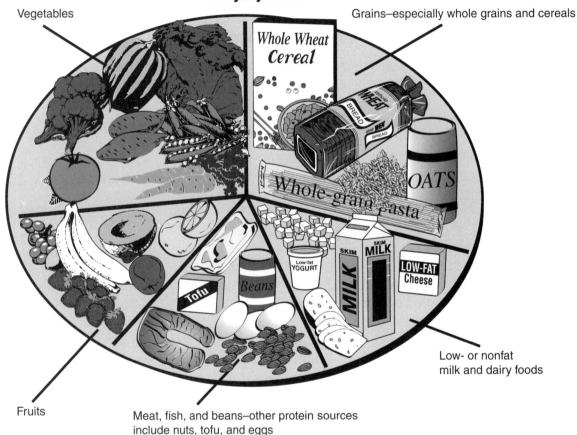

Everyday foods

Vegetables

Grains–especially whole grains and cereals

Fruits

Meat, fish, and beans–other protein sources include nuts, tofu, and eggs

Low- or nonfat milk and dairy foods

"Sometimes" foods

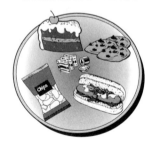

The key to a balanced diet is to recognize that grains (especially whole grains), vegetables, and fruits are needed in greater proportion than are the foods from the meat, fish, and beans and milk groups.

From L.W.Y. Cheung, H. Dart, S. Kalin, and S.L. Gortmaker, 2007, *Eat Well & Keep Moving,* 2nd ed. (Champaign, IL: Human Kinetics).

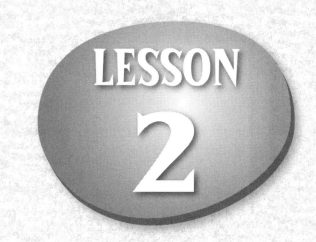

Carb Smart

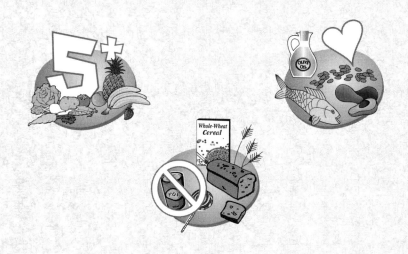

BACKGROUND

The foods we eat contain many kinds of nutrients. Nutrients are the chemical substances in food that your body uses to keep healthy. Macronutrients (carbohydrate, fat, and protein) are the major food components. Micronutrients (vitamins and minerals) are the nutrients that you need in very small amounts and are present in many foods. Both groups of nutrients are important for a healthy body.

All foods contain 1, 2, or all 3 of the macronutrients. Let's look at the functions of each macronutrient:

Protein provides the body with the building blocks for making and repairing tissue (like muscle, bone, hair, and skin) and helps your body grow. Enzymes that control all the body processes from growth to digestion are also made of protein.

Fat helps the body transport certain vitamins and is a rich source of energy.

Carbohydrate provides the body with the quickest source of energy. It is the only nutrient that can be readily used for energy in every single cell in the body, and it is the preferred source of energy for the brain. Carbohydrate is found in all of the five food groups. But not all types of carbohydrate are healthy choices. Some are better than others.

In the grains group, the healthiest carbohydrate choices are whole grains, the less processed the better. Examples of whole grains include whole wheat, barley, brown rice, buckwheat, millet, whole oats, quinoa, and whole rye; these grains can be served on their own or made into whole-grain breads, cereals, pasta, and other products. Whole grains contain fiber, vitamins, and minerals; however, the refining process strips away many of these beneficial nutrients. Even though refined grains (such as white bread, white rice, and white pasta) are fortified with vitamins and minerals, fortification does not replace all of the lost nutrients. Another problem with refined grains is that they get digested and absorbed very quickly, which can cause sugar levels in the blood to spike. In response, the body quickly takes up sugar from the blood and puts it into storage (in muscle, fat and the liver) to bring sugar levels down to normal. Working so quickly, though, the body may overshoot things a bit, making blood sugar levels a bit low; this can cause feelings of false hunger (even after a big meal) and tiredness.

Fruits and many vegetables are excellent sources of carbohydrate, and they are also rich in fiber, vitamins, and minerals. Other good carbohydrate sources include low-fat (1%) or skim milk and low-fat or nonfat yogurt from the milk group and dried beans (legumes) from the meat, fish, and beans group. (Other foods in these groups are not high in carbohydrate.)

Drinks and foods with added sugar, such as soft drinks, energy drinks, punches, cookies, and candy, also provide carbohydrate. But unfortunately, these drinks basically contain just sugar and water, and these foods typically have sugar as one of their main ingredients. (For more information on sugar-sweetened beverages, see lesson 7, Sugar Water.) These types of foods are said to be filled with empty calories because they contain mostly sugar, and they provide many calories but few of the nutrients the body needs to stay healthy and grow strong. Eating too much of these foods makes it difficult to meet other nutrient needs without eating excessive calories. Like refined grains, these sugary foods are quickly absorbed by the body and cause blood sugar levels to spike. These foods are not the best carbohydrate choices; they should be eaten only in small amounts and only once in a while. Similarly, whole-grain cereals and snack bars, fruited yogurts, and flavored milks may contain large amounts of added sugar. On a regular basis, choose whole-grain and dairy products that have little or no added sugar.

In summary, to be carb smart, keep the following tips in mind:

▶ Choose whole grains whenever possible, making sure that at least half of your servings of grains each day come from whole grains.

▶ When selecting foods made with whole grains (breads, breakfast cereals, crackers, pasta, muffins), choose products that list whole wheat, whole oats, whole rye, or other whole grains as the first ingredient and that have little or no added sugar. Also, choose foods that keep the grain as intact as possible (e.g., choose coarsely ground steel-cut oatmeal rather than instant oatmeal for breakfast).

▶ Brightly colored fruits and vegetables make great carbohydrate choices, as do dry beans (legumes), and plain (unflavored and unsweetened) low-fat (1%) and nonfat milk and yogurt.

▶ Make soft drinks, energy drinks, cookies, doughnuts, and other foods with large amounts of added sugar, saturated fat, and trans fat "sometimes" foods instead of everyday foods.

ESTIMATED TEACHING TIME AND RELATED SUBJECT AREA

Estimated teaching time: 50 minutes
Related subject area: health

OBJECTIVES

1. Students will be introduced to the role of carbohydrate in the diet.
2. Students will understand that following the Principles of Healthy Living (particularly the guidelines to choose whole grains and limit foods and drinks with added sugar) will help them select healthy sources of carbohydrate. (For more information on the Principles of Healthy Living, see lesson 1.)

MATERIALS

1. Five food groups name pages (provided)
2. Strong tape
3. Food picture cards (the National Dairy Council produces cutout models of approximately 200 foods and beverages that can be ordered by calling 1-800-426-8271 or by contacting your local Dairy Council) or pictures of food cut out from magazines (be sure to include vegetables, fruits, whole-grain breads and cereals, and low-fat (1%) or nonfat milk and yogurt, which are all high in carbohydrate)
4. Worksheet 1, Which Group?

5. Worksheet 2, Fueling Up the Body
6. Worksheet 3, Going for the Whole Grain
7. Teacher resource page 1, Carbohydrate Foods
8. Teacher resource page 2, Low-Carbohydrate Foods
9. Solutions to worksheet 1
10. Solutions to worksheet 2
11. Teacher transparency 1, The Balanced Plate for Health
12. Teacher transparency 2, Principles of Healthy Living

PROCEDURE

1. Explain to the students that food gives us energy and that this lesson introduces a good energy source: carbohydrate. Carbohydrate is one of three kinds of nutrients found in foods that provide us with energy, and it is used by every cell in the body. Fat and protein are the other two sources of energy. Most foods contain a blend of nutrients, and some foods have more carbohydrate than others have. Whole-grain breads and cereals, dry beans or legumes, fruits, vegetables, and low-fat (1%) or nonfat milk and yogurt are good sources of carbohydrate. Protein foods such as fish, poultry, meat, or eggs and fat sources such as oil do not provide carbohydrate.

   Teacher resource page 1 lists foods that are healthy sources of carbohydrate and foods that are not healthy sources of carbohydrate (e.g., foods that contain refined grains, added sugar, saturated fat, or trans fat). Use these lists to ensure that students select the healthiest high-carbohydrate foods in their worksheets and in the classroom activity. Teacher resource page 2 lists foods that are not rich in carbohydrate.

2. Distribute worksheet 1, Which Group? Review the food groups with the students, using teacher transparency 1, The Balanced Plate for Health. Have the students identify the food groups for each of the foods listed on the worksheet by writing each of the foods in the spaces provided; sweets (not a food group) go in a separate box.

3. Place the five food groups name pages on the wall (either in the front of the room or around the room to allow for more movement) and spread the food picture cards on the floor or a large table. Have students individually select foods that are healthy sources of carbohydrate and tape them next to the appropriate food group on the wall. Try having students take turns at finding a food from each food group (the first student finds a grain food, the second student finds a fruit, and so on) so that foods from all groups are represented.

4. Point out that there are carbohydrate-containing foods in each food group. Ask the students to tell you whether all foods that are high in carbohydrate are healthy choices. Discuss what might make a food a healthy choice, and talk about which foods are not the best choices. Remind the students of the Principles of Healthy Living (particularly the ones related to whole grains, added sugars, fruits and vegetables, and healthy fat). If students still have

their Building Block for Healthy Living cubes from lesson 1, use these as a reminder, or use teacher transparency 2, Principles of Healthy Living.

5. Have the class stand up and do "the wave" (raising and lowering the arms, as you might do at a sporting event). Explain that this is what happens in our bodies when we eat white bread or white rice (or other refined grains): There is a quick rise in blood sugar, giving us energy, but our bodies work quickly to pull that sugar out of the blood and into storage (in our muscles). That is why the quick boost of energy we feel after eating refined grains does not last.

6. Discuss better ways to get quick energy that lasts for a long time so that the body's energy levels do not shoot up and down. Healthy carbohydrate in whole-grain foods, fruits, and vegetables provides a longer boost because the sugar and starch in the foods take longer to be digested and enter the blood stream. These foods also provide fiber and many vitamins and minerals. Low-fat and nonfat milk and low-fat or nonfat yogurt also naturally contain carbohydrate and are a good source of protein and calcium.

7. Review the list of foods that have been categorized by food group (worksheet 1). Instruct the students to circle the foods that contain healthy carbohydrate (remind students that these foods will have vitamins, minerals, and fiber with little or no added sugar). All food groups will have some foods circled, since there are healthy, high-carbohydrate choices available in each group.

8. Notice that some foods listed in the sweets column (which is not a food group) do contain carbohydrate, but none of them make good everyday choices. Explain that sweets do contain carbohydrate, and so they do give the body energy. Discuss with the students why these foods do not make the healthiest choices and should be considered "sometimes" choices rather than everyday choices (see the background section at the beginning of this lesson).

9. Have the students form groups and complete worksheet 2, Fueling Up the Body, which involves planning a menu for a physically active individual of their choice. They can choose an Olympic athlete, a professional dancer, a basketball star, a friend who plays a lot of sports, or even themselves.

10. Distribute worksheet 3, Going for the Whole Grain. Have students write a paragraph explaining why it is important to eat whole grains and naming a few whole grain foods that they like to eat.

EXTENSION ACTIVITY

1. Assess the types of snacks served at a school-based or community-based sporting event (e.g., a Little League, football, or hockey game). Snacks may include foods served at the concession stand or provided on the sidelines by the team coaches.

2. Do the athletes have access to a healthy variety of energy foods? Are they drinking water or some type of sweetened beverage? Do the spectators have healthy snack choices? What recommendations could you make to the coach?

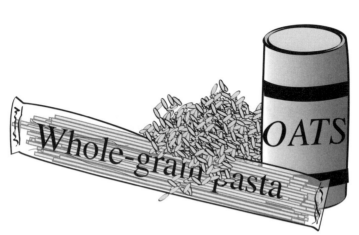

Grain

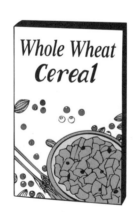

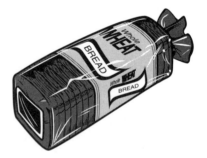

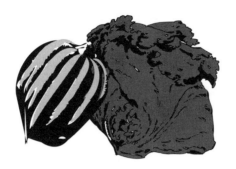

Vegetable

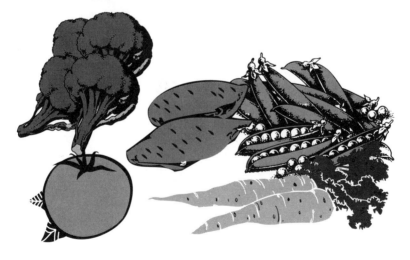

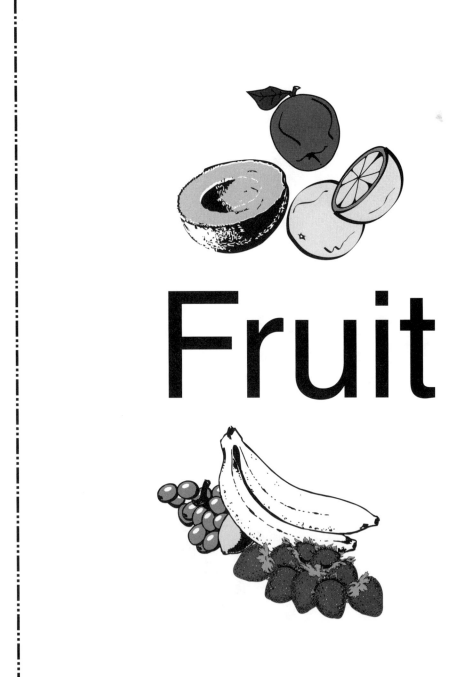

Fruit

Meat, chicken, fish, and beans

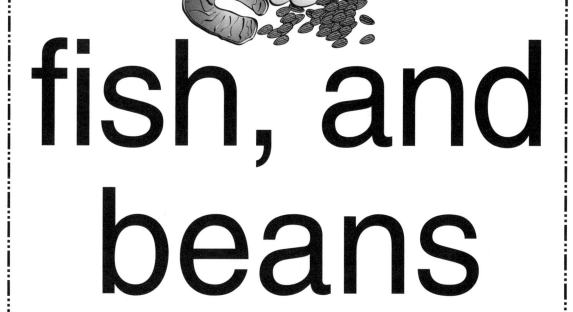

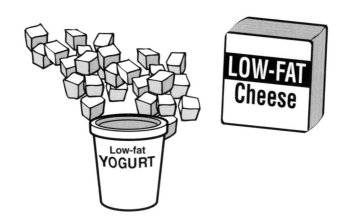

Milk, yogurt and cheese

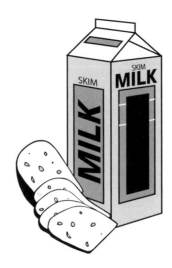

From L.W.Y. Cheung, H. Dart, S. Kalin, and S.L. Gortmaker, 2007, *Eat Well & Keep Moving*, 2nd ed. (Champaign, IL: Human Kinetics).

Which Group?

Directions

Place each of the foods in the Food List table (table 2.1) into the appropriate food group in the Serve It Up table (table 2.2). Place sweets in the appropriate box. You will need to put more than one item in each box, so please write small enough to include many food items.

▶TABLE 2.1   Food List

Bananas	Sweet potatoes	Macaroni	Sunflower seeds
Apples	Broccoli	String cheese	Whole-grain rolls
Brown rice	Winter squash	Hummus	Pineapple
Whole wheat bread	Whole wheat spaghetti	Low-fat cottage cheese	Low-fat chocolate milk
Pancakes	Peaches	Candy	Cabbage
Low-fat milk	Low-fat pudding	Greens	Nonfat milk
Tuna	Salmon	Kale	Grapes
Coca-Cola	Cheerios	Baked beans	Chicken
Oatmeal	Black beans	Spinach	Kool-Aid
Kiwi fruit	Barley pilaf	Blueberries	Carrots
Peanut butter	Oranges	Turkey	Eggs
Black-eyed peas	Tuna	Lettuce	Plums
Frozen yogurt	Lean roast beef	Jelly beans	Beets
Low-fat plain yogurt	Peaches canned in heavy syrup	Apple Jacks cereal	Low-fat ricotta cheese
Raisins	Mashed potatoes	Walnuts	Tofu
Blueberry muffin	Lentils	Gatorade	Corn

From L.W.Y. Cheung, H. Dart, S. Kalin, and S.L. Gortmaker, 2007, *Eat Well & Keep Moving*, 2nd ed. (Champaign, IL: Human Kinetics).

(continued)

▶ TABLE 2.2   Serve It Up

Grains	Vegetables	Fruits	Meat, fish, and beans	Milk
		Example: bananas		

Sweets

From L.W.Y. Cheung, H. Dart, S. Kalin, and S.L. Gortmaker, 2007, *Eat Well & Keep Moving*, 2nd ed. (Champaign, IL: Human Kinetics).

Fueling Up the Body

My name:_____

Other group members: _____

Directions

As a group, pick an athlete or a very active person who needs a lot of energy. You do not have to pick a super-athlete; the person can be someone's friend or family member. Next, plan a day's menu for the person. Remember to choose a lot of healthy carbohydrate foods as well as a variety of foods from each food group. As someone with an active lifestyle, this person will follow the Principles of Healthy Living.

Person's name: _____

Breakfast

Lunch

Snack

Dinner

Snack

From L.W.Y. Cheung, H. Dart, S. Kalin, and S.L. Gortmaker, 2007, *Eat Well & Keep Moving*, 2nd ed. (Champaign, IL: Human Kinetics).

Name _____

Going for the Whole Grain

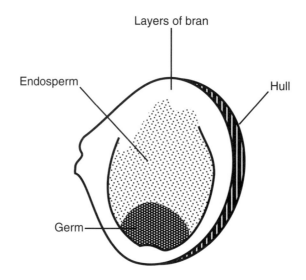

Layers of bran

Endosperm

Hull

Germ

Directions

Write a paragraph explaining why it is important to eat whole grains. Name at least two whole grain foods that you like to eat.

_____

_____

_____

_____

_____

_____

_____

_____

_____

_____

_____

Carbohydrate Foods

Best-Choice Carbohydrate Foods

Best-choice carbohydrate foods are filled with vitamins, minerals, and often fiber; they have little or no added sugars, little or no saturated fat, and no trans fat. Making healthy carbohydrate choices helps avoid spikes in blood sugar. Examples of these nutritious carbohydrate sources include the following:

Grains: Whole grains (the less processed the better) such as barley, brown rice, buckwheat, bulgur, millet, whole oats, quinoa, or whole wheat; whole wheat (or other whole-grain) breads, bagels, rolls, English muffins, pitas, or tortillas; hot whole-grain cereals such as steel-cut oatmeal and kasha; whole-grain ready-to-eat cereals such as shredded wheat or oat squares;* whole wheat spaghetti or pasta; home-popped or air-popped popcorn; whole-grain crackers;** whole-grain pancakes or waffles (without syrup)

Fruits: Fresh fruit, frozen fruit, or fruit canned in its own juice, including oranges, grapefruit, pineapple, blackberries, raspberries, blueberries, cantaloupe, honeydew, kiwi, mango, papaya, raisins and other dried fruit (prunes), peaches, nectarines, bananas, apples, pears

Vegetables: Fresh, frozen, or canned vegetables without added saturated fat or trans fat, including sweet potatoes, winter squash, corn, and parsnips (other vegetables that are healthy choices but have smaller amounts of carbohydrate are beets, turnips, green beans, kale, spinach, carrots, tomatoes)

Meat, fish, and beans: Dry beans without added unhealthy saturated fat or trans fat, such as black beans, kidney beans, chickpeas, pinto beans, lentils, black-eyed peas

Milk: Low-fat (1%) or nonfat milk, plain low-fat or nonfat yogurt

Refined grains (e.g., white bread, white rice, white pasta, and other products made with white flour) may be fortified with vitamins and minerals, but they are still not as healthy as whole-grain foods. Potatoes are high in carbohydrate, but they are digested quickly and are similar to refined grains in their effect on blood sugar. These foods are not best choices; they should only be eaten, at most, a few times a week, and in small portions.

*Make sure that sugar is not one of the first three ingredients.

**Make sure to choose products that contain no trans fat and are low in saturated fat; for more information on choosing healthy fat, see lessons 5 and 6.

From L.W.Y. Cheung, H. Dart, S. Kalin, and S.L. Gortmaker, 2007, *Eat Well & Keep Moving,* 2nd ed. (Champaign, IL: Human Kinetics). Adapted from National Heart, Lung, and Blood Institute, We Can! (n.d.). Go, Slow, and Whoa Foods. Retrieved March 14, 2007, from www.nhlbi.nih.gov/health/public/heart/obesity/wecan/downloads/gswtips.pdf.

(continued)

"Sometimes" Carbohydrate Foods

Some carbohydrate-containing foods have few vitamins and minerals, are low in fiber, and contain large amounts of added sugar or added saturated fat and trans fat. While sweetened breakfast cereals and milk products do contain vitamins and minerals, they often have large amounts of added sugar or contain unhealthy fat. These foods should only be eaten once in a while, if at all. Examples of these less nutritious carbohydrate sources include the following:

▶ **Grains:** Doughnuts, pastries, fruit and cereal bars, sugar-sweetened cereals

▶ **Fruit:** Fruit canned in heavy syrup, fruit punches or -ades (lemonade), fruit leather, dried sweetened fruit

▶ **Milk:** Chocolate milk (or other sweetened, flavored milk drinks), ice cream, frozen yogurt, pudding

▶ **Sweets:** Candy, cookies, cakes, soft drinks, sports drinks,* fruit punches, other sweetened beverages

---

*During most types of physical activity, children can get adequate hydration and energy by drinking water and having a healthy snack (such as orange slices). Most sports drinks are designed for endurance athletes who compete for more than an hour at high intensity. Save sports drinks for when children are participating in high-intensity, long-duration sports competitions (greater than 1 hour), or for when children are vigorously active for a long time in the heat.

From L.W.Y. Cheung, H. Dart, S. Kalin, and S.L. Gortmaker, 2007, *Eat Well & Keep Moving*, 2nd ed. (Champaign, IL: Human Kinetics). Adapted from National Heart, Lung, and Blood Institute, We Can! (n.d.). Go, Slow, and Whoa Foods. Retrieved March 14, 2007, from www.nhlbi.nih.gov/health/public/heart/obesity/wecan/downloads/gswtips.pdf.

Low-Carbohydrate Foods

Many protein foods such as meat, poultry, fish, and cheese do not contain carbohydrate, while some vegetables contain only minimal amounts. Examples of foods that are low in carbohydrate include the following:

Meat	Nuts
Fish	Sunflower seeds
Hamburgers (without bun)	Greens
Eggs	Lettuce
Hot dogs (without bun)	Cucumbers
Cheese	Mushrooms
Chicken or turkey	Celery

From L.W.Y. Cheung, H. Dart, S. Kalin, and S.L. Gortmaker, 2007, *Eat Well & Keep Moving,* 2nd ed. (Champaign, IL: Human Kinetics).

Which Group?

The foods are correctly sorted in table 2.3.

▶ **TABLE 2.3 Serve It Up Solutions**

Grains	Vegetables	Fruits	Meat, fish, and beans	Milk
Brown rice	**Sweet potatoes**	**Bananas**	Peanut butter	**Low-fat milk**
Whole wheat bread	Broccoli*	**Apples**	**Black-eyed peas**	**Low-fat plain yogurt**
Pancakes	**Winter squash**	**Raisins**	**Hummus**	Frozen yogurt
Whole wheat spaghetti	Mashed potatoes	**Peaches**	**Black beans**	Low-fat pudding
Cheerios	Lettuce*	**Oranges**	Lean roast beef	Low-fat cottage cheese
Barley pilaf	Greens*	**Blueberries**	**Lentils**	**Nonfat milk**
Blueberry muffin	Kale*	**Kiwi fruit**	**Baked beans**	Low-fat chocolate milk
Macaroni	Spinach*	**Pineapple**	Turkey	Low-fat ricotta cheese
Apple Jacks cereal	Cabbage*	Peaches canned in heavy syrup	Walnuts	String cheese
Whole-grain rolls	Carrots*	**Grapes**	Chicken	
	Corn	**Plums**	Eggs	
	Beets*		Salmon	
			Tuna	
			Tofu	

Teacher note: Best-choice carbohydrate foods are bolded.

*While these vegetables are not high in carbohydrate, they are nutritious choices (high in fiber, vitamins, and minerals).

Sweets		
Candy	Coca-Cola	Jelly beans
Gatorade	Kool-Aid	

From L.W.Y. Cheung, H. Dart, S. Kalin, and S.L. Gortmaker, 2007, *Eat Well & Keep Moving,* 2nd ed. (Champaign, IL: Human Kinetics).

Fueling Up the Body

Person's name: Tiger Woods

Breakfast: Steel-cut oatmeal with raisins, 1 banana, 1 slice of whole wheat toast spread with peanut butter, low-fat milk

Lunch: Turkey sandwich on whole wheat roll with lettuce, sliced tomato and hummus spread, carrot sticks, plain low-fat yogurt with fresh strawberries, 1 apple, whole wheat pita chips, water

Snack: Whole-grain fig bars, sunflower seeds, water

Dinner: Large plate of whole wheat spaghetti with tomato sauce and small amount of parmesan cheese, whole wheat French bread, large helping of steamed broccoli, green salad with white beans in olive oil dressing, low-fat milk

Snack: Half a cantaloupe

The overall plan provides plenty of whole grains, more than 5 servings of fruits and vegetables (including a variety of colors such as deep green and orange), healthy sources of fat (peanut butter, hummus, olive oil, sunflower seeds), and low-fat dairy selections.

From L.W.Y. Cheung, H. Dart, S. Kalin, and S.L. Gortmaker, 2007, *Eat Well & Keep Moving,* 2nd ed. (Champaign, IL: Human Kinetics).

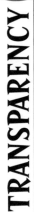

The Balanced Plate for Health

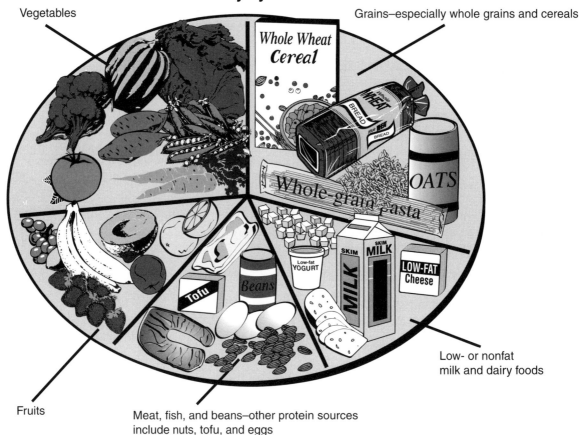

Everyday foods

Vegetables

Grains–especially whole grains and cereals

Low- or nonfat milk and dairy foods

Fruits

Meat, fish, and beans–other protein sources include nuts, tofu, and eggs

"Sometimes" foods

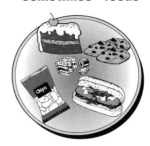

The key to a balanced diet is to recognize that grains (especially whole grains), vegetables, and fruits are needed in greater proportion than are the foods from the meat, fish, and beans and milk groups.

From L.W.Y. Cheung, H. Dart, S. Kalin, and S.L. Gortmaker, 2007, *Eat Well & Keep Moving,* 2nd ed. (Champaign, IL: Human Kinetics).

Principles of Healthy Living

Go for 5 Fruits and Veggies—More Is Better!

Eat 5 or more servings of fruits and vegetables each day! Eat a variety of colors—try red, orange, yellow, green, blue, and purple.

Get Whole Grains and Sack the Sugar!

Choose healthy whole grains for flavor, fiber, and vitamins. Limit sweets. Candy, soft drinks, and other sugary drinks have almost nothing in them that is good for you—no vitamins or minerals or other healthy things. They contain just sugar.

Keep the Fat Healthy!

We need fat in our diets, but not all types of fat are good for us. Our bodies like the healthy fat that tends to come from plants and is liquid at room temperature. Examples are olive oil, canola oil, vegetable oil, and peanut oil. Our bodies do not like unhealthy fat, which is solid at room temperature. Examples include saturated fat (usually found in animal products, such as meat and whole milk) and trans fat (found in fast-food fries and store-bought cookies). Of the unhealthy fats, trans fat is the worst and should rarely, if ever, be eaten.

Start Smart With Breakfast!

Eating breakfast helps you focus on schoolwork and gives you energy to play. Breakfast is a great meal for adding whole grains, fruit, and low-fat or nonfat milk to your day!

Keep Moving!

Being active is a very important part of healthy living. Do what you like most, and keep your body moving for at least an hour a day!

Freeze the Screen!

Watching TV, playing video games, or playing on the computer keeps your body still. Keep screen time as low as it can go, and never let it add up to more than 2 hours per day.

From L.W.Y. Cheung, H. Dart, S. Kalin, and S.L. Gortmaker, 2007, *Eat Well & Keep Moving,* 2nd ed. (Champaign, IL: Human Kinetics).

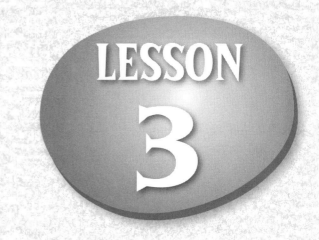

The Safe Workout: An Introduction

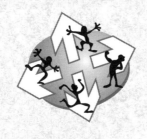

BACKGROUND

The human body can do amazing things. However, in order for the body to perform well, it must be taken care of. To keep the body healthy, we must choose good foods, exercise regularly, stay away from harmful substances (such as tobacco and other drugs), and get plenty of sleep. The body needs good food to give it energy, to help it grow, and to allow it to repair itself. Exercising regularly also helps keep the body healthy. Some exercises make the heart, lungs, and blood vessels stronger, while others help with flexibility and the body's ability to bend. The body needs all kinds of exercise. This lesson teaches students the safe way to exercise and at the same time reviews the five basic food groups.

This lesson also introduces the five parts of a safe workout. The five parts of the safe workout help prevent injuries while exercising. These five parts are (1) the warm-up, (2) the stretch, (3) the fitness activity, (4) the cool-down, and (5) the cool-down stretch. Each part will be introduced by stating why it is important and how to do it correctly. Because of time constraints, the parts of the lesson workout are shorter than what they normally should be in an actual workout. For example, the lesson warm-up is only 1 to 2 minutes, when ideally the warm-up should last at least 5 minutes. What's important is that the students learn that a warm-up is the first part of a safe workout and that it should be done whenever they get ready for active sports or play. For instance, they should warm up at home before they ride bikes or play basketball.

Children should get at least 60 minutes of physical activity every day; this should include moderate- and vigorous-intensity activities and can be accumulated throughout the day in sessions of 15 minutes or longer. But exercising and doing the five parts of a safe workout is only half of the story! In addition to being physically active, eating right is the other half of the winning combination that keeps our bodies healthy. In this lesson the students will be learning about the food groups and how to choose foods wisely while moving!

This lesson is a classroom-based activity that can be used as a practice run for the other physical activity lessons that will be taught in the gymnasium, community room, or cafeteria.

OVERVIEW

This lesson introduces students to the various parts of a safe workout. Together as a class, the students review the different workout components, and then they form groups, with each group presenting a different part of the workout to the entire class. At the heart of this lesson is a fitness activity in which students gather foods based on the five food groups. The lesson concludes with the Stay Healthy Corner, a time for discussion of some of the Principles of Healthy Living. (For more information on these principles, see lesson 1.) You can set up a specific area of the classroom for the Stay Healthy Corner and decorate it with pictures or student drawings that represent the Principles of Healthy Living (e.g., healthy foods, children engaged in physical activity, and so on). Or you can simply set aside time for discussion at the end of the lesson.

ESTIMATED TEACHING TIME AND RELATED SUBJECT AREA

Estimated teaching time: 1 hour, 20 minutes
Related subject area: physical education

OBJECTIVES

1. Students will be able to identify and sequence the components of a safe and healthy workout.
2. Students will be able to discuss and demonstrate each component of a safe workout.
3. Students will be able to demonstrate awareness of the food groups and healthy foods within each group.

MATERIALS

1. Pictures of various foods (the National Dairy Council produces cutout models of approximately 200 foods and beverages that can be ordered by calling 800-426-8271 or by contacting your local Dairy Council)
2. Stretch and Strength Fitness Diagrams (see appendix A, pages 565-569)
3. Safe workout component cards and food group information cards (provided)
4. Tape
5. Safe workout and fitness terms sentence strips (provided)
6. Portable CD player or radio to play music during the warm-up (optional)
7. Five hula hoops or paper grocery bags
8. Teacher resource page 1, What Belongs in Each Food Group?
9. Transparency 1, Principles of Healthy Living (optional)

PROCEDURE

1. Each component of the safe workout is written on an individual sentence strip.
   Warm-up (1-2 minutes)
   Stretch (1-2 minutes)
   Fitness activity (15-20 minutes)
   Cool-down (1 minute)
   Cool-down stretch (1 minute)
2. Tape the sentence strips with the components of the safe workout on the left side of the blackboard, scattering them in random order.
   Warm-up—The first part of the safe workout, in which slow movements get your body ready for stretching and the fitness activity.

> Stretch—The part of the safe workout in which you do exercises that improve flexibility fitness and get the body ready for the fitness activity.
>
> Fitness activity—The part of a safe workout in which strength and endurance fitness exercises are performed.
>
> Cool-down—The part of the safe workout in which your body slows down and recovers from the fitness activity.
>
> Cool-down stretch—The last part of the safe workout, in which you do exercises that improve flexibility fitness.

3. On the right side of the blackboard, tape the sentence strips that contain key fitness terms relating to the components of the workout.

> Pacing—Maintaining a comfortable speed so that you can perform your exercise for an extended time.
>
> Flexibility fitness—The part of fitness that stretches the muscles and areas around the muscles to get your body ready for action.
>
> Strength fitness—The part of fitness that makes your muscles, except the heart muscle, stronger and healthier.
>
> Endurance fitness—The part of fitness that improves the heart muscle, lungs, and blood vessels (builds cardiorespiratory fitness).

4. As a class, read aloud all the terms on the board.

5. Ask the students, "Who knows the first step of a safe workout?" Have a student come to the board to answer the question. After the student gives the correct answer, let the student select the Warm-Up sentence strip and place it on an open part of the blackboard.

6. Continue by asking, "What is the second step of a safe workout?" Another student answers, picks the Stretch strip, and puts it on the board in the correct order—just after the Warm-Up strip. Repeat this process for the remaining components of the workout.

7. After the workout is in order, discuss the terms *flexibility fitness, strength fitness, endurance fitness,* and *pacing.* Ask the students where they think each term should be placed in the workout (for example, flexibility fitness belongs with the stretch component of the workout). Have the students provide the answer and then place the term next to the appropriate component of the workout.

8. Briefly introduce the lesson. Tell the students, "In our lesson on the Principles of Healthy Living, we learned that our bodies need the right amounts and kinds of food daily and that they need to move and get regular physical activity. Specifically, we learned that we should eat a variety of foods from each of the food groups and that we should choose carefully to make sure we get all of the nutrients that we need without eating unnecessary sugar or unhealthy fat. Making the right choices about the food we eat affects the health of our bodies. By eating balanced meals, our bodies stay healthy, grow, and perform physical activities like playing and dancing.

   "Regular, moderate to vigorous physical activity is also important to our body's health—we should get at least an hour of physical activity every day. The safe workout steers us in the right direction so that we exercise and participate in physical activities in ways that are good for our bodies. Today we will learn about the components of a safe workout."

9. Have the class form five groups, and give each group the name of one of the five food groups. Give each group the food group information card with the name and example foods in their food group. Equal numbers of students will be represented in the grain group; fruit group; vegetable group; milk group; and meat, fish, and beans group.

   Grain group: whole grains (barley, brown rice, buckwheat, bulgur, millet, quinoa, wheat), breads (whole wheat or rye bread, whole-grain rolls, stone-ground corn or whole wheat tortillas, whole wheat pitas), cereals (oatmeal, seven-grain hot cereal, ready-to-eat cereals made with whole oats, whole wheat, or other whole grains), pasta (whole wheat noodles, soba noodles), crackers (whole wheat crackers, whole rye crispbread), pancakes (whole wheat or buckwheat)

   Vegetable group: collard greens, mustard greens, spinach, kale, chard, bok choy, napa cabbage, red cabbage, winter squash, summer squash, zucchini, sweet potatoes, broccoli, carrots, tomatoes, corn, turnips, string beans, lettuce, onions, okra , beets, cauliflower, brussels sprouts, dry beans and peas (kidney beans, black beans, soybeans, chickpeas, lentils, black-eyed peas)

   Fruit group: peaches, nectarines, cantaloupe, watermelon, grapefruit, raisins, apples, pears, oranges, bananas, strawberries, tangerines, grapes, pineapple, mangoes, blueberries, cherries, figs, kiwi fruits, avocados

   Meat, fish, and beans group: fish (salmon, trout, cod, shrimp, crab, scallops, light tuna, sardines), nuts and nut butters (peanut butter, almonds, hazelnuts, walnuts), seeds (sunflower, pumpkin), dry beans and peas (kidney beans, black beans, soybeans, chickpeas, lentils, black-eyed peas), chicken, turkey, meat (beef, pork, ham), eggs, tofu and other high-protein vegetarian alternatives (tempeh, falafel, vegetable burgers)

   Milk group: low-fat (1%) or nonfat plain milk, low-fat flavored milk, string cheese (reduced-fat mozzarella sticks), low-fat cottage cheese, low-fat cheddar cheese, plain low-fat or nonfat yogurt

   For a list of what belongs in each food group, and the best choices in each group, see teacher resource 1.

   Tell the students, "When eating, we must be sure to put the different combinations of foods together in a particular way so that we can have a balanced and nutritious meal. When doing physical activity, we must do different kinds of things so that we can have a safe and beneficial workout. The safe workout can be broken into five parts. We will discuss and go through each of these parts so that you understand what they are and how and when they should be done."

10. Randomly give each group of students a safe workout component card. Each card names a component of the safe workout, explains why it is important, and gives an example of an exercise that could be done to represent that component. The cards for the first three components—the warm-up card, the stretch card, and the two fitness cards (one for strength fitness and one for endurance fitness)—can be distributed as they are, one to each of four groups; the cards for the last two components—the cool-down card and the cool-down stretch card—can be handed to one group.

11. Allow students 3 to 5 minutes to review their workout component and the other information on their card. Explain that a speaker from each of the groups will introduce the entire class to the component and lead the class in doing the exercises for the first three components (warm-up, stretch, and fitness activity).

12. Following the order of the safe workout, have a student from the warm-up group and a student from the stretching group introduce their individual component and lead the class in the appropriate exercises. Be sure the speaker from the warm-up group presents before the speaker from the stretching group.

a. Warm-up

1. Benefits of warming up
   - Helps prevent injuries
   - Increases body temperature
   - Gets the body ready for the rest of the workout
2. How to warm up
   - Perform a series of slow movements for 5 to 10 minutes.
   - Examples include slow jogging in place and slow jumping jacks.

b. Stretch

1. Benefits of stretching
   - Improves flexibility fitness
   - Improves the ability of muscles to work
   - Improves the body's ability to move
   - Decreases the number of injuries
2. How to stretch (see appendix A, pages 565-567)
   - Hold each stretch for 10 or more seconds (count out loud: 1 Mississippi, 2 Mississippi . . . 10 Mississippi).
   - Don't bounce—hold the stretch gently.
   - Stretch slowly.
   - Use proper form to avoid injuries.
   - Examples include the neck stretch, butterfly, and quad burner (thigh stretch).

13. After the warm-up and stretching exercises are finished, explain to the students that they are now prepared to complete the fitness components of the workout.

14. Have the next two groups introduce the two fitness components and lead the entire class in the exercises.

a. Strength fitness (see appendix A, pages 568-569)

1. Benefits of strength fitness
   - Improves the ability of your muscles to move or resist a force or workload
   - Helps you perform your daily tasks without tiring
   - Helps prevent injuries
   - Improves your skills in games and sports, such as jumping rope, playing dodgeball, or shooting a basketball
2. How to improve strength fitness
   - Make your muscles work more than they are used to—make them go faster, work longer, or lift heavier objects, or exercise more often.
   - Train, don't strain.
   - Don't do too much too soon or too often.

Note: You may use the CD player or radio to play music during the warm-up (optional).

b. Endurance fitness

   1. Benefits of endurance fitness

- Improves health of heart, lungs, and blood vessels (builds cardio-respiratory fitness)
- Gives you energy

   2. How to improve endurance fitness

- Do nonstop, continuous movement activities such as bike riding, walking, or rope jumping (students may jog or walk in place to demonstrate endurance activities in class).
- Find a pace (speed) you can do for a long time—"Pace, don't race!"
- Find endurance activities that you like so you will want to do them.
- Mix up your workout—ride your bike to the park, play ball, and then ride your bike home again.

During this time you should walk around the class and correct students as they perform these exercises.

15. After you have reviewed the fitness components, lead the class in the shopping fitness activity.

16. The purpose of the game is to determine if each student in a group knows which food items fit into her food group. Tell the students, "We are also playing this game to become fit and learn how to pace ourselves so that we can make our bodies stronger and able to do an activity for a certain length of time without becoming tired."

   a. Keep the students in their five food groups and ask each group to form a line (see figure 3.1). The formation used will depend on the layout and space of the room.

   b. Using a cone or distinguishable line, designate a place where the first person in each line can stand. The second person in line will move to this place after the first student has left the position.

   c. Point out to the students an area in the room where numerous and various pictures of foods from the different food groups are scattered. This is the grocery store. (You can put pictures into place before class begins.)

   d. Place a hula hoop or large paper bag to the right of each line of students. This hula hoop can be called a *plate* or a *refrigerator* (as noted in figure 3.1; alternative arrangements are noted in figure 3.2).

   e. Explain the path the students will take so that there is no confusion and students can perform the tasks safely. Explain to the students, "Each of you will go to the grocery store to shop for a food that is found in your food group. When you reach the front of the line and it is your turn, jog in a straight path until you get to the grocery store. Once there, select the correct food for your group, pick it up, and jog back to the refrigerator (or plate) and deposit the food picture in it. Then jog to the back of your line and jog in place until every member of every group has taken at least two trips to the grocery store." Remind the students, "This is not a race or a competition between groups."

17. The students should be actively engaged when doing the fitness activity. Each team will have to jog lightly throughout the entire activity as individuals from each group go one at a time to the pile of food pictures, and fellow team members continue to jog while they wait their turn (spend 15 minutes maximum on this activity). You may modify the movement by having students skip to the store or hop in place.

Gym line formation
for shopping fitness activities

[**X** = one student]

The purpose of the game is to determine if each student in a group knows which food items fit into their food group. We are also playing this game so that we can become fit and learn how to pace ourselves so that we can make our bodies stronger and able to do an activity for a certain length of time without becoming tired.

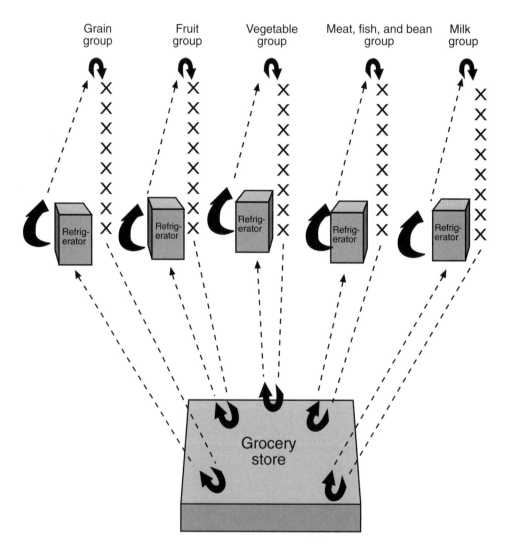

▶ Figure 3.1   Gym line formation for shopping fitness activity.

18. When the fitness activity is completed, have the group with the last two components of the safe workout present the cool-down and cool-down stretches, respectively.

   a. Cool-down

      1. Benefits of cooling down

         • Lets the body slow down or recover from the fitness activity

         • Helps prevent injuries and muscle soreness

Option #1

Option #2

Option #3

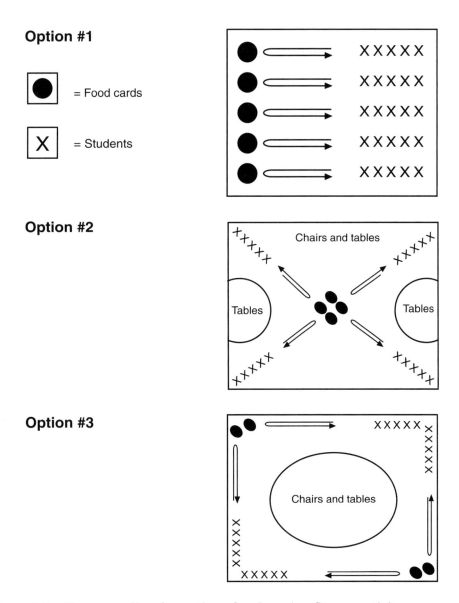

▶ Figure 3.2   Classroom line formations for shopping fitness activity.

  2. How to cool down
     • Walk slowly.
     • Walk in place slowly.
 b. Cool-down stretch (see appendix A, pages 565-567)
     1. Benefits of the cool-down stretch
        • Helps prevent soreness
        • Improves flexibility fitness
     2. How to do the cool-down stretch
        • Hold each stretch for 10 or more seconds (count out loud: 1 Mississippi, 2 Mississippi . . . 10 Mississippi).
        • Examples include the neck stretch, butterfly, and quad burner (thigh stretch).

19. When the cool-down stretch has been completed, have all the groups reassemble for the Stay Healthy Corner discussion.

20. Stress that, while it is important to eat from all of the food groups, it is also important to select a variety of foods from within each group. We need various nutrients—protein, carbohydrate, fat, minerals, and vitamins—to help us grow, give us energy, and repair our bodies. Since no one food contains everything we need, we want to eat different foods each day (eating different foods also makes our meals more interesting). Have each group look at their food selections again and notice how many different types of foods they can choose from each group. (You may also invite groups to walk around to look at the variety in each of the other food groups.) Ask each group to consider the Principles of Healthy Living, especially the ones regarding whole grains, fruits and vegetables, and healthy fat. Then, have them select 2 or 3 foods from the pile that would make particularly good food choices. (Optional: You may display transparency 1 or give the students copies of the transparency.) Examples may include whole wheat bread, low-fat milk, peanut butter, or fish. Remind students that they should eat 5 or more servings of fruits and vegetables each day and that they should include green and orange vegetables in their diet for maximum nutrient intake.

21. Review any combination foods that may have been selected. Remind students that mixed dishes often provide them with delicious options for eating vegetables. Have students name some dishes that contain at least two different food groups. Focus on those that contain vegetables, such as bean chili, vegetable pizza, or chicken stir-fry.

22. Close the lesson by reminding students to get at least 1 hour of physical activity every day. It is okay to get that activity a little bit at a time—through 15 minutes of walking to school, 20 minutes of playing tag—just so long as it adds up to an hour a day. Mix it up to keep it fun.

SAFE WORKOUT COMPONENT CARDS

Warm-Up

Benefits of Warming Up

- ▶ Helps prevent injuries
- ▶ Increases body temperature
- ▶ Gets the body ready for the rest of the workout

How to Warm Up

- ▶ Perform a series of slow movements for 5 to 10 minutes.
- ▶ Examples include slow jogging in place and slow jumping jacks.

Stretch

Benefits of Stretching

- ▶ Improves flexibility fitness
- ▶ Improves the ability of muscles to work
- ▶ Improves the body's ability to move
- ▶ Decreases the number of injuries

How to Stretch

- ▶ Hold each stretch for 10 or more seconds (count out loud: 1 Mississippi, 2 Mississippi . . . 10 Mississippi).
- ▶ Don't bounce—hold the stretch gently.
- ▶ Stretch slowly.
- ▶ Use proper form to avoid injuries.
- ▶ Examples include the neck stretch, butterfly, and quadriceps burner (thigh stretch).

From L.W.Y. Cheung, H. Dart, S. Kalin, and S.L. Gortmaker, 2007, *Eat Well & Keep Moving*, 2nd ed. (Champaign, IL: Human Kinetics).

(continued)

Strength Fitness

Benefits of Strength Fitness

▶ Improves the ability of your muscles to move or resist a force or workload

▶ Helps you perform your daily tasks without getting tired

▶ Helps prevent injuries

▶ Improves your skills in games and sports, such as jumping rope, playing dodgeball, or shooting a basketball

How to Improve Strength Fitness

▶ Make your muscles work more than they are used to— make them go faster, work longer, or lift heavier objects, or exercise more often.

▶ Train, don't strain.

▶ Don't do too much too soon too often.

Endurance Fitness

Benefits of Endurance Fitness

▶ Improves the health of your heart, lungs, and blood vessels (builds cardiorespiratory fitness)

▶ Gives you energy

How to Improve Endurance Fitness

▶ Do nonstop, continuous movement activities such as bike riding, walking, or rope jumping (students may jog or walk in place to demonstrate endurance activities in class).

▶ Find a pace (speed) you can do for a long time—"Pace, don't race!"

▶ Find endurance activities that you like so you will want to do them.

▶ Mix up your workout—ride your bike to the park, play ball, and then ride your bike home again.

From L.W.Y. Cheung, H. Dart, S. Kalin, and S.L. Gortmaker, 2007, *Eat Well & Keep Moving,* 2nd ed. (Champaign, IL: Human Kinetics).

(continued)

Cool-Down

Benefits of Cooling Down

▶ Lets the body slow down or recover from the fitness activity

▶ Helps prevent injuries and muscle soreness

How to Cool Down

▶ Walk slowly.

▶ Walk in place slowly.

Cool-Down Stretch

Benefits of the Cool-Down Stretch

▶ Helps prevent soreness

▶ Improves flexibility fitness

How to Do the Cool-Down Stretch

▶ Hold each stretch for 10 or more seconds (count out loud: 1 Mississippi, 2 Mississippi . . . 10 Mississippi).

▶ Examples include the neck stretch, butterfly, and quad burner (thigh stretch).

From L.W.Y. Cheung, H. Dart, S. Kalin, and S.L. Gortmaker, 2007, *Eat Well & Keep Moving,* 2nd ed. (Champaign, IL: Human Kinetics).

FOOD GROUP INFORMATION CARDS

Grain Group

Includes whole grains (barley, brown rice, buckwheat, bulgur, millet, oats, quinoa, whole wheat), breads (whole wheat or rye bread, whole-grain rolls, stone-ground corn or whole wheat tortillas, whole wheat pitas), cereals (oatmeal, seven-grain hot cereal, ready-to-eat cereals made with whole oats, whole wheat, or other whole grains), pasta (whole wheat noodles, soba noodles), crackers (whole wheat crackers, whole rye crispbread), pancakes (whole wheat or buckwheat)

Vegetable Group

Includes collard greens, mustard greens, spinach, kale, chard, bok choy, napa cabbage, red cabbage, winter squash, summer squash, zucchini, sweet potatoes, broccoli, carrots, tomatoes, corn, turnips, string beans, lettuce, onions, okra, beets, cauliflower, brussels sprouts, dry beans and peas (kidney beans, black beans, soybeans, chickpeas, lentils, black-eyed peas)

Fruit Group

Includes peaches, nectarines, cantaloupe, watermelon, grapefruit, raisins, apples, pears, oranges, bananas, strawberries, tangerines, grapes, pineapple, mangoes, blueberries, cherries, figs, kiwi fruits, avocados

From L.W.Y. Cheung, H. Dart, S. Kalin, and S.L. Gortmaker, 2007, *Eat Well & Keep Moving,* 2nd ed. (Champaign, IL: Human Kinetics).

(continued)

Meat, Fish, and Beans Group

Includes fish (salmon, trout, cod, shrimp, crab, scallops, light tuna, sardines), nuts and nut butters (peanut butter, almonds, hazelnuts, walnuts), seeds (sunflower, pumpkin), dry beans and peas (kidney beans, black beans, soybeans, chickpeas, lentils, black-eyed peas), chicken, turkey, meat (beef, pork, ham), eggs, tofu and other high-protein vegetarian alternatives (tempeh, falafel, veggie burgers)

Milk Group

Includes low-fat (1%) or nonfat plain milk, low-fat flavored milk, string cheese (reduced-fat mozzarella sticks), low-fat or nonfat cottage cheese, low-fat cheddar cheese, plain low-fat or nonfat yogurt, low-fat frozen yogurt

From L.W.Y. Cheung, H. Dart, S. Kalin, and S.L. Gortmaker, 2007, *Eat Well & Keep Moving,* 2nd ed. (Champaign, IL: Human Kinetics).

COMPONENTS OF A SAFE WORKOUT

Sentence Strips

Warm-up—The first part of the safe workout, in which slow movements get the body ready for stretching and the fitness activity.

Stretch—The part of the safe workout in which you do exercises that improve flexibility fitness and get the body ready for the fitness activity.

Fitness activity—The part of the safe workout in which you perform strength and endurance fitness exercises.

Cool-down—The part of the safe workout in which your body slows down and recovers from the fitness activity.

Cool-down stretch—The last part of the safe workout, in which you do exercises that improve flexibility fitness.

SAFE WORKOUT TERMS

Sentence Strips

Pacing—Maintaining a comfortable speed so that you can perform your exercise over an extended time.

Flexibility fitness—The part of fitness that stretches the muscles and body parts around the muscles to get your body ready for action.

Strength fitness—The part of fitness that makes your muscles (except the heart muscle) stronger and healthier.

Endurance fitness—The part of fitness that improves the heart muscle, lungs, and blood vessels (builds cardiorespiratory fitness).

From L.W.Y. Cheung, H. Dart, S. Kalin, and S.L. Gortmaker, 2007, *Eat Well & Keep Moving,* 2nd ed. (Champaign, IL: Human Kinetics).

What Belongs in Each Food Group?

Table 3.1 provides examples of foods from each food group. For combination foods, students may estimate which food group makes up the majority of the mixed dish. For instance, if a student in the grain group selects spaghetti and meatballs, he may decide that spaghetti is the primary ingredient while also recognizing that this dish contains vegetable (tomato sauce) and meat (meatballs).

▶ **TABLE 3.1   Food Items From Each Food Group**

Food group	Food items	Best choices*
Grains	Whole grains (barley, brown rice, buckwheat, bulgur, millet, quinoa, wheat), breads (whole wheat or rye bread, whole-grain rolls, stone-ground corn or whole wheat tortillas, whole wheat pitas), cereals (oatmeal, seven-grain hot cereal, ready-to-eat cereals made with whole oats, whole wheat, or other whole grains), pasta (whole wheat noodles, soba noodles), crackers (whole wheat crackers, whole rye crispbread), pancakes (whole wheat or buckwheat)	• Choose whole grains or foods made with minimally processed whole grains. • Choose foods that list a whole grain as the first ingredient.
Vegetables	Collard greens, mustard greens, spinach, kale, chard, bok choy, green cabbage, red cabbage, winter squash, summer squash, zucchini, sweet potatoes, broccoli, carrots, tomatoes, corn, turnips, string beans, lettuce, onions, okra, beets, cauliflower, brussels sprouts, dry beans and peas (kidney beans, black beans, soybeans, chickpeas, lentils, black-eyed peas)	• Choose a rainbow of colors, especially dark green and orange. • Choose dry beans and peas.**
Fruits	Peaches, nectarines, cantaloupe, watermelon, grapefruit, raisins, apples, pears, oranges, bananas, strawberries, tangerines, grapes, pineapple, mangoes, blueberries, cherries, figs, kiwi fruits, avocados	• Choose a rainbow of colors. • Choose whole fruits or sliced fruits (rather than fruit juices).
Meat, fish, and beans	Fish (salmon, trout, cod, shrimp, crab, scallops, light tuna, sardines), nuts (almonds, hazelnuts, walnuts), nut butters (peanut butter, almond butter), seeds (sunflower, pumpkin), dry beans and peas (kidney beans, black beans, soybeans, chickpeas, lentils, black-eyed peas), chicken, turkey, meat (beef, pork, ham), eggs, tofu and other high-protein vegetarian alternatives (tempeh, falafel, vegetable burgers)	• Choose dry beans and peas,** fish, poultry, nuts, and high-protein vegetarian alternatives more often than meat. • When eating meat, choose lean cuts.
Milk	Plain milk (nonfat or 1%), low-fat flavored milk, string cheese (reduced-fat mozzarella sticks), low-fat or nonfat cottage cheese, low-fat cheddar cheese, plain low-fat or nonfat yogurt, low-fat or nonfat frozen yogurt	• Choose plain low-fat (1%) or nonfat milk, yogurt, and other dairy foods.***

*Best-choice foods contain the most nutrients and contribute to overall health.

**Dry beans and peas can also be considered part of the vegetable group.

***Students who cannot drink milk can choose lactose-free milk or calcium-fortified nondairy alternatives such as unflavored and unsweetened rice milk or soy milk.

From L.W.Y. Cheung, H. Dart, S. Kalin, and S.L. Gortmaker, 2007, *Eat Well & Keep Moving,* 2nd ed. (Champaign, IL: Human Kinetics).

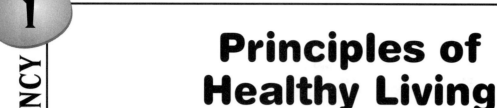

Principles of Healthy Living

Go for 5 Fruits and Veggies—More Is Better!

Eat 5 or more servings of fruits and vegetables each day! Eat a variety of colors—try red, orange, yellow, green, blue, and purple.

Get Whole Grains and Sack the Sugar!

Choose healthy whole grains for flavor, fiber, and vitamins. Limit sweets. Candy, soft drinks, and other sugary drinks have almost nothing in them that is good for you—no vitamins or minerals or other healthy things. They contain just sugar.

Keep the Fat Healthy!

We need fat in our diets, but not all types of fat are good for us. Our bodies like the healthy fat that tends to come from plants and is liquid at room temperature. Examples are olive oil, canola oil, vegetable oil, and peanut oil. Our bodies do not like unhealthy fat, which is solid at room temperature. Examples include saturated fat (usually found in animal products such as meat and whole milk) and trans fat (found in fast-food fries and store-bought cookies). Of the unhealthy fats, trans fat is the worst and should rarely, if ever, be eaten.

Start Smart With Breakfast!

Eating breakfast helps you focus on schoolwork and gives you energy to play. Breakfast is a great meal for adding whole grains, fruit, and low-fat or nonfat milk to your day!

Keep Moving!

Being active is a very important part of healthy living. Do what you like most, and keep your body moving for at least an hour a day!

Freeze the Screen!

Watching TV, playing video games, or playing on the computer keeps your body still. Keep screen time as low as it can go, and never let it add up to more than 2 hours per day.

From L.W.Y. Cheung, H. Dart, S. Kalin, and S.L. Gortmaker, 2007, *Eat Well & Keep Moving,* 2nd ed. (Champaign, IL: Human Kinetics).

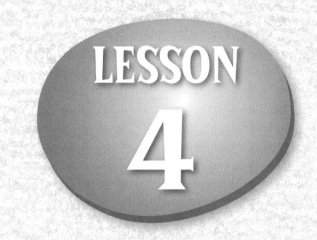
Balancing Act

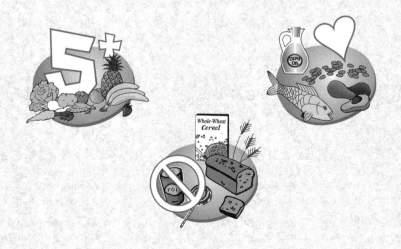

BACKGROUND

A balanced diet is important because different foods contain different combinations of nutrients. No single food can supply all the nutrients needed to maintain good health. For example, oranges provide vitamin C but not vitamin B_{12}, while low-fat cheese provides vitamin B_{12} but not vitamin C. Foods in one food group cannot replace those in another. Similarly, not all foods in the same group contain the same nutrients. Oranges, for instance, do not contain much vitamin A, but cantaloupe is a good source of this vitamin. Choosing foods from all the food groups and choosing a variety of foods within each food group every day will make your diet interesting as well as balanced.

Nutrition surveys have found that American children are eating a bit too much saturated fat and not enough fruits, vegetables, and calcium-rich foods. Foods from all of the food groups are important. To make the best choices within each food group, remember these guidelines from the Principles of Healthy Living (see lesson 1):

▶ Eat 5 or more servings of fruits and vegetables each day.

▶ Choose whole-grain foods and limit foods and beverages with added sugar.

▶ Choose healthy fat, limit saturated fat, and avoid trans fat.

The Get 3 At School and 5⁺ A Day promotion, which encourages students to eat more fruits and vegetables, can be used as an extension to this lesson. See lesson 28 in part III, Promotions for the Classroom, for details.

ESTIMATED TEACHING TIME AND RELATED SUBJECT AREAS

Estimated teaching time: 80 minutes

Related subject areas: science, math

OBJECTIVES

1. Students will learn to value a balanced diet and be able to assess and create a healthy and balanced menu.

2. Students will be able to examine menus and learn to identify and link sources of nutrients with specific foods.

MATERIALS

1. Handout 1, Food, Nutrients, and You

2. Worksheet 1, Runner's Balanced Diet

3. Worksheet 2, Now You Create a Balanced Meal!

4. Solutions to worksheet 1

5. Solutions to worksheet 2
6. Transparency 1, Principles of Healthy Living
7. Transparency 2, The Balanced Plate for Health
8. Transparency 3, Maria's Menu—Food Choices
9. Solutions to transparency 3

PROCEDURE

1. Ask students to discuss the meaning of the word *balance.* Possible student responses include the following:
   * Balance represents equality, fairness.
   * Balance means to remain upright, avoid falling.
   * Balance means to be stable, steady.
   * Balance means that one side equals the other side. There is not too much or too little on either side.

2. Ask the students how the definition of *balance* relates to the term *balanced diet.*

   The key idea is that having a balanced diet means eating a variety of healthy foods from each food group. Possible student responses include the following:
   * People need to eat different kinds of foods for the body to obtain an assortment of vitamins, minerals, carbohydrate, protein, fat, and water.
   * If you eat one food all the time, you won't get enough of the nutrients provided by other food choices, and so you won't be balanced.

3. Project transparency 1, Principles of Healthy Living, and review the key messages with the students, especially the principles that relate to fruits and vegetables, whole grains, and healthy fat. Next, project transparency 2, The Balanced Plate for Health, and review the importance of choosing foods from all the food groups, as well as choosing a variety of foods from each food group every day. Next, project transparency 3, Maria's Menu—Food Choices, and have the students examine Maria's menu to see whether it meets the healthy living guidelines. Together, the students will complete the table to assess Maria's diet using these considerations:
   * Are her grain choices whole grains?
   * Did she eat at least 5 servings of fruits and vegetables?
   * Did she choose healthy fat sources, such as olive oil, or foods that contain healthy fat, such as peanut butter and fish?
   * Did she limit her intake of added sugar and sugar-sweetened beverages?

   Ask the students, "Is Maria's diet balanced or unbalanced?" The answer is that her diet is somewhat balanced. She selected foods from each food group, but she could make some healthier choices and have a more varied menu. For example, Maria could do the following:
   * **Fruits:** Rather than choose a banana at both breakfast and lunch, she could choose sliced strawberries in place of a banana at one of the meals. Also, she could add grapes or apple slices at dinner to get another healthy fruit into her diet.

- **Vegetables:** French fries are not healthy vegetables, plus Maria had them for both lunch and dinner. She needs to eat more healthy vegetables (especially ones that are dark green and deep orange); she could choose baked sweet potato fries, steamed broccoli, or cauliflower sautéed in olive oil.
- **Grains:** She gets no whole grains. She needs to choose 100% whole wheat breads and buns as well as grains that have little or no added sugar (choose oatmeal or unsweetened shredded wheat rather than Frosted Flakes).
- **Sugar-sweetened beverages:** Rather than drink Kool-Aid and chocolate milk, better choices for Maria would be water, 100% fruit juice (no more than 8 ounces, or 250 milliliters, per day), or plain 1% or nonfat milk. To make it easier to stay within the 8-ounce fruit juice limit, Maria could dilute a small amount of 100% fruit juice (4 ounces) with sparkling water.
- **Unhealthy fat:** Whole milk, bacon, and cheeseburgers are high in saturated fat. It would be better for Maria to choose 1% or nonfat milk and a dinner entrée that is lower in saturated fat, such as baked chicken without the skin. French fries are high in trans fat, which should generally be avoided.

4. Review the meaning of the term *eating balanced meals.* Discuss the following key points:
   - A balanced diet gives your body what it needs to be healthy and to grow strong. The key to a balanced diet is choosing a variety of healthy foods from each food group.
   - Each food group provides a unique mix of nutrients the body needs, so it is important to eat foods from each group every day. We do not need the same amount of food from each group. The key to a balanced diet is to recognize that we need a greater proportion of grains (especially whole grains), vegetables, and fruits than we do foods from the meat, fish, and beans and milk groups. (To reinforce this point and the next point, display transparency 2, The Balanced Plate for Health.)
   - A balanced, healthy diet also contains a variety of foods from within each food group. Just as each food group offers a different mix of nutrients, so too do individual foods within a food group. By choosing many different types of foods within a group, you are helping make sure that your body gets the nutrients it needs to thrive. Plus, eating a variety of foods also keeps your meals interesting and full of flavor.
   - Sweets (including soft drinks and other sweet beverages) and foods that are high in unhealthy fat are not a necessary part of a balanced, healthy diet. In fact, they are often the main foods that make a diet unbalanced and unhealthy, since they can take the place of more nutritious choices. Choose these foods only sometimes to make sure that what you eat stays balanced and healthy.

5. Distribute handout 1, Food, Nutrients, and You, and briefly discuss the six types of nutrients, their functions, and their food sources.

6. Have students form pairs or small groups. Distribute worksheet 1, and read "A Runner's Story" aloud.

A Runner's Story

A long-distance runner has been training hard for the past month. She has been running every day and has been eating a balanced diet. She is racing and runs hard toward the finish line. Her training and her balanced diet help her win the race.

7. After reading the story, have the students discuss in their pairs or small groups how specific foods and their related nutrients would help the runner successfully train and complete the race. Have them fill in the blanks on the chart, including what the runner might have eaten to get each nutrient. Discuss the group's ideas and list their food choices on the board, along with the nutrients and benefits provided. (Refer to the solutions for worksheet 2 for ideas.)

8. Display the Principles of Healthy Living transparency once again and relate student answers back to this guide. Do the foods that they picked for the Runner's Balanced Diet worksheet come from all food groups? Do their food selections follow the Principles of Healthy Living (specifically, to eat whole grains, 5 or more servings of fruit and vegetables, and healthy fat)?

SUMMARY

1. Distribute worksheet 2, Now You Create a Balanced Meal! Have students work individually, in their pairs, or small groups to create a balanced menu and their own Balanced Plate for Health. A solutions worksheet is provided as an example of a balanced meal.

2. When the pairs or small groups have finished, ask them to share their balanced meals with the class. Post each group's meal on a bulletin board for everyone to view.

3. Encourage the students to ensure that their meals are as balanced as possible each day so they will get all the nutrients they need to grow and be healthy.

Name _____

Food, Nutrients, and You

▶ **TABLE 4.1   Food, Nutrients, and You**

Nutrients and their functions	Food sources
Water • Helps cool your body when it is working hard • Helps you digest your food • Helps nutrients get to different parts of the body	• Water, other beverages,* fruit, vegetables, soup
Carbohydrate • Gives you energy quickly • Can be stored as energy for later use • Gives sweetness and texture to foods	• Whole grains, fruit, starchy and root vegetables (like yams and sweet potatoes), legumes and dry beans (like kidney beans or black-eyed peas), low-fat or nonfat milk, low-fat or fat-free yogurt
Protein • Builds and repairs muscles • Helps your body grow • Gives you energy	• Lean meat, poultry, fish, dry beans, nuts, low-fat and skim milk and milk products, eggs, tofu
Fat • Gives you energy, especially for long-term use • Makes you feel less hungry • Makes food taste good • Helps keep your skin smooth	• Vegetable oil, olive oil, canola oil, peanut oil, nuts, seeds, and fish are rich in healthy fat. • Fatty meats and milk products are high in unhealthy fat; choose lean meats and low-fat or nonfat milk products instead.
Minerals • Help your blood carry oxygen and nutrients to your muscles and other body parts (iron) • Help build strong bones and teeth (calcium)	• Lean meat, some vegetables (spinach), whole grains and fortified cereals, legumes (navy or black beans, iron) • Low-fat or skim milk, low-fat cheese, low-fat or fat-free yogurt, dark-green vegetables (broccoli, kale), tofu, fortified 100% orange juice, fortified nondairy milk (calcium)
Vitamins • Help you to see better at night (vitamin A) • Help your body get energy from the food you eat (B vitamins) • Help your body heal cuts and bruises (vitamin C) • Help you fight off infections (vitamin C)	• Vegetables (especially dark green and orange), fruit, low-fat or nonfat milk (vitamin A) • Whole grains, fish, poultry, lean meat, low-fat or nonfat milk (B vitamins) • Fruit (especially citrus), and vegetables (vitamin C)

*Best choices do not have caffeine or sugar.

From L.W.Y. Cheung, H. Dart, S. Kalin, and S.L. Gortmaker, 2007, *Eat Well & Keep Moving,* 2nd ed. (Champaign, IL: Human Kinetics).

Runner's Balanced Diet

A Runner's Story

A long-distance runner has been training hard for the past month. She has been running every day and has been eating a balanced diet. She is racing and runs hard toward the finish line. Her training and her balanced diet help her win the race.

Why does the runner need to eat a balanced diet, and how did it help her to win? Use worksheet 1, Food, Nutrients, and You, to fill out the following chart:

▶TABLE 4.2   Runner's Balanced Diet

Nutrient in her balanced diet	How nutrient helps her	What she might have eaten
Carbohydrate		
Protein		
Fat		
Minerals		
Vitamins		
Water		

From L.W.Y. Cheung, H. Dart, S. Kalin, and S.L. Gortmaker, 2007, *Eat Well & Keep Moving,* 2nd ed. (Champaign, IL: Human Kinetics).

WORKSHEET 1

Name _____

Now You Create a Balanced Meal!

Directions

Create a balanced meal that you would enjoy. Pick a food from each food group and then write down the nutrients that each food gives you.

▶ **TABLE 4.3   Now You Create a Balanced Meal!**

Food group	Your food choice	Nutrients the food gives you
Grains		
Fruits		
Vegetables		
Meat, fish, and beans		
Milk		

From L.W.Y. Cheung, H. Dart, S. Kalin, and S.L. Gortmaker, 2007, *Eat Well & Keep Moving,* 2nd ed. (Champaign, IL: Human Kinetics).

(continued)

Mark the appropriate box to answer Yes or No to the following questions:

▶TABLE 4.4 Did You Meet the Healthy Living Goals?

	Yes	No
Did you include healthy fat?		
Did you include whole grains?		
Did you include sweetened beverages or sweets?		
Did you include fruits and vegetables?		

Create your own Balanced Plate for Health: In each section of the plate below, list healthy foods that you like.

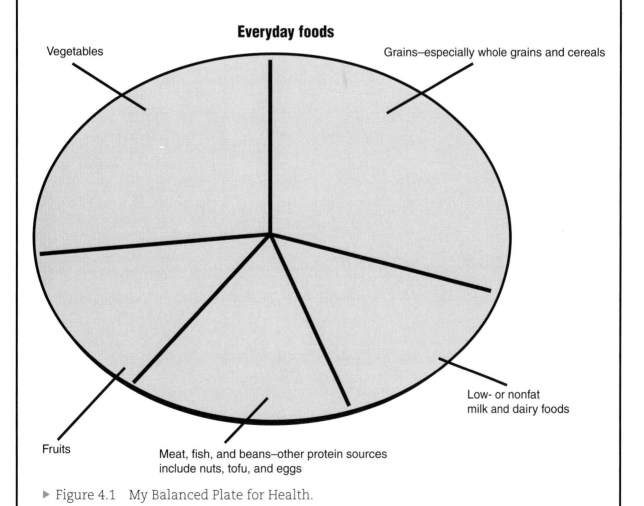

Everyday foods

Vegetables

Grains—especially whole grains and cereals

Low- or nonfat milk and dairy foods

Fruits

Meat, fish, and beans—other protein sources include nuts, tofu, and eggs

▶ Figure 4.1 My Balanced Plate for Health.

Runner's Balanced Diet

A Runner's Story

A long-distance runner has been training hard for the past month. She has been running every day and has been eating a balanced diet. She is racing and runs hard toward the finish line. Her training and her balanced diet help her win the race.

Why does the runner need to eat a balanced diet, and how did it help her to win? Use worksheet 1, Food, Nutrients, and You, to fill out the following chart:

▶ **TABLE 4.5   Example of a Runner's Balanced Diet Solution**

Nutrient in her balanced diet	How nutrient helps her	What she might have eaten
Carbohydrate	• Gives her quick energy	Whole wheat pasta, whole-grain bread, chickpeas and other beans, bananas and other fruits
Protein	• Helps her build up and repair muscles	1% or skim milk, chicken, fish, beans
Fat	• Gives her long-term energy	Vegetable oil (in salad dressing and cooking), nuts
Minerals	• Give her strong bones • Help her blood carry oxygen to muscles	1% or skim milk, low-fat or fat-free yogurt, chicken, lean meat, whole-grain bread, fortified cereal
Vitamins	• Help her see at night • Help her get energy from food	Carrots, broccoli, spinach, oranges, whole grains, 1% or skim milk
Water	• Helps her stay cool while she is running hard	Water, fruit juice, vegetable juice, soups, fresh fruit

Now You Create a Balanced Meal!

Directions

Create a balanced meal that you would enjoy. Pick a food from each food group and then write down the nutrients that each food gives you.

▶ **TABLE 4.6   Now You Create a Balanced Meal! Solution Example**

Food group	Your food choice	Nutrients the food gives you
Grains	Whole wheat bread	Carbohydrate, vitamins, minerals
Fruits	Orange wedges	Water, carbohydrate, vitamins, minerals
Vegetables	Spinach salad and olive oil dressing	Vitamins, minerals, carbohydrate, fat
Meat, fish, and beans	Peanut butter	Protein, vitamins, minerals, fat
Milk	Nonfat milk	Water, protein, carbohydrate, vitamins, minerals

Mark the appropriate box to answer Yes or No to the following questions:

▶ **TABLE 4.7   Did You Meet the Healthy Living Goals? Solution**

	Yes	No
Did you include healthy fat?	✓	
Did you include whole grains?	✓	
Did you include sweetened beverages or sweets?		✓
Did you include fruits and vegetables?	✓	

From L.W.Y. Cheung, H. Dart, S. Kalin, and S.L. Gortmaker, 2007, *Eat Well & Keep Moving*, 2nd ed. (Champaign, IL: Human Kinetics).

Principles of Healthy Living

Go for 5 Fruits and Veggies—More Is Better!

Eat 5 or more servings of fruits and vegetables each day! Eat a variety of colors—try red, orange, yellow, green, blue, and purple.

Get Whole Grains and Sack the Sugar!

Choose healthy whole grains for flavor, fiber, and vitamins. Limit sweets. Candy, soft drinks, and other sugary drinks have almost nothing in them that is good for you—no vitamins or minerals or other healthy things. They contain just sugar.

Keep the Fat Healthy!

We need fat in our diets, but not all types of fat are good for us. Our bodies like the healthy fat that tends to come from plants and is liquid at room temperature. Examples are olive oil, canola oil, vegetable oil, and peanut oil. Our bodies do not like unhealthy fat, which is solid at room temperature. Examples include saturated fat (usually found in animal products such as meat and whole milk) and trans fat (found in fast-food fries and store-bought cookies). Of the unhealthy fats, trans fat is the worst and should rarely, if ever, be eaten.

Start Smart With Breakfast!

Eating breakfast helps you focus on schoolwork and gives you energy to play. Breakfast is a great meal for adding whole grains, fruit, and low-fat or nonfat milk to your day!

Keep Moving!

Being active is a very important part of healthy living. Do what you like most, and keep your body moving for at least an hour a day!

Freeze the Screen!

Watching TV, playing video games, or playing on the computer keeps your body still. Keep screen time as low as it can go, and never let it add up to more than 2 hours per day.

From L.W.Y. Cheung, H. Dart, S. Kalin, and S.L. Gortmaker, 2007, *Eat Well & Keep Moving*, 2nd ed. (Champaign, IL: Human Kinetics).

The Balanced Plate for Health

Everyday foods

Vegetables

Grains—especially whole grains and cereals

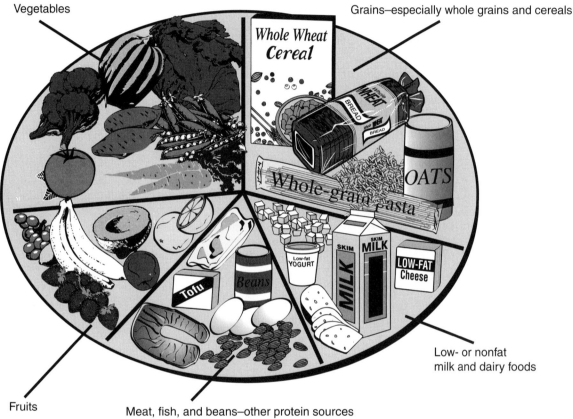

Low- or nonfat
milk and dairy foods

Fruits

Meat, fish, and beans—other protein sources
include nuts, tofu, and eggs

"Sometimes" foods

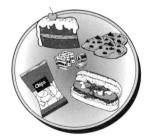

The key to a balanced diet is to recognize
that grains (especially whole grains), vegetables, and fruits are needed in greater
proportion than are the foods from the
meat, fish, and beans and milk groups.

From L.W.Y. Cheung, H. Dart, S. Kalin, and S.L. Gortmaker, 2007, *Eat Well & Keep Moving,* 2nd ed. (Champaign, IL: Human Kinetics).

Maria's Menu—Food Choices

▶TABLE 4.8   Maria's Menu—Food Choices

Breakfast	Lunch	Dinner
Frosted Flakes with banana slices Whole milk	Turkey sandwich on 2 slices of white bread with mayonnaise French fries Low-fat chocolate milk Banana	Bacon cheeseburger on white bun French fries Fruit punch 2 small cookies

▶TABLE 4.9   Does Maria's Menu Meet the Goal?

Healthy living goals	Does Maria's menu meet the goal?	What would you recommend?
Choose a variety of foods from every food group.		
Get whole grains and sack the sugar.		
Eat 5 or more servings of fruits and vegetables each day—more is better.		
Keep the fat healthy.		

Maria's Menu—Food Choices

▶TABLE 4.10 Maria's Menu—Food Choices Solution

Breakfast	Lunch	Dinner
Frosted Flakes with banana slices Whole milk	Turkey sandwich on 2 slices of white bread with mayonnaise French fries Low-fat chocolate milk Banana	Bacon cheeseburger on white bun French fries Fruit punch 2 small cookies

▶TABLE 4.11 Does Maria's Menu Meet the Goal? Solution

Healthy eating goals	Does Maria's menu meet the goal?	What would you recommend?
Choose a variety of foods from every food group.	No, she has food from all the food groups but not a lot of variety within each group.	Instead of having a banana for both breakfast and lunch, she could have strawberries with breakfast; instead of choosing bread at lunch and dinner, she could choose a whole-grain side dish, such as tabbouleh or brown rice.
Get whole grains and sack the sugar.	No, she has not chosen any whole grains, and she has several foods with added sugar (Frosted Flakes, chocolate milk, fruit punch, cookies).	She could choose whole-grain cereal with little or no added sugar (e.g., oatmeal, shredded wheat) for breakfast, whole wheat bread for lunch, and a whole-grain bun for dinner; she could have plain low-fat or nonfat milk for lunch and water or a small glass of 100% fruit juice with dinner; she could choose fruit (apple slices, orange wedges, grapes) for dessert.
Eat 5 or more servings of fruits and vegetables each day—more is better.	No, she does not have enough vegetables (French fries don't count as part of the 5+ servings).	She could add romaine lettuce and sliced tomato to her sandwich at lunch and choose raw carrot sticks or bell pepper slices instead of French fries; she could eat steamed broccoli, sautéed spinach, roasted sweet potatoes, or other vegetables with dinner.
Keep the fat healthy.	No, whole milk, bacon, and cheeseburgers are high in saturated fat. French fries are high in trans fat, which should generally be avoided.	Maria could drink 1% or nonfat milk and choose a dinner entrée that is lower in saturated fat, such as baked chicken without the skin, a veggie burger with reduced-fat cheese, or grilled fish. She could eat baked sweet potato fries (made with canola oil) rather than French fries.

From L.W.Y. Cheung, H. Dart, S. Kalin, and S.L. Gortmaker, 2007, *Eat Well & Keep Moving*, 2nd ed. (Champaign, IL: Human Kinetics).

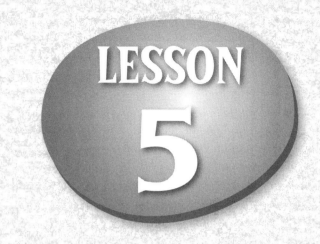

Fast-Food Frenzy

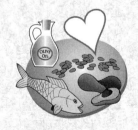

BACKGROUND

Fat is a necessary part of our diets. Fat makes food taste good, and it helps the body absorb and transport fat-soluble vitamins, such as vitamins A, D, E, and K. Fat is the primary way energy is stored in the body, and body fat cushions and protects our internal organs. In addition, components of fat are also involved in other important body functions such as maintaining healthy skin and hair.

The problem is that most Americans consume too much unhealthy fat (namely, saturated fat and trans fat), which increases the risk of heart disease and stroke. The good news is that eating less unhealthy fat and eating more healthy fat (namely, polyunsaturated fat and monounsaturated fat) help reduce the risk of heart disease.

FAT FACTS

Healthy fat, meaning monounsaturated and polyunsaturated fat, can decrease the risk of heart disease. These types of fat are liquid at room temperature. Examples of foods high in monounsaturated fat include olive, canola, and peanut oils; almonds; and avocados. Nuts (such as walnuts) and soybean, corn, and cottonseed oils are rich in polyunsaturated fat. Fatty ocean fish contain a special type of polyunsaturated fat (omega-3 fat) that is also very healthy.

Unhealthy fat, meaning saturated and trans fat, can increase the risk of heart disease. Saturated fat is solid at room temperature and comes mainly from animal-based foods. Examples include full-fat dairy products (such as whole milk, cream, butter, and ice cream), fatty cuts of meat, poultry skin, and lard, as well as palm oil and coconut oil. One way to minimize intake of unhealthy fat is to choose lean meats, remove poultry skin, select low-fat or nonfat dairy products, and replace saturated fat with unsaturated fat in food preparation (for instance, sautéing vegetables in olive oil instead of butter).

Trans fat is formed when polyunsaturated vegetable fat is partially hydrogenated. This process turns the normally liquid oils into solid or semisolid fat. Trans fat content is now listed on food labels. Common sources of trans fat in the U.S. diet include fast foods (such as French fries, chicken nuggets, or onion rings), packaged snacks (biscuits, some crackers, etc.), baked goods (such as cookies, piecrusts, doughnuts, pastries, and cakes), hard stick margarines, vegetable shortening, and other foods made with partially hydrogenated vegetable oil.

The *Dietary Guidelines for Americans* recognizes the importance of reducing saturated fat intake and sets a daily limit of 10% of total daily calories from saturated fat. The American Heart Association recommends an even lower limit for saturated fat—7% of total daily calories. The *Dietary Guidelines for Americans* also advises keeping trans fat consumption as low as possible, and research suggests that it is most prudent to avoid consuming trans fat from partially hydrogenated oils.

This lesson will help students recognize that many of their favorite fast foods may be high in saturated and trans fat. Students will use nutrient information to assess fast-food menus and identify items that are high in saturated and trans fat.

The % Daily Value (% DV) can help you find out whether a food is relatively high or low in a nutrient (the % DV is listed on the Nutrition Facts label, and it is available for fast foods through restaurants' nutrition information in their brochures or on their Web sites). The Daily Value (DV) is a guideline for how much of each nutrient should be consumed each day. The % DV is based on a diet of 2,000 calories per day; for each nutrient, it tells us what percentage of the recommended DV is found in 1 serving of food. Note that a person's actual daily caloric needs vary depending on age, gender, and level of activity; for more information on caloric needs, see lesson 15, Keeping the Balance.

The % DV for saturated fat is particularly important. If a food's % DV for saturated fat is 5 or less, the food is considered low in saturated fat. The more foods chosen that have a % DV of 5 or less for saturated fat, the easier it is to eat a healthier daily diet. A food that has a DV of 20% or more for saturated fat is considered high in saturated fat. Eating too many of these foods makes it easy to exceed the daily limit for saturated fat. The overall daily goal is to select foods that together contain less than 100% of the DV for saturated fat.

Since saturated fat should contribute no more than 10% of total daily calories, a person who requires 2,000 calories per day should not consume more than 200 calories of saturated fat. Since 1 gram of fat contains 9 calories, 200 calories translates to no more than 22 grams of saturated fat (2,000 calories $\times$ .10 = 200 calories from saturated fat, and 200 calories $\div$ 9 calories per gram = 22 grams of saturated fat).

There is no % DV for trans fat, because it is unclear if there is any safe level of intake.

HOW IS % DAILY VALUE FOR SATURATED FAT CALCULATED?

Although all food labels provide % DV for nutrients, it is good to know how to calculate the % DV for saturated fat.

To calculate % DV for a particular food, divide the number of grams of saturated fat per serving by 22 and multiply by 100 (22 is used because it is recommended that a person eating a 2,000-calorie daily diet consume no more than 22 grams of saturated fat each day, as described previously).

For example, a cup of whole milk has 5 grams of saturated fat; (5 $\div$ 22) $\times$ 100 = 23%. While 5 grams may not sound like much, just 1 cup of whole milk contains 23% of the DV for saturated fat for a person who eats 2,000 calories a day.

ESTIMATED TEACHING TIME AND RELATED SUBJECT AREAS

Estimated teaching time: 65 minutes

Related subject areas: language arts, math, science, visual arts

OBJECTIVES

1. Students will be able to assess the saturated and trans fat content of their favorite fast-food meals.
2. Students will be able to design a fast-food meal that is low to moderate in saturated fat (less than or equal to 34% of the DV for saturated fat) and has 0 grams of trans fat.

MATERIALS

1. Worksheet 1, Adding Up the Saturated and Trans Fat
2. Solutions to worksheet 1
3. Large sheets of paper
4. Nutrition information on menu items from fast-food restaurants, collected from fast-food restaurants or their Web sites (optional)

PROCEDURE

1. Ask the students to raise their hands if they like to eat at fast-food restaurants.
2. Have students tell you their favorite fast-food eating places.
3. Explain that in today's lesson, students will have a chance to learn about the nutrition of some of their favorite fast foods, especially about the types of fat these foods contain. Tell the students about the differences between healthy fat and unhealthy fat:
   - Healthy fat—monounsaturated and polyunsaturated fat—is liquid at room temperature; it comes from plant sources, such as olive oil, canola oil, peanut oil, corn oil, safflower oil, nuts, peanut butter, and avocados; and it is also found in fish. Healthy fat can help reduce the risk of heart disease.
   - Unhealthy fat—saturated fat and trans fat—is solid at room temperature; it often comes from animal sources or from oils that have been partially hydrogenated (a chemical process that turns liquid oil into a solid), and it increases the risk of heart disease.
   - Explain that many fast foods are high in unhealthy saturated fat and trans fat. Saturated fat should be limited in a healthy eating plan, and trans fat from partially hydrogenated oils should be avoided.

4. Have each student write down all the foods that make up his favorite fast-food meal, including side orders like French fries, salads and salad dressings, other sauces, drinks, and desserts, if he usually orders them.
5. Review with students the concept of % Daily Value (% DV). Explain that the % DV lets them find out whether a food is high or low in a nutrient. Regarding saturated fat, if the % DV is 5 or less, then the food is considered low in saturated fat. If the % DV is 20 or more, then that food is considered high in saturated fat. The more foods chosen that have a % DV of 5 or less for fat, the easier it is to eat a healthier daily diet.
6. The overall daily goal (for all the foods you eat in a day) is to select foods that together contain less than 100% of the DV for saturated fat. For a meal like lunch or dinner, a good goal is to keep the total % DV for saturated fat less than 34% (34% is approximately a third of the daily 100% DV—see the note on this page). There is no % DV for trans fat; the goal is to avoid trans fat.
7. Distribute worksheet 1, Adding Up the Saturated and Trans Fat, and have each student determine the total % DV for saturated fat in her favorite fast-food meal, along with the total grams of trans fat. Students who cannot find an item from their meal on the list should use the saturated fat and trans fat

The use of 34% as the DV for saturated fat for a meal like lunch or dinner is simply an approximation of what someone might eat for lunch or dinner. The 34% was picked to help provide a standard for the class activity and is not a recommendation. Remind students that they need to focus on the overall recommendation to select foods throughout the day that together contain less than 100% of the DV for saturated fat and to avoid trans fat.

information from an item very similar to the one they chose. Alternatively, most fast-food restaurants have nutrition information available to those who ask. Such information is also often available on the restaurants' Web sites.

8. Explain to the students that a healthy lunch or dinner should not (on average) contain more than 34% of the DV for saturated fat (both hidden in foods and added to foods), and less is even better. Trans fat should be avoided.

Also tell the students that, although fast-food eating places are favorites of many young people, most fast foods are also high in salt and refined carbohydrate as well as low in fiber. This is the opposite of the diet recommended for staying healthy and lowering the risk of diseases such as heart disease and cancer. (Remind them of the Principles of Healthy Living covered in lesson 1.)

9. Ask the students whether their fast-food meals contained less than 34% of the DV for saturated fat and 0 grams of trans fat. If any did, list the items from those meals on the board.

10. Have the students form pairs or small groups. Ask them to create a healthy lunch that is low in saturated fat (less than 34% of the DV) and has 0 grams of trans fat and that most of them would enjoy. Students can create the healthy lunch by selecting foods that are low in saturated fat and have 0 grams of trans fat from the fast-food selections (found on worksheet 1, Adding Up the Saturated and Trans Fat). Have students write down their choices on large sheets of paper, including each menu choice and the % DV for saturated fat and the grams of trans fat it contains.

11. Post the healthier menus and ask the groups to share their menus with the class. Encourage the students to think of these lower saturated fat and lower trans fat items when they eat at a fast-food restaurant.

Optional: Have the class create a histogram that graphs the saturated fat and trans fat content in each group's menu selection.

12. Stress that students should not be fearful of fat. Remind them to enjoy foods with healthy fat, such as olive, canola, and other plant oils; nuts and peanut butter; avocados; and fish. It is OK to occasionally eat a small serving of a food that is high in saturated fat (also known as a *"sometimes" food).* But on a regular basis, they should choose foods that are low in saturated fat and avoid trans fat.

13. Follow-up activities may include the following:

   • Have the students create an advertisement that would appeal to others their age for a healthier meal (one that is low in saturated fat and trans fat) at a fast-food restaurant. This ad may be designed for a magazine or billboard (poster), for television (skit, jingle), or for radio (dialogue, jingle).

   • Review the nutrition information provided in worksheet 1, Adding Up the Saturated and Trans Fat, and try to create a menu that meets the healthy living goals (for instance, a meal that includes fruits, vegetables, and whole grains; has limited amounts of saturated fat and avoids trans fat; and limits sugar-sweetened beverages and added sugar).

   • Have students write a paragraph in their classroom journals about five important things they should consider when choosing foods at a restaurant or fast-food chain.

Name _____

Adding Up the Saturated and Trans Fat

How much saturated fat and trans fat do the most common foods at your favorite fast-food restaurant contain? This activity will help you find out.

Directions

1. Look at the foods you chose for your favorite fast-food meal. Find those foods on the following lists. If one of your foods isn't in the lists, find one that seems like it.

2. Find the % Daily Value (% DV) for saturated fat and the grams of trans fat contained in the different foods. Circle these for each of the foods you chose.

3. Add up the % DV for saturated fat that you circled. Write the number in the answer box on page 89.

4. Decide whether the total is greater than, equal to, or less than 34%. Circle the correct choice in the answer box.

5. Add up all of the grams of trans fat that you circled. Record that number in the answer box.

▶ TABLE 5.1   Percent Daily Values of Saturated Fat and Grams of Trans Fat for Fast Food

Burgers	% DV saturated fat	Grams of trans fat
Burger King Whopper	55	1.5
Jack-in-the-Box Jumbo Jack	55	1.5
McDonald's Big Mac	51	1.5
Wendy's Old-Fashioned Burger	35	1
McDonald's Quarter Pounder	37	1
McDonald's Quarter Pounder with cheese	61	1.5
Burger King Double Whopper with cheese	120	2.5
Burger King Whopper Junior	30	0.5
Wendy's double with cheese	73	2.5
McDonald's plain hamburger	16	0.5
Burger King Veggie Burger	13	0

(continued)

From L.W.Y. Cheung, H. Dart, S. Kalin, and S.L. Gortmaker, 2007, *Eat Well & Keep Moving*, 2nd ed. (Champaign, IL: Human Kinetics).

(continued)

TABLE 5.1 *(continued)*

Fish	% DV saturated fat	Grams of trans fat
Long John Silver's fish sandwich	20	4.5
McDonald's Filet-O-Fish	20	1
Burger King fish filet	30	2.5

Pizza, tacos, chili	% DV saturated fat	Grams of trans fat
Wendy's chili	11	0
14" Pizza Hut Thin 'n Crispy, supreme (2 slices)	70	1
14" Pizza Hut standard, cheese (2 slices)	70	0
Jack-in-the-Box taco	15	1
Taco Bell bean burrito	13	0.5
Taco Bell beef burrito	40	1
Taco Bell beef Enchirito	45	1
Taco Bell taco	15	0

Other fast food items	% DV saturated fat	Grams of trans fat
French fries, medium	23	4.5
Onion rings, medium	20	3.5
Jack-in-the-Box shake, medium	140	2
Kentucky Fried Chicken biscuit	10	3.5
Burger King TenderCrisp chicken Caesar salad with dressing	50	3.5
Burger King TenderGrill chicken garden salad with lite dressing	23	0
McDonald's grilled chicken Caesar salad with dressing	32	0
McDonald's Crispy Chicken Southwest salad with dressing	25	1.5
Long John Silver's coleslaw	11	0
Wendy's side salad	7	0

Sandwiches	% DV saturated fat	Grams of trans fat
Arby's Roast Beef	40	1
Arby's Roast Beef with cheese	25	1
Arby's Roast Beef sub	50	1.5
Arby's turkey sub	27	0.5
Subway meatball sub	50	1
Subway chicken breast sub	7	0
Subway roast beef sub	9	0
Subway tuna salad sub	32	0.5

(continued)

From L.W.Y. Cheung, H. Dart, S. Kalin, and S.L. Gortmaker, 2007, *Eat Well & Keep Moving,* 2nd ed. (Champaign, IL: Human Kinetics).

(continued)

TABLE 5.1   *(continued)*

Desserts	% DV saturated fat	Grams of trans fat
McDonald's apple or cherry pie	16	5
McDonald's chocolate chip cookies	12	1.5
McDonald's hot fudge sundae	35	0
McDonald's Fruit 'n Yogurt Parfait	5	0
McDonald's Apple Dippers	0	0
Dairy Queen banana split	50	0
Dairy Queen medium chocolate chip cookie dough Blizzard	100	4
Dairy Queen Oreo Brownie Earthquake	75	0
Dairy Queen ice cream sandwich	12	0.5
Wendy's mandarin oranges	0	0

Drinks	% DV saturated fat	Grams of trans fat
100% orange juice (8 oz., 250 ml)	0	0
1% milk (8 oz., 250 ml)	8	0
Nonfat milk (8 oz., 250 ml)	0	0
Water	0	0

Chicken	% DV saturated fat	Grams of trans fat
Kentucky Fried Chicken Snacker	14	0
McDonald's McNuggets (6)	16	1.5
Kentucky Fried Chicken Crispy Strips (3)	19	0
Burger King Chicken Tenders (6)	18	2.5
McDonald's grilled chicken sandwich	11	0

Combination dishes	% DV saturated fat	Grams of trans fat
Panda Express beef with broccoli	6	0
Panda Express vegetable fried rice	14	0
Panda Express orange chicken	25	1
Pizza Hut spaghetti with meat sauce	35	0
Pizza Hut spaghetti with tomato sauce	8	0
Kentucky Fried Chicken macaroni and cheese	18	1

From L.W.Y. Cheung, H. Dart, S. Kalin, and S.L. Gortmaker, 2007, *Eat Well & Keep Moving,* 2nd ed. (Champaign, IL: Human Kinetics). Data from J.A. Pennington and J.S. Douglas, 2004, *Bowes and Church's food values of portions commonly used,* 18th (Philadelphia: Lippincott, Williams, and Wilkins). Nutrition information on fast foods obtained from restaurant company Web sites. Retrieved June 25, 2007:

Arby's, www.arbys.com/nutrition/; Burger King, www.bk.com/#menu=3,-1,-1; Dairy Queen, www.dairyqueen.com/NCPublic/DQComNutrition-Calculator.htm; Jack-in-the-Box, www.jackinthebox.com/ourfood/dynamic/nutrition.php?b; Kentucky Fried Chicken, www.yum.com/nutrition/menu.asp?brandID_Abbr=2_KFC; Long John Silver's, www.ljsilvers.com/nutrition/default.htm; McDonald's, www.mcdonalds.com/usa/eat/nutrition_info.html; Panda Express, www.pandaexpress.com/menu/nutrition.aspx; Pizza Hut, www.pizzahut.com/menu/Nutrition.aspx; Subway, www.subway.com/applications/NutritionInfo/index.aspx; Taco Bell, www.yum.com/nutrition/menu.asp?brandID_Abbr=5_TB; Wendy's, www.wendys.com/food/NutritionLanding.jsp.

(continued)

Answer Box

1. What % DV for saturated fat does your meal contain?

2. Into which of the following categories does your answer to question 1 belong? (Circle one.)

- Greater than 34%
- Equal to 34%
- Less than 34%

3. How many grams of trans fat does your meal contain?

Calculation of % DV for saturated fat is based on a person needing 2,000 calories per day. There is currently no % DV for trans fat; it is important to regularly avoid foods that contain trans fat.

From L.W.Y. Cheung, H. Dart, S. Kalin, and S.L. Gortmaker, 2007, *Eat Well & Keep Moving,* 2nd ed. (Champaign, IL: Human Kinetics).

Adding Up the Saturated and Trans Fat

How much saturated fat and trans fat do the most common foods at your favorite fast-food restaurant contain? This activity will help you find out.

Directions

1. Look at the foods you chose for your favorite fast-food meal. Find those foods on the following lists. If one of your foods isn't in the lists, find one that seems very like it.

2. Find the % Daily Value (% DV) for saturated fat and the grams of trans fat contained in the different foods. Circle these for each of the foods you chose.

3. Add up the % DV for saturated fat that you circled. Write the number in the answer box.

4. Decide whether the total is greater than, equal to, or less than 34%. Circle the correct choice in the answer box on page 93.

5. Add up all of the grams of trans fat that you circled. Record that number in the answer box.

▶ **TABLE 5.2** **Percent Daily Values of Saturated Fat and Grams of Trans Fat for Fast Food**

Burgers	% DV saturated fat	Grams of trans fat
Burger King Whopper	(55)	(1.5)
Jack-in-the-Box Jumbo Jack	55	1.5
McDonald's Big Mac	51	1.5
Wendy's Old-Fashioned Burger	35	1
McDonald's Quarter Pounder	37	1
McDonald's Quarter Pounder with cheese	61	1.5
Burger King Double Whopper with cheese	120	2.5
Burger King Whopper Junior	30	0.5
Wendy's double with cheese	73	2.5
McDonald's plain hamburger	16	0.5
Burger King Veggie Burger	13	0

(continued)

From L.W.Y. Cheung, H. Dart, S. Kalin, and S.L. Gortmaker, 2007, *Eat Well & Keep Moving*, 2nd ed. (Champaign, IL: Human Kinetics).

(continued)

TABLE 5.2 *(continued)*

Fish	% DV saturated fat	Grams of trans fat
Long John Silver's fish sandwich	20	4.5
McDonald's Filet-O-Fish	20	1
Burger King fish filet	30	2.5

Pizza, tacos, chili	% DV saturated fat	Grams of trans fat
Wendy's chili	11	0
14" Pizza Hut Thin 'n Crispy, supreme (2 slices)	70	1
14" Pizza Hut standard, cheese (2 slices)	70	0
Jack-in-the-Box taco	15	1
Taco Bell bean burrito	13	0.5
Taco Bell beef burrito	40	1
Taco Bell beef Enchirito	45	1
Taco Bell taco	15	0

Other fast food items	% DV saturated fat	Grams of trans fat
French fries, medium	(23)	(4.5)
Onion rings, medium	20	3.5
Jack-in-the-Box shake, medium	140	2
Kentucky Fried Chicken biscuit	10	3.5
Burger King TenderCrisp chicken Caesar salad with dressing	50	3.5
Burger King TenderGrill chicken garden salad with lite dressing	23	0
McDonald's grilled chicken Caesar salad with dressing	32	0
McDonald's Crispy Chicken Southwest salad with dressing	25	1.5
Long John Silver's coleslaw	11	0
Wendy's side salad with Caesar dressing	20	0

Sandwiches	% DV saturated fat	Grams of trans fat
Arby's Roast Beef	40	1
Arby's Roast Beef with cheese	25	1
Arby's Roast Beef sub	50	1.5
Arby's turkey sub	27	0.5
Subway meatball sub	50	1
Subway chicken breast sub	7	0
Subway roast beef sub	9	0
Subway tuna salad sub	32	0.5

(continued)

From L.W.Y. Cheung, H. Dart, S. Kalin, and S.L. Gortmaker, 2007, *Eat Well & Keep Moving*, 2nd ed. (Champaign, IL: Human Kinetics).

(continued)

TABLE 5.2   *(continued)*

Desserts	% DV saturated fat	Grams of trans fat
McDonald's apple or cherry pie	16	5
McDonald's chocolate chip cookies	12	1.5
McDonald's hot fudge sundae	35	0
McDonald's Fruit 'n Yogurt Parfait	5	0
McDonald's Apple Dippers	0	0
Dairy Queen banana split	50	0
Dairy Queen medium chocolate chip cookie dough Blizzard	100	4
Dairy Queen Oreo Brownie Earthquake	75	0
Dairy Queen ice cream sandwich	12	0.5
Wendy's mandarin oranges	0	0

Drinks	% DV saturated fat	Grams of trans fat
100% fruit juices	0	0
1% milk (8 oz., 250 ml)	(8)	(0)
Nonfat milk (8 oz., 250 ml)	0	0
Water	0	0

Chicken	% DV saturated fat	Grams of trans fat
Kentucky Fried Chicken Snacker	14	0
McDonald's McNuggets (6)	16	1.5
Kentucky Fried Chicken Crispy Strips (3)	19	0
Burger King Chicken Tenders (6)	18	2.5
McDonald's grilled chicken sandwich	11	0

Combination dishes	% DV saturated fat	Grams of trans fat
Panda Express beef with broccoli	6	0
Panda Express vegetable fried rice	14	0
Panda Express orange chicken	25	1
Pizza Hut spaghetti with meat sauce	35	0
Pizza Hut spaghetti with tomato sauce	8	0
Kentucky Fried Chicken macaroni and cheese	18	1

From L.W.Y. Cheung, H. Dart, S. Kalin, and S.L. Gortmaker, 2007, *Eat Well & Keep Moving,* 2nd ed. (Champaign, IL: Human Kinetics). Data from J.A. Pennington and J.S. Douglas, 2004, *Bowes and Church's food values of portions commonly used,* 18th (Philadelphia: Lippincott, Williams, and Wilkins). Nutrition information on fast foods obtained from restaurant company Web sites. Retrieved June 25, 2007:

Arby's, www.arbys.com/nutrition/; Burger King, www.bk.com/#menu=3,-1,-1; Dairy Queen, www.dairyqueen.com/NCPublic/DQComNutrition-Calculator.htm; Jack-in-the-Box, www.jackinthebox.com/ourfood/dynamic/nutrition.php?b; Kentucky Fried Chicken, www.yum.com/nutrition/menu.asp?brandID_Abbr=2_KFC; Long John Silver's, www.ljsilvers.com/nutrition/default.htm; McDonald's, www.mcdonalds.com/usa/eat/nutrition_info.html; Panda Express, www.pandaexpress.com/menu/nutrition.aspx; Pizza Hut, www.pizzahut.com/menu/Nutrition.aspx; Subway, www.subway.com/applications/NutritionInfo/index.aspx; Taco Bell, www.yum.com/nutrition/menu.asp?brandID_Abbr=5_TB; Wendy's, www.wendys.com/food/NutritionLanding.jsp.

(continued)

Answer Box (Example)

1. What is the total % Daily Value (DV) for saturated fat?

86%

2. Into which of the following categories does your answer to question 1 belong? (Circle one.)

- (• Greater than 34%)
- • Equal to 34%
- • Less than 34%

3. How many grams of trans fat does your meal contain?

6

Calculation of % DV for saturated fat is based on a person needing 2,000 calories per day. There is currently no % DV for trans fat; it is important to regularly avoid foods that contain trans fat.

From L.W.Y. Cheung, H. Dart, S. Kalin, and S.L. Gortmaker, 2007, *Eat Well & Keep Moving,* 2nd ed. (Champaign, IL: Human Kinetics).

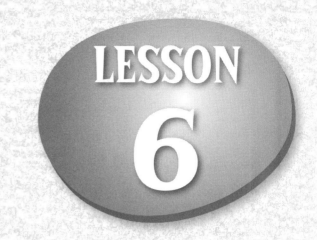

Snack Attack

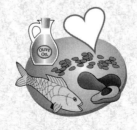

BACKGROUND

For children in the United States, snacks contribute roughly 25% of daily energy intake and roughly 20% of intake of other nutrients. Unfortunately, many popular snack foods are high in unhealthy fat (saturated and trans fat), added sugar, and salt. Ideally we should eat only limited amounts of these "sometimes" kinds of foods and regularly eat more nutrient-rich foods such as fruits, vegetables, whole grains, and low-fat or nonfat dairy selections.

This lesson helps students make healthier snack choices, primarily by choosing snack foods with more healthy fat and less unhealthy fat. Healthy fat, meaning monounsaturated and polyunsaturated fat, may decrease the risk of heart disease; most plant oils are excellent sources of healthy fat, as are nuts, seeds, and fish. Unhealthy fat, meaning saturated and trans fat, can increase the risk of heart disease. Saturated fat is found mainly in animal products (such as full-fat dairy products, fatty cuts of meat, poultry skin, and lard) and in tropical oils (palm oil and coconut oil). Trans fat is formed when polyunsaturated vegetable oils are partially hydrogenated, a process that turns the normally liquid oils into solid or semisolid fat. (For more details on healthy and unhealthy fat, see lesson 5, Fast-Food Frenzy.)

Reading food labels is an effective way to compare the fat and nutrient content of various snack foods. The place to find out whether a food is relatively high or low in a nutrient is the % Daily Value (% DV) column on the Nutrition Facts label. The Daily Value (DV) is a guideline for how much of each nutrient we should consume each day. The % DV is based on a diet of 2,000 calories per day; for each nutrient, it tells us what percentage of the recommended Daily Value is found in 1 serving of food.

The % DV for saturated fat is particularly important when selecting snack or other foods. If a food's % DV for saturated fat is 5 or less, the food is considered low in saturated fat. Foods that have a % DV of 20 or more are considered high in saturated fat. (To learn how to calculate % DV for saturated fat, see How Is % Daily Value for Saturated Fat Calculated? in lesson 5, page 83.) The more foods chosen that have a % DV of 5 or less for saturated fat, the easier it is to stay within the healthy fat limits. The overall daily goal is to select foods that together contain less than 100% of the DV for saturated fat. For vitamins, fiber, calcium, and iron, however, the goal is get 100% of the DV.

There is no % DV for trans fat because it is unclear if there is any safe level of intake; the consumption of trans fat is strongly associated with increased risk of coronary heart disease, sudden death, and possibly diabetes. The *Dietary Guidelines for Americans* advises keeping trans fat consumption as low as possible. Research suggests it may be prudent to limit trans fat consumption from partially hydrogenated oils to no more than 0.5% of total energy intake per day. For a diet of 2,000 calories per day, that means limiting trans fat intake from partially hydrogenated oils to roughly 1 gram per day. For practical purposes, that means avoiding trans fat from partially hydrogenated oils.

Food labels list the number of grams of trans fat per serving. Keep in mind that products made with partially hydrogenated oils can still claim "0 grams trans fat" if the product contains less than 0.5 grams of trans fat per serving. These small amounts of trans fat can add up over the day. So make sure to watch out for the words *partially hydrogenated vegetable oil* in the ingredients list. Switch to an alternative product that does not contain partially hydrogenated oil, especially if it is a product you consume regularly.

Fast-food chains, sit-down restaurants, bakeries, and other commercial food establishments are not required to give nutrition information on the foods they serve. Many large chains offer this information on their Web sites. One strategy for minimizing trans fat consumption in restaurants is to avoid deep-fried foods, since many restaurants still use partially hydrogenated oils for deep-frying. Consumers can also become advocates and ask their favorite restaurants to switch from partially hydrogenated oils to healthy oils.

ESTIMATED TEACHING TIME AND RELATED SUBJECT AREAS

Estimated teaching time: 1 hour, 30 minutes

Related subject areas: science, math, art

OBJECTIVES

1. Students will describe why they should select healthful snacks.
2. Students will learn how to choose healthier snacks by analyzing food labels to locate information on unhealthy fat content.

MATERIALS

1. Transparency 1, Reading Food Labels
2. Worksheet 1, Be Fat Wise
3. Snack Food Information Cards (for use with worksheet 1)
4. Worksheet 2, Snacking the Fast-Food Way
5. Worksheet 3, What's in a Snack?
6. Solutions to worksheet 1
7. Solutions to worksheet 2 (create a transparency of worksheet 2)
8. A variety of empty snack food packages (students may bring these in)

PROCEDURE

1. Have students make a list of their 10 favorite snack foods or beverages, and then have them identify items that meet the Principles of Healthy Living (you may display the overhead transparency 1 from lesson 1, page 23; focus on the guidelines related to healthy fat, whole grains, fruits and vegetables, and added sugars). Discuss the importance of regularly choosing foods that are low in saturated fat and the importance of avoiding trans fat. Eating snacks high in saturated fat is OK every once in a while. But on a regular basis, choose foods that are low in saturated fat and avoid trans fat.

2. Have students complete Be Fat Wise (worksheet 1) individually, in pairs, or in groups of three. Distribute one Snack Food Information Card to each student, pair, or group of three students and instruct students to graph the

unhealthy fat content (saturated plus trans fat) in each of the three food choices. Have them identify the healthiest and unhealthiest snack choices and explain why. Review the answers (see worksheet solutions). Discuss what the healthy snack options all have in common and what the unhealthy snack options all have in common.

3. Distribute worksheet 2, Snacking the Fast-Food Way, and have students work in pairs to make an educated guess about which food of the two choices has the lowest amount of saturated and trans fat. Display the solutions as an overhead transparency and discuss them.

4. Show the Reading Food Labels transparency and explain the labeled information. Highlight that reading labels is the way to determine the saturated fat content of the foods we eat and also to determine whether a food is high in saturated fat (20% or more of DV) or low in saturated fat (5% or less of DV). Food labels also tell us about trans fat content.

5. Distribute food packages of popular snack foods. Have students locate and record on the What's in a Snack? worksheet (worksheet 3) the serving size, the amount of saturated fat grams per serving, the % DV for saturated fat, and the amount of trans fat grams listed on the food label. For those foods listing 0 grams of trans fat, have students also look at the ingredients list for partially hydrogenated vegetable oils (this ingredient indicates that there is a small amount of trans fat in the product). Remind students that small amounts of trans fat can add up throughout the day, so it is best to choose snacks that do not contain any trans fat or partially hydrogenated oils.

6. Ask students to determine which snacks can be combined to add up to 100% of the recommended daily maximum of saturated fat (the % DVs of the different snacks add up to 100). (Students can do this individually or in groups, or this may be done as a class.) It may take only 3 to 5 snacks, depending on their saturated fat content. Explain that just those snacks alone contain a person's daily maximum allowance of saturated fat. (See table 6.1 for an example.)

Remind students of the following: "The % Daily Value (based on a 2,000-calorie diet) can help you follow nutrition experts' advice not to eat more

▶**TABLE 6.1   Examples of Foods That Total to 100% DV for Saturated Fat**

Snack foods	% DV for saturated fat
Potato sticks (2/3 cup)	20%
Chocolate cupcake	27%
Reese's Peanut Butter Cups	30%
Reduced-fat string cheese (1 stick)	16%
Peanut butter and cracker sandwiches	7%
Total	100%

Nutrition information on Reese's Peanut Butter Cups retrieved from company Web site on March 18, 2007: Hershey's, www.hersheys.com/products/details/reesespeanutbuttercups.asp.

than 10% of your calories from saturated fat. All you need to do is add up the % DV for saturated fat in all the foods you eat in a day. Your goal is to eat less than 100% of the DV for saturated fat."

7. Explain to students that snacks that have a lot of saturated fat can be eaten once in a while and should be considered as "sometimes" foods. Most of the time, however, students should choose foods that contain healthy (unsaturated) plant fat (such as peanut butter, nuts, avocados, and olive oil) or whole grains, fruits, and vegetables. Remind students that they should avoid foods that have trans fat or partially hydrogenated oils.

EXTENSION ACTIVITIES

1. Have students create an Eat Well Snack List (see table 6.2) that shows healthy snack choices (based on type of fat and considering other aspects such as low in added sugars) in each of the food groups. Display or copy and distribute transparency 2 from lesson 1, the Balanced Plate for Health (p. 24), to illustrate the food groups (optional).

▶ TABLE 6.2   Example of Eat Well Snack List

Food group	Eat well examples
Grains	Whole wheat pretzels, whole-grain rye crispbread, whole wheat crackers, tabbouleh (bulgur salad), air-popped popcorn (or home-popped popcorn in vegetable oil)
Vegetables	Baby carrots, pepper slices, broccoli trees, celery sticks, cherry tomatoes, edamame, zucchini spears
Fruits	Apples, grapes, orange slices, strawberries, melon wedges, dried apricots, raisins
Milk	Low-fat or nonfat plain yogurt, reduced-fat cheese sticks
Meat, fish, and beans	Bean spread (such as hummus), almonds, walnuts, sunflower seeds, peanut butter, tahini, sliced turkey

2. Have students design a snack food label for a snack food that is low in saturated fat and has 0 grams trans fat and that would appeal to their peers.

3. Research the link between saturated and trans fat and heart disease.

4. Have students identify snack foods that are high in added sugar (e.g., cupcakes, candy bars, soft drinks) or salt (e.g., chips, cheese curls). Explain that the amount of sugar (in grams) is listed on the label and that the different types of added sugar are found in the ingredients list (see lesson 7 for a list of commonly added sugars). Sodium has a % DV that follows the rules for saturated fat: If a product has 20% or more of the DV for sodium it is considered high in salt. Have students think of healthier snack alternatives (e.g., combine slices of four favorite fruits in a bowl, toast whole wheat pita bread strips, or dip tortilla chips free of partially hydrogenated oils in salsa).

5. Have students write a formal letter to the school food service director or the manager of their favorite restaurant asking her to stop cooking with partially hydrogenated oils and to use healthy vegetable oils (such as olive or canola oil) instead.

Reading Food Labels

Nutrition Facts

Serving Size (1 cup) (228g) —————————————— | Serving size |

Servings Per Container (2) —————————————— | Servings per container |

Amount Per Serving

Calories 250   Calories from Fat 120

% Daily Value*

Total Fat 13g	**20%**
Saturated Fat (3g)	(15%)
Trans Fat (3g)	
Cholesterol 31mg	**10%**
Sodium 470mg	**20%**
Total Carbohydrate 31g	**10%**
Dietary Fiber 0g	**0%**
Sugars 5g	
Protein 5g	

Vitamin A 4%	•	Vitamin C 2%	
Calcium 15%	•	Iron 4%	

Saturated fat per serving

Trans fat per serving: Choose foods that have 0g of *trans* fat

% DV of saturated fat: Foods with a DV for saturated fat of 5 or less are low in saturated fat. Foods with a % DV for saturated fat of 20 or more are high in saturated fat. The daily goal is to choose foods that together contain less than 100% of the DV for saturated fat.

*Percent Daily Values are based on a 2,000 calorie diet. Your daily values may be higher or lower depending on your calorie needs:

	Calories	2,000	2,500
Total Fat	Less than	65g	80g
Sat. Fat	Less than	20g	25g
Cholesterol	Less than	300mg	300mg
Sodium	Less than	2,400mg	2,400mg
Total Carbohydrate		300g	375g
Dietary Fiber		25g	30g

Calories per gram:
Fat 9 • Carbohydrate 4 • Protein 4

Name _____

Be Fat Wise

Directions

Graph the saturated fat and trans fat content for each snack food on the list provided by your teacher. Use different colored pencils to graph the saturated fat and the trans fat in each food. Then use this information to identify the best and worst snack choices in the group.

1. Which food is the healthiest choice?

   Why?

2. Which food is the unhealthiest choice?

   Why?

From L.W.Y. Cheung, H. Dart, S. Kalin, and S.L. Gortmaker, 2007, *Eat Well & Keep Moving*, 2nd ed. (Champaign, IL: Human Kinetics).

(continued)

Grams	Saturated + trans fat	Saturated + trans fat	Saturated + trans fat	Saturated + trans fat
15				
14				
13				
12				
11				
10				
9				
8				
7				
6				
5				
4				
3				
2				
1				
	Example: snack cake	Food 1:	Food 2:	Food 3:

Example: The snack cake contains 2.5g of saturated fat and 2.5g of trans fat.

From L.W.Y. Cheung, H. Dart, S. Kalin, and S.L. Gortmaker, 2007, *Eat Well & Keep Moving,* 2nd ed. (Champaign, IL: Human Kinetics).

SNACK FOOD INFORMATION CARDS

Group 1

Vanilla ice cream (5g saturated fat, 0g trans fat)

Low-fat soft-serve vanilla frozen yogurt (1g saturated fat, 0g trans fat)

Plain nonfat yogurt with banana slices (0g saturated fat, 0g trans fat)

Group 2

Apple (0g saturated fat, 0g trans fat)

Snack-size packaged apple pie (7g saturated fat, 8g trans fat)

Apple cinnamon Pop-Tart (2g saturated fat, 0g trans fat)

Group 3

Whole wheat toast (1 slice) with natural peanut butter (1 tbsp.) (1 g saturated fat, 0 g trans fat)

Peanut butter cracker sandwich pack (1 package of 6 sandwiches) (0.5g saturated fat, 2g trans fat)

Peanut butter sandwich crème cookies (5g saturated fat, 3g trans fat)

From L.W.Y. Cheung, H. Dart, S. Kalin, and S.L. Gortmaker, 2007, *Eat Well & Keep Moving*, 2nd ed. (Champaign, IL: Human Kinetics). Nutrition information for brand-name foods retrieved from company Web sites on July 6, 2007:

PopTart, www2.kelloggs.com/brand/brand.aspx?brand=202&cat=poptarts.

(continued)

Group 4

Trail mix with raisins and nuts (1g saturated fat, 0g trans fat)

Chocolate crème-filled doughnut (3g saturated fat, 4g trans fat)

Blueberry muffin (3g saturated fat, 0g trans fat)

Group 5

Potato chips (3g saturated fat, 0g trans fat)

Combos pepperoni pizza cracker snacks (5g saturated fat, 0g trans fat)

Whole wheat crackers (1g saturated fat, 0g trans fat)

Group 6

Bologna (2g saturated fat, 0g trans fat)

Lunchables pizza (5g saturated fat, 0g trans fat)

Roast turkey (0g saturated fat, 0g trans fat)

Snacking the Fast-Food Way

Directions

Using what you know about the sources of saturated and trans fat, look at each set of foods below and place an (X) in the box next to the food that you believe contains more saturated and trans fat.

▶ **TABLE 6.3   Snacking the Fast-Food Way**

❏ McDonald's apple pie ❏ McDonald's Apple Dippers (skip the caramel dip to cut down on sugar)	❏ Side salad with Italian vinaigrette ❏ Medium French fries
❏ 1 cheeseburger ❏ 1 veggie burger	❏ Burger King Whopper with cheese ❏ Burger King TenderGrill chicken sandwich with honey mustard
❏ 1 cup 1% chocolate milk ❏ 1 chocolate milkshake	❏ KFC baked beans ❏ KFC macaroni and cheese
❏ 1 beef taco ❏ 1 cup turkey chili	❏ Subway 6" meatball sub ❏ Subway 6" turkey breast sub

From L.W.Y. Cheung, H. Dart, S. Kalin, and S.L. Gortmaker, 2007, *Eat Well & Keep Moving,* 2nd ed. (Champaign, IL: Human Kinetics).

WORKSHEET

2

Name _____

What's in a Snack?

Look at the snack food labels to find the serving size, the amount of saturated fat grams per serving, the % DV for saturated fat, and the amount of trans fat grams per serving. Record this information in the table.

For foods listing 0 grams of trans fat, look at the ingredients list to see whether the food contains any partially hydrogenated oil or shortening. Record the information in the table.

▶**TABLE 6.4   What's In a Snack?**

Product name	Serving size	Servings per container	Saturated fat (grams)	% DV for saturated fat	Trans fat (grams)	Partially hydrogenated oil (yes or no)

From L.W.Y. Cheung, H. Dart, S. Kalin, and S.L. Gortmaker, 2007, *Eat Well & Keep Moving,* 2nd ed. (Champaign, IL: Human Kinetics).

Be Fat Wise

The best and worst choices, along with the total grams of unhealthy fat and comments for discussion, are listed in table 6.5.

▶ **TABLE 6.5   Be Fat Wise Solutions**

Group	Best choice (grams saturated + trans fat)	Worst choice (grams saturated + trans fat)	Comments
Group 1	Plain nonfat yogurt with banana slices (0g)	Vanilla ice cream (5g)	The amount of saturated fat in ice cream varies by brand and can be 15g or more per serving.
Group 2	Apple (0g)	Packaged apple pie (15g)	Commercially prepared pies likely contain unhealthy trans fat, but even home-made pie crusts and other flaky pastries often contain unhealthy fat.
Group 3	Whole wheat toast with peanut butter (1.5g)	Peanut butter sandwich crème cookies (8g)	Whole wheat toast provides fiber and peanut butter provides healthy monoun-saturated fat and is low in saturated fat; the cookies are high in saturated and trans fat.
Group 4	Trail mix (1g)	Chocolate crème-filled doughnut (7g)	Trail mix contains healthy fat from nuts and is low in saturated fat (choose varieties that do not add sugar or salt). Doughnuts are high in saturated and trans fat.
Group 5	Whole wheat crackers (1g)	Combos pepperoni pizza cracker snacks (5g)	Whole wheat crackers contain fiber and are low in saturated fat. Some chips, crackers, and other snacks contain partially hydrogenated vegetable oils but in a small enough quantity that the nutrition label says "0 grams trans fat." Even a small amount of trans fat can raise the risk of heart disease, so make sure to read the ingredients list and choose foods that do not contain partially hydrogenated oils.
Group 6	Turkey (0g)	Lunchables pepperoni pizza (5g)	Packaged lunch mixes have much more saturated fat than lean meat purchased from the deli has.

From L.W.Y. Cheung, H. Dart, S. Kalin, and S.L. Gortmaker, 2007, *Eat Well & Keep Moving,* 2nd ed. (Champaign, IL: Human Kinetics). Nutrition information for brand-name foods retrieved from company Web sites on July 6, 2007:

Combos, www.combos.com; Lunchables, http://kraftfoods.com/main.aspx?s=product&m=product/product_catalog.

Snacking the Fast-Food Way

An (X) is marked next to the food that contains more saturated and trans fat in each set of food choices. The grams of saturated and trans fat for each food are also listed.

▶**TABLE 6.6** Snacking the Fast-Food Way

☒ McDonald's apple pie (3.5g saturated fat, 5g trans fat) ☐ McDonald's Apple Dippers (skip the caramel dip to cut down on sugar) (0g saturated fat, 0g trans fat)	☐ Side salad with Italian vinaigrette (2g saturated fat, 0g trans fat) ☒ Medium French fries (3.5g saturated fat, 5g trans fat)
☒ 1 cheeseburger (6g saturated fat, 1g trans fat) ☐ 1 veggie burger (2.5g saturated fat, 0g trans fat)	☒ Burger King Whopper with cheese (8g saturated fat, 1g trans fat) ☐ Burger King TenderGrill chicken sandwich with honey mustard (2g saturated fat, 0g trans fat)
☐ 1 cup 1% chocolate milk (2.5g saturated fat, 0g trans fat) ☒ 1 chocolate milkshake (6g saturated fat, 0.5g trans fat)	☐ KFC baked beans (0g saturated fat, 0g trans fat) ☒ KFC macaroni and cheese (3.5g saturated fat, 1g trans fat)
☒ 1 beef taco (4g saturated fat, 1g trans fat) ☐ 1 cup turkey chili (1g saturated fat, 0g trans fat)	☒ Subway 6" meatball sub (11g saturated fat, 1g trans fat) ☐ Subway 6" turkey breast sub (1.5g saturated fat, 0g trans fat)

From L.W.Y. Cheung, H. Dart, S. Kalin, and S.L. Gortmaker, 2007, *Eat Well & Keep Moving*, 2nd ed. (Champaign, IL: Human Kinetics). Nutrition information on brand-name fast foods retrieved from company Web sites on June 25, 2007:

Burger King, www.bk.com/#menu=3,-1,-1; Kentucky Fried Chicken, www.yum.com/nutrition/menu.asp?brandID_Abbr=2_KFC; McDonald's, www.mcdonalds.com/usa/eat/nutrition_info.html; Subway, www.subway.com/applications/NutritionInfo/index.aspx.

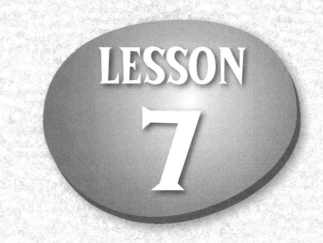

Sugar Water: Think About Your Drink

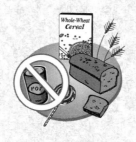

BACKGROUND

A major source of sugar in the American diet is sugar-sweetened beverages such as soft drinks, fruit punch, energy drinks, sweetened iced teas, and sports drinks. Children's consumption of soft drinks is rising. Studies have found that children are starting to consume them in infancy. By adolescence, 32% of girls and 52% of boys drink 24 ounces (780 milliliters) or more of soft drinks each day.

The steady climb in children's intake of sugar-sweetened beverages is troubling for many reasons. As children's soft drink consumption has increased, their milk consumption has decreased. That is a worrisome trend, given that adolescence is a time of rapid bone development and increased calcium needs. Teenagers who do not maximize bone development during these crucial years (by getting enough calcium and regular physical activity) may increase their risk of osteoporosis in late adulthood.

*During most types of physical activity, children can get adequate hydration and energy by drinking water and having a healthy snack (such as orange slices). Most sports drinks are designed for endurance athletes who compete for more than an hour at high intensity. Save sports drinks for when children are participating in high-intensity, long-duration sports competitions (greater than 1 hour) or for when children are vigorously active for a long time in the heat.

Sugar-sweetened beverages are said to be filled with empty calories because they basically contain just sugar and water, and they provide many calories but few of the nutrients the body needs to stay healthy and grow strong. A growing body of research strongly suggests that sugar-sweetened beverage consumption is associated with excess weight gain in children and adults. One study found that middle school students who increased their consumption of sugar-sweetened beverages gained excess weight; for each additional 12-ounce (375-milliliter) serving of sugar-sweetened beverage consumed per day, the odds of becoming obese increased by 60%. Reducing or avoiding empty calories from sugar-sweetened beverages may help with weight control: Another study found that when overweight teenagers reduced their consumption of sugar-sweetened beverages by replacing those beverages with calorie-free ones, they lost about 1 pound (0.5 kilogram) per month. Other research connects the consumption of sugar-sweetened beverages with a risk for type 2 diabetes.

**Choose soy or other nondairy drinks that have no more than 12 grams of sugar per 8-ounce (250-milliliter) serving.

A healthy eating plan includes few if any beverages with added sugar. The Harvard Prevention Research Center recommends that children consume no more than 2 8-ounce glasses of sugar-sweetened beverages per week. This includes soft drinks, fruit punches, sweetened ice teas, sports drinks,* and energy drinks. Children should also avoid consuming artificially-sweetened beverages, since the long-term effects of artificial sweetener consumption are unknown and since artificial sweeteners may encourage a taste for sweetness. Children should be encouraged to select healthier beverages such as water for quenching thirst or low-fat and skim milk for calcium; calcium-fortified soy drinks** and calcium-fortified 100% orange juice are also good sources of calcium. Consumption of 100% fruit juice should be limited to no more than 8 ounces (250 milliliters) per day. Juice contains vitamins and minerals, but it naturally contains a large amount of fruit sugar (fructose) and lacks the fiber found in fresh whole fruit. To make it easier to stay within the 8-ounce fruit juice limit, dilute a small amount of 100% fruit juice (4 ounces) with sparkling water.

ESTIMATED TEACHING TIME AND RELATED SUBJECT AREAS

Estimated teaching time: 1 hour, 15 minutes

Related subject areas: math, health, language arts (vocabulary)

OBJECTIVES

1. Students will measure the amount of sugar consumed from soft drinks and evaluate the results.
2. Students will identify the different forms of sugar added to beverages.
3. Students will demonstrate how the body responds to sugary drinks.
4. Students will learn to replace soft drinks and other sugar-sweetened beverages with healthy drinks.

MATERIALS

1. Sugar (5-pound bag, or 2 kilograms)
2. Measuring teaspoons
3. Small paper cups or clear plastic cups
4. Worksheet 1, Sugar Count
5. Worksheet 2, Find the Sugar
6. Drink labels that students have brought in from home (optional)
7. Solutions to worksheet 2

PROCEDURE

PART I: EVALUATE SUGAR INTAKE

1. Introduce the lesson by asking students to say what they think about the word *sugar.* Ask them to list the foods and drinks that they consume that contain sugar. What is the most common food or beverage listed?

2. Explain that soft drinks represent a major source of sugar intake in the diets of older children and teenagers. Distribute worksheet 1 (Sugar Count) to students and instruct them to complete the Soft Drink Count table by recording the number of 12-ounce (375-milliliter) cans and 20-ounce (600-milliliter) bottles of soft drink they consumed the previous day. Then have the students calculate the total number of teaspoons of sugar consumed from the soft drinks.

3. Have students evaluate their sugar intake (part II of worksheet 1). Distribute the paper cups. Instruct the students to measure out a teaspoon of sugar for each teaspoon of sugar they consumed from soft drinks the previous day and to pour the sugar into their cups to visualize the amount of sugar consumed. Alternatively, to minimize the amount of sugar used for this activity, choose a few students to measure out their sugar intake and demonstrate it to the class.

   Discuss the students' observations—were they surprised at the amount of sugar they consumed?

   a. A child who consumes just 1 can of soft drink per day (10 teaspoons of sugar) may consume 70 teaspoons of sugar over 1 week, which translates to about 3 pounds (1 kilogram) of sugar each month (using the simple calculation of 4 weeks in a month) and 36 pounds (16 kilograms) of sugar each year.

You may need to assist students in estimating the amount of soft drink they consumed if they consumed something other than a can or bottle. This exercise is not meant to be an exact record but rather a rough estimate of the amount of sugar consumed from soft drinks.

Students who did not drink soft drinks the previous day may fill out the sheet based on what they drink on a typical day; if several students did not drink soft drinks the previous day or some students rarely drink soft drinks because of household rules, it may be more effective to conduct this activity in groups.

There are 24 teaspoons in 1/2 cup.

b. To demonstrate what 3 pounds (1 kilogram) feels like, pass around the bag of sugar. While not exact (your bag of sugar will be close to 5 pounds, or 2 kilograms), it will give students an idea about the volume and weight of sugar consumed via soft drinks. Remind students that, like soft drinks, the bag is full of sugar but has no other nutrients. There are no vitamins or minerals in sugar— just empty calories (meaning energy without any other benefits for the body).

c. Remind students that a soft drink is not the only beverage that contains added sugars. Review the list created by the students at the start of this lesson and point out the other drinks that contain large amounts of added sugar (e.g., sports drinks, energy drinks, fruit punches, lemonade, sweetened iced teas).

4. Discuss beverages that provide students with a health benefit, such as water, low-fat or nonfat milk, and 100% fruit juice (in moderation). Complete part III of worksheet 1 (Calcium Switch) to calculate the amount of calcium each child would consume if she chose low-fat or skim milk instead of soft drinks. For this exercise, students will calculate the total ounces of soft drinks consumed the previous day and determine the amount of calcium that they would have consumed if all of the soft drink was low-fat or nonfat milk.

If a child replaces 1 can of soft drink with 12 ounces (375 milliliters) of low-fat or skim milk, he takes in 455 milligrams of calcium, which meets almost 40% of the total daily calcium requirement.

Adapted by permission, from J. Carter et al., 2007, *Planet Health,* 2nd ed. (Champaign, IL: Human Kinetics).

PART II: IDENTIFY SUGAR IN DRINKS

1. Distribute worksheet 2 (Find the Sugar) so that students may identify other words for sugar (in part I of worksheet 2). Next, have students find some of these words in the drink ingredients lists provided in part II of worksheet 2. Explain that many drinks that sound healthy actually contain a lot of added sugar (ask students to name some fruit drinks or energy drinks that they like, since many fruit drinks and energy drinks have a lot of added sugar; see worksheet 2 for an example). This sugar often hides itself because the ingredient lists on food labels use other names for sugar.

In addition to containing large amounts of sugar, energy drinks often contain caffeine, herbs, and other additives that may not be healthy for children.

----

a. For an optional math extension, review the Nutrition Facts labels from worksheet 2 and ask the students, "Where does the label list the amount of sugar?" Explain how to convert grams of sugar to teaspoons of sugar (1 teaspoon for every 4 grams).

b. Calculate the teaspoons of sugar in popular drinks either by using the Nutrition Facts labels provided or by asking students to bring in labels from drinks they have at home.

2. Remind students of the healthy living goal to limit sugary drinks. Soft drinks and other sweet drinks (e.g., sports drinks, energy drinks, fruit punches, lemonade, sweetened iced teas) contain high amounts of sugar and usually nothing else that is good for us—they basically contain just sugar and water. That's why we say that sugar-sweetened drinks give us empty calories.

PART III: APPLICATION AND EXTENSION OF INFORMATION

1. Ask students to describe why we might want or need sugar. Explain that sugar provides the body with a quick source of energy that tastes good. The problem with consuming sugary drinks or snacks is that the energy boost from these sources does not last.

2. Have the class stand up and do the wave (raising and lowering their arms, as you might do at a sporting event). Explain that this is what happens in our bodies when we drink a whole can of sugary drink all at once (or eat sugary foods, like a pack of jelly beans): There is a quick rise in blood sugar, giving us energy, but our bodies work quickly to pull that sugar out of the blood and into storage (in our muscles). That is why the quick boost of energy we feel after drinking a sugary drink does not last.

Adapted by permission, from J. Carter et al., 2007, *Planet Health,* 2nd ed. (Champaign, IL: Human Kinetics).

3. Discuss better ways to get quick energy that lasts for a long time, so that the body's energy levels do not shoot up and down. Healthy carbohydrate in whole-grain foods, fruits, and vegetables provides a longer boost because the sugar and starch in the foods take longer to be digested and enter the blood stream. These foods also provide fiber and many vitamins and minerals. Low-fat and nonfat milk and low-fat or nonfat yogurt also naturally contain carbohydrate and are a good source of protein and calcium. To sustain energy levels, choose snacks that combine healthy sources of carbohydrate (e.g., whole grains, fruits, and vegetables) with healthy sources of protein (e.g., nuts, hummus, and low-fat cheese). (For more information on choosing healthy carbohydrate, see lesson 2, Carb Smart.)

4. If time allows, invite students to create a list of healthy drink options and discuss the best choices according to their health benefits. For example, the students might list

- plain or sparkling water (alleviates thirst and promotes hydration),
- nonfat or low-fat milk (provides calcium for strong bones and teeth), and
- 100% fruit juice (offers vitamins and minerals); note that consumption of 100% fruit juice should be limited to no more than 8 ounces per day.

EXTENSION ACTIVITIES

1. Ask students to calculate how much sugar they would consume from soft drinks in a year if they continued to drink as much as they drank yesterday. (Multiply answer 3 from worksheet 1 by 365.)

2. Discuss the advertisements that they see on television or in print for sugary drinks. Ask the students to pick one ad that is familiar and discuss what they think about the ad. Have them describe the ad, the actors in the ad (for instance, are the children happy or athletic?), and the way the ad makes them feel about the product. (See lesson 18, worksheet 2, What's Up With This Ad?, page 272, for a worksheet that may be used for this activity.) For more information about assessing advertisements and the media, visit the Center for Media Literacy at www.medialit.org, an organization that provides resources for educators.

3. Create posters that advertise healthy beverage choices and post them near the cafeteria.

Name _____

Sugar Count

Part I: What's Your Soft Drink Count?

Fill in the Soft Drink Count table (table 7.1) with the number of 12-ounce (375-milliliter) cans and 20-ounce (600-milliliter) bottles of soft drink you drank yesterday.

- -

You may need to estimate the amounts that you drank and round to a whole number. For instance, if you opened a 20-ounce (600-milliliter) bottle but only drank half of it, you consumed approximately one 12-ounce (375-milliliter) can of soft drink.

▶TABLE 7.1   Soft Drink Count

	12 oz. (375 ml) can of soft drink (10 tsp. of sugar)	20 oz. (600 ml) bottle of soda (17 tsp. of sugar)
How many did you drink yesterday?		

Calculate the total teaspoons of sugar you consumed from soft drinks.

1. How many teaspoons of sugar did you consume from 12-ounce (375-milliliter) cans of soft drink? _____ For example, if you drank 2 cans, then 2 cans × 10 teaspoons = 20 teaspoons of sugar.

2. How many teaspoons of sugar did you consume from 20-ounce (600-milliliter) bottles of soft drink? _____ For example, if you drank 2 bottles, then 2 bottles × 17 teaspoons = 34 teaspoons of sugar.

3. Add the results (sugar from soft drinks in a can and sugar from soft drinks in a plastic bottle) to determine the total teaspoons of sugar you consumed yesterday from soft drinks (add the answers from question 1 and question 2):

From L.W.Y. Cheung, H. Dart, S. Kalin, and S.L. Gortmaker, 2007, *Eat Well & Keep Moving,* 2nd ed. (Champaign, IL: Human Kinetics).

(continued)

Part II: How Much Sugar Is This?

Using the sugar provided, measure out the amount of sugar that you consumed from soft drinks yesterday. How would you describe the amount of sugar consumed?

Part III: Calcium Switch

Soft drinks and other sweet drinks contain high amounts of sugar and usually nothing else that is good for us—they basically contain just sugar and water. That's why we say that sugar-sweetened drinks give us empty calories. Determine how much calcium you could consume if you drank low-fat or skim milk in place of the soft drinks you drank yesterday.

   1. How much soft drink did you drink yesterday?

   Number of cans of soft drink ___ × 12 ounces per can = ___ ounces of soft drink from cans

   Number of bottles of soft drink ___ × 20 ounces per bottle = ___ ounces of soft drink from plastic bottles

   Add the ounces of soft drink from cans and plastic bottles to get the total ounces of soft drink consumed: _____.

Note that there are 30 milliliters in one ounce.

   2. Each ounce (30 milliliters) of low-fat or skim milk contains 38 milligrams of calcium. How much calcium would you have consumed by drinking milk instead of soft drinks yesterday?

Note that children need 1,300 milligrams of calcium each day.

From L.W.Y. Cheung, H. Dart, S. Kalin, and S.L. Gortmaker, 2007, *Eat Well & Keep Moving,* 2nd ed. (Champaign, IL: Human Kinetics).

Name _____

Find the Sugar

Part I: Word Find

Figure 7.1 lists various names for sugar. Find each of these words in the puzzle. Words may appear forward, backward, diagonally, horizontally, and vertically.

```
S S R E O Y G S R M R O E G E U R A T
S V Y S S O D R S R E S H O N E Y T G
C P X O U O U O N P E R A X U G U M H
S U C T O O C Y E S A E S L S S O A A
A R U C P G O A E G S E R M L T O E M
O Y O U M R O A U O U U E A R S N O F
L S C R H H R S R G R G S L U L S E T
R N N F S E O C N S D U H T N N G X O
O R G E N O U S C T E N P O E O O S C
A O S T E S U O M M S O O S C G D E E
S C O O O E O M O L A S S E S C S S E
E U U U A S O S T R E E G O O R U L E
E R O O M R E U S E R E M N L E U U R
T C T G L U C O S E O F C N R U G A S
A O E R R S E S O R T X E D N P Y S E
E R O U L D A P Y U O T A A R C C U O
```

Find these words for sugar in the puzzle:

Fructose	Dextrose	Sugar
Corn syrup	Honey	Maltose
Glucose	Sucrose	Molasses

▶ FIGURE 7.1   Find the Sugar puzzle.

From L.W.Y. Cheung, H. Dart, S. Kalin, and S.L. Gortmaker, 2007, *Eat Well & Keep Moving,* 2nd ed. (Champaign, IL: Human Kinetics).

(continued)

Part II: What's In Your Drink?

Circle the words for sugar in the ingredient lists that follow. Which drink has the most types of added sugar? Next, circle the grams of sugar in each food label. Which drink has the most grams of sugar? Note which drinks are sold in bottles that contain more than one serving.

Capri Sun Fruit Punch Ingredients

High fructose corn syrup, pear and grape juice from concentrate, citric acid, water extracted orange and pineapple juice concentrates, ascorbic acid, vitamin E acetate, natural flavor

Nutrition Facts

Serving Size 6.75 fl oz (200 ml)

Amount Per Serving	% DV*
Calories 90	
Total Fat 0g	0%
Sodium 15mg	1%
Total Carbohydrate 24g	8%
Sugars 24g	
Protein 0g	

Vitamin C 0%

Not a significant source of calories from fat, saturated fat, trans fat, cholesterol, dietary fiber, vitamin A, calcium, or iron.
*Percent Daily Values are based on a 2,000 calorie diet. Your daily values may be higher or lower depending on your calorie needs.

Hi-C Blast in Berry Blue Flavor Ingredients

Pure filtered water, high fructose corn syrup, pear juice from concentrate, less than 0.5% raspberry juice from concentrate, vitamin C (ascorbic acid), natural flavors, citric acid (for tartness), modified corn starch, glycerol ester of wood rosin, sodium hexametaphosphate and sodium benzoate, potassium sorbate, calcium disodium EDTA (to protect taste), blue #1

Nutrition Facts

Serving Size 8 fl oz (250 ml)

Amount Per Serving	% DV*
Calories 170	
Total Fat 0g	0%
Sodium 110mg	5%
Total Carbohydrate 46g	15%
Sugars 44g	
Protein 0g	

Vitamin C 100%

Not a significant source of calories from fat, saturated fat, trans fat, cholesterol, dietary fiber, vitamin A, calcium, or iron.
*Percent Daily Values are based on a 2,000 calorie diet. Your daily values may be higher or lower depending on your calorie needs.

From L.W.Y. Cheung, H. Dart, S. Kalin, and S.L. Gortmaker, 2007, *Eat Well & Keep Moving*, 2nd ed. (Champaign, IL: Human Kinetics). Nutrition information obtained from company Web sites, retrieved July 6, 2007:

Capri Sun Fruit Punch, www.kraftfoods.com/CapriSun/1_1_CS_Base.html; Hi-C, www.minutemaid.com/productsMain.jsp?group=Other.

(continued)

Orange Juice (Minute Maid) Ingredients

100% pure squeezed orange juice from concentrate (pure filtered water, premium concentrate orange juice)

Note: This drink may be sold in bottles that contain more than one serving. A 10-ounce bottle contains 30 grams of sugar.

Nutrition Facts

Serving Size 8 fl oz (250 ml)

Amount Per Serving		% DV*
Calories 110		
Total Fat 0g		0%
Sodium 15mg		1%
Potassium 450 mg		13%
Total Carbohydrate 27g		15%
Sugars 24g		
Protein 2g		

Vitamin C	70%	B$_6$	4%
Thiamin	10%	Niacin	2%
Folate	15%	Calcium	2%

Magnesium 6%

Not a significant source of calories from fat, saturated fat, trans fat, cholesterol, dietary fiber, vitamin A, calcium, or iron.
* Percent Daily Values are based on a 2,000 calorie diet. Your daily values may be higher or lower depending on your calorie needs.

Gatorade Thirst Quencher Ingredients

Water, sucrose syrup, glucose–fructose syrup, citric acid, natural and artificial flavors, salt, sodium citrate, monopotassium phosphate, vegetable juice (for color), ester gum

Note: This drink is sold in bottles that contain more than one serving. A 24-ounce bottle contains 42 grams of sugar.

Nutrition Facts

Serving Size 8 fl oz (250 ml)

Amount Per Serving		% DV*
Calories 50		
Total Fat 0g		0%
Sodium 110mg		5%
Potassium 30 mg		1%
Total Carbohydrate 14g		5%
Sugars 14g		
Protein 0g		

Not a significant source of calories from fat, saturated fat, trans fat, cholesterol, dietary fiber, vitamin A, vitamin C, calcium, or iron.
*Percent Daily Values are based on a 2,000 calorie diet. Your daily values may be higher or lower depending on your calorie needs.

From L.W.Y. Cheung, H. Dart, S. Kalin, and S.L. Gortmaker, 2007, *Eat Well & Keep Moving*, 2nd ed. (Champaign, IL: Human Kinetics). Nutrition information obtained from company Web sites, retrieved March 18, 2007:

Gatorade, www.gatorade.com/products/gatorade_thirst_quencher/; Minute Maid, www.minutemaid.com/productsMain.jsp?group=Variety_Juices_and_Drinks.

(continued)

Lipton Iced Tea, Peach Flavor Ingredients

Water, high fructose corn syrup, tea, citric acid (provides tartness), hexametaphosphate (to protect flavor), natural flavors, malic acid, phophoric acid, sodium benzoate and potassium sorbate (preserves freshness), caramel color, calcium disodium EDTA (to protect flavor), red 40

Note: This drink is sold in bottles that contain more than one serving. A 20-ounce bottle contains 45 grams of sugar.

Nutrition Facts
Serving Size 8 fl oz (250 ml)

Amount Per Serving		% DV*
Calories 70		
Total Fat 0g		0%
Sodium 70mg		0%
Potassium 0 mg		0%
Total Carbohydrate	19g	6%
Sugars 18g		
Protein 0g		

Not a significant source of calories from fat, saturated fat, trans fat, cholesterol, dietary fiber, vitamin A, vitamin C, calcium, or iron.
*Percent Daily Values are based on a 2,000 calorie diet. Your daily values may be higher or lower depending on your calorie needs.

Arizona Caution Extreme Energy Shot Performance Drink Ingredients

Carbonated water, sucrose, high fructose corn syrup, pear and apple and peach juice concentrate, mango puree, orange honey, taurine, citric acid, D-ribose, L-carnitine, guarana, inositol, *Panax ginseng,* natural flavors, caffeine, glucuronolactone, monopotassium phosphate, ascorbic acid, beta-carotene (for color), milk thistle, gum acacia, pantothenic acid, vitamin B_6, vitamin B_{12}

Note: This drink is sold in bottles that contain more than one serving. A 16-ounce bottle contains 64 grams of sugar.

Nutrition Facts
Serving Size 8.3 fl oz (250 ml)

Amount Per Serving		% DV*
Calories 130		
Total Fat 0g		0%
Sodium 25mg		1%
Potassium 0mg		0%
Total Carbohydrate 34g		11%
Sugars 33g		
Protein 0g		

Not a significant source of calories from fat, saturated fat, trans fat, cholesterol, dietary fiber, vitamin A, vitamin C, calcium, or iron.
*Percent Daily Values are based on a 2,000 calorie diet. Your daily values may be higher or lower depending on your calorie needs.

From L.W.Y. Cheung, H. Dart, S. Kalin, and S.L. Gortmaker, 2007, *Eat Well & Keep Moving,* 2nd ed. (Champaign, IL: Human Kinetics). Nutrition information obtained from company Web sites, retrieved July 6, 2007:

Arizona Extreme Energy Shot, www.arizonabev.com/csr/Products.asp; Lipton Iced Tea, www.lipton.com/our_products/iced_tea/index.asp.

Find the Sugar

Part I: Word Find

Figure 7.2 lists various names for sugar. Find each of these words in the puzzle. Words may appear forward, backward, diagonally, horizontally, and vertically.

```
S S R E O Y G S R M R O E G E U R A T
S V Y S S O D R S R E S H O N E Y T G
C P X O U O U O N P E R A X U G U M H
S U C T O O C Y E S A E S L S S O A A
A R U C P G O A E G S E R M L T O E M
O Y O U M R O A U O U U E A R S N O F
L S C R H H R S R G R G S L U L S E T
R N N F S E O C N S D U H T N N G X O
O R G E N O U S C T E N P O E O O S C
A O S T E S U O M M S O O S C G D E E
S C O O O E O M O L A S S E S C S S E
E U U U A S O S T R E E G O O R U L E
E R O O M R E U S E R E M N L E U U R
T C T G L U C O S E O F C N R U G A S
A O E R R S E S O R T X E D N P Y S E
E R O U L D A P Y U O T A A R C C U O
```

Find these words for sugar in the puzzle:

Fructose	Dextrose	Sugar
Corn syrup	Honey	Maltose
Glucose	Sucrose	Molasses

▶ FIGURE 7.2   Find the sugar puzzle solution.

Part II: What's In Your Drink?

Circle the words for sugar in the ingredient lists that follow. Which drink has the most types of added sugar? Next, circle the grams of sugar in each food label. Which drink has the most grams of sugar?

(continued)

Capri Sun Fruit Punch Ingredients

Water, **high fructose corn syrup,** pear and grape juice from concentrate, citric acid, water extracted orange and pineapple juice concentrates, ascorbic acid, vitamin E acetate, natural flavor

Nutrition Facts

Serving Size 6.75 fl oz (200 ml)

Amount Per Serving	% DV*
Calories 100	
Total Fat 0g	**0%**
Sodium 15mg	**1%**
Total Carbohydrate 27g	**8%**
Sugars 27g	
Protein 0g	

Vitamin C 0%

Not a significant source of calories from fat, saturated fat, trans fat, cholesterol, dietary fiber, vitamin A, calcium, or iron.
*Percent Daily Values are based on a 2,000 calorie diet. Your daily values may be higher or lower depending on your calorie needs.

Hi-C Blast in Berry Blue Flavor Ingredients

Pure filtered water, **high fructose corn syrup,** pear juice from concentrate, less than 0.5% raspberry juice from concentrate, vitamin C (ascorbic acid), natural flavors, citric acid (for tartness), modified corn starch, glycerol ester of wood rosin, sodium hexametaphosphate and sodium benzoate, potassium sorbate, calcium disodium EDTA (to protect taste), blue #1

Nutrition Facts

Serving Size 8 fl oz (250 ml)

Amount Per Serving	% DV*
Calories 170	
Total Fat 0g	**0%**
Sodium 110mg	**5%**
Total Carbohydrate 46g	**15%**
Sugars 44g	
Protein 0g	

Vitamin C 100%

Not a significant source of calories from fat, saturated fat, trans fat, cholesterol, dietary fiber, vitamin A, calcium, or iron.
*Percent Daily Values are based on a 2,000 calorie diet. Your daily values may be higher or lower depending on your calorie needs.

From L.W.Y. Cheung, H. Dart, S. Kalin, and S.L. Gortmaker, 2007, *Eat Well & Keep Moving*, 2nd ed. (Champaign, IL: Human Kinetics). Nutrition information obtained from company Web sites, retrieved July 6, 2007:

Capri Sun Fruit Punch, www.kraftfoods.com/CapriSun/1_1_CS_Base.html; Hi-C, www.minutemaid.com/productsMain.jsp?group=Other.

(continued)

Orange Juice (Minute Maid)
Ingredients

100% pure squeezed orange juice from concentrate (pure filtered water, premium concentrate orange juice)

Note: This drink may be sold in bottles that contain more than one serving. A 10-ounce bottle contains 30 grams of sugar.

Nutrition Facts

Serving Size 8 fl oz (250 ml)

Amount Per Serving	% DV*
Calories 110	
Total Fat 0g	0%
Sodium 15mg	1%
Potassium 450 mg	13%
Total Carbohydrate 27g	15%
Sugars (24g)	
Protein 2g	

Vitamin C	120%	B$_6$	4%
Thiamin	10%	Niacin	2%
Folate	15%	Calcium	2%

Magnesium 6%

Not a significant source of calories from fat, saturated fat, trans fat, cholesterol, dietary fiber, vitamin A, calcium, or iron.
*Percent Daily Values are based on a 2,000 calorie diet. Your daily values may be higher or lower depending on your calorie needs.

Gatorade Thirst Quencher
Ingredients

Water, (sucrose syrup,) (glucose–fructose syrup,) citric acid, natural and artificial flavors, salt, sodium citrate, monopotassium phosphate, vegetable juice (for color), ester gum

Note: This drink may be sold in bottles that contain more than one serving. A 24-ounce bottle contains 42 grams of sugar.

Nutrition Facts

Serving Size 8 fl oz (250 ml)

Amount Per Serving	% DV*
Calories 50	
Total Fat 0g	0%
Sodium 110mg	5%
Potassium 30 mg	1%
Total Carbohydrate 14g	5%
Sugars (14g)	
Protein 0g	

Not a significant source of calories from fat, saturated fat, trans fat, cholesterol, dietary fiber, vitamin A, vitamin C, calcium, or iron.
*Percent Daily Values are based on a 2,000 calorie diet. Your daily values may be higher or lower depending on your calorie needs.

From L.W.Y. Cheung, H. Dart, S. Kalin, and S.L. Gortmaker, 2007, *Eat Well & Keep Moving*, 2nd ed. (Champaign, IL: Human Kinetics). Nutrition information obtained from company Web sites, retrieved March 18, 2007:

Gatorade, www.gatorade.com/products/gatorade_thirst_quencher/; Minute Maid, www.minutemaid.com/productsMain.jsp?group=Variety_Juices_and_Drinks.

(continued)

Lipton Iced Tea, Peach Flavor Ingredients

Water, **high fructose corn syrup,** tea, citric acid (provides tartness), hexametaphosphate (to protect flavor), natural flavors, malic acid, phosphoric acid, sodium benzoate and potassium sorbate (preserves freshness), caramel color, calcium disodium EDTA (to protect flavor), red 40

Note: This drink is sold in bottles that contain more than one serving. A 20-ounce bottle contains 45 grams of sugar.

Nutrition Facts

Serving Size 8 fl oz (250 ml)

Amount Per Serving	% DV*
Calories 70	
Total Fat 0g	0%
Sodium 0mg	0%
Potassium 0 mg	0%
Total Carbohydrate 26g	9%
Sugars 26g	
Protein 0g	

Not a significant source of calories from fat, saturated fat, trans fat, cholesterol, dietary fiber, vitamin A, vitamin C, calcium, or iron.
*Percent Daily Values are based on a 2,000 calorie diet. Your daily values may be higher or lower depending on your calorie needs.

Arizona Caution Extreme Energy Shot Performance Drink Ingredients

Carbonated water, **sucrose, high fructose corn syrup,** pear and apple and peach juice concentrate, mango puree, **orange honey,** taurine, citric acid, D-ribose, L-carnitine, guarana, inositol, *Panax ginseng,* natural flavors, caffeine, glucuronolactone, monopotassium phosphate, ascorbic acid, beta-carotene (for color), milk thistle, gum acacia, pantothenic acid, vitamin B_6, vitamin B_{12}

Note: This drink is sold in bottles that contain more than one serving. A 16-ounce bottle contains 64 grams of sugar.

Nutrition Facts

Serving Size 8.3 fl oz (250 ml)

Amount Per Serving	% DV*
Calories 130	
Total Fat 0g	0%
Sodium 25mg	1%
Potassium 0mg	0%
Total Carbohydrate 34g	11%
Sugars 33g	
Protein 0g	

Not a significant source of calories from fat, saturated fat, trans fat, cholesterol, dietary fiber, vitamin A, vitamin C, calcium, or iron.
*Percent Daily Values are based on a 2,000 calorie diet. Your daily values may be higher or lower depending on your calorie needs.

Teacher Notes

High fructose corn syrup is the sugar added to all drinks except orange juice, which has no added sugars.

Sucrose syrup and glucose–fructose syrup are added to Gatorade, and the Extreme Energy drink contains honey.

The Extreme Energy drink contains three types of added sugar (sucrose, high fructose corn syrup, and orange honey). Note that energy drinks also contain caffeine and several other additives that may not be healthy for children.

Hi-C Berry Blast punch contains the most sugar at 44 grams per 8-ounce (250-milliliter) serving (this is equivalent to 11 teaspoons, or 55 milliliters, of sugar).

From L.W.Y. Cheung, H. Dart, S. Kalin, and S.L. Gortmaker, 2007, *Eat Well & Keep Moving,* 2nd ed. (Champaign, IL: Human Kinetics). Nutrition information obtained from company Web sites, retrieved July 6, 2007:

Arizona Extreme Energy Shot, www.arizonabev.com/csr/Products.asp; Lipton Iced Tea, www.lipton.com/our_products/iced_tea/index.asp.

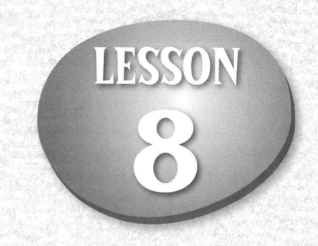

The Safe Workout: Snacking's Just Fine, If You Choose the Right Kind

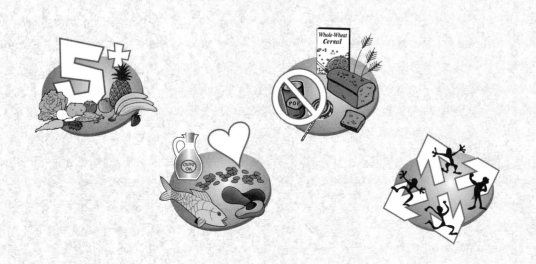

BACKGROUND

This lesson teaches students the importance of movement and eating well for a healthy body. The lesson includes the five parts of a safe workout, the different parts of fitness, and a nutrition concept (healthful snacks). The exciting part of this lesson is that the students will be moving while they are learning!

Snacks can be an important part of a child's diet. For students, snacks (if chosen wisely) can help provide the calories and nutrients that they need for growth, development, and physical activity.

Students should learn how to choose healthful snacks. Often, they choose highly processed snacks that are high in salt, refined grains, added sugar, saturated fat, and trans fat. These snacks are high in calories and low in useful nutrients (like vitamins and minerals) and are said to be filled with empty calories—calories that are not accompanied by healthful nutrients. Snacks like fruit, low-fat yogurt, and whole wheat bread, on the other hand, are nutrient dense—they contain calories that are accompanied by vitamins and minerals. However, children on average are not eating enough fruits and vegetables. They need to understand why they should choose nutrient-dense snacks rather than snacks filled with empty calories. Recommend fruits, vegetables, whole-grain products, low-fat dairy foods, nuts, or seeds as snacks.

OVERVIEW

This lesson reviews the different parts of a safe workout and includes an endurance fitness activity in which students shop for healthful snacks.

ESTIMATED TEACHING TIME AND RELATED SUBJECT AREA

Estimated teaching time: 1 hour
Related subject area: health

OBJECTIVES

1. Students will discuss and demonstrate each component of a safe workout.
2. Students will understand the importance of getting at least 60 minutes of physical activity every day as part of a healthy lifestyle.
3. Students will understand the benefits of choosing healthful snacks over less healthful snacks.

MATERIALS

1. Pictures of various snack foods (the National Dairy Council produces cutout food models of approximately 200 foods and beverages that can be ordered by calling 800-426-8271 or by contacting your local Dairy Council)—you may also want to use food wrappers or packages collected for lesson 6

2. Stretch and Strength Fitness Diagrams (see appendix A, pages 565-569)
3. Portable CD player/radio (optional)
4. Five hula hoops, boxes, or paper grocery bags

PROCEDURE

PART I: VOCABULARY TERMS REVIEW

Warm-up—The first part of the safe workout, in which slow movements get the body ready for stretching and the fitness activity.

Stretch—The part of the safe workout in which you do exercises that improve flexibility fitness and get the body ready for the fitness activity.

Fitness activity—The part of the safe workout in which strength and endurance fitness exercises are performed.

Cool-down—The part of the safe workout in which your body slows down and recovers from the fitness activity.

Cool-down stretch—The last part of the safe workout, in which you do exercises that improve flexibility fitness.

Pacing—Maintaining a comfortable speed so that you can perform your exercise over an extended time.

Flexibility fitness—The part of fitness that stretches the muscles and areas around the muscles to get your body ready for action; the ability to bend.

Strength fitness—The part of fitness that makes your muscles stronger and healthier.

Endurance fitness—The part of fitness that improves the heart muscle, lungs, and blood vessels.

PART II: SMART SNACKS

1. Ask the students, "What is a snack? Should we eat snacks?"
2. Discuss with students what they eat for snacks.
3. Ask students what they think of the phrase *Snacking is just fine, if you choose the right kind.*
4. Ask the students, "Which food groups contain healthful kinds of snacks?" (Possible answers include the following: All groups contain healthful snack foods; fruits and vegetables, whole grains, low-fat dairy foods, nuts and seeds, and lean meat all make good snack choices.)
5. Discuss with students why fruits, vegetables, whole grains, low-fat dairy foods, and nuts or seeds and even lean meats are the right kind of snacks. (They contain healthful nutrients that our bodies need, like vitamins and minerals. Snacking on fruits and vegetables can help you meet your goal of 5 or more servings each day. The Principles of Healthy Living encourage us to choose fruits and vegetables, whole grains, and healthy fats and to limit foods with added sugar.)

6. Have students name snacks from each of the following food groups:

Grains: whole wheat toast, whole wheat crackers (without trans fat), whole wheat pita bread

Fruits: apples, oranges, grapes, kiwi, pears, 100% fruit juice (no more than 8 ounces per day), raisins

Vegetables: carrots, leafy green salad, broccoli, cauliflower, celery, cucumber slices

Milk: nonfat milk, low-fat (1%) milk, low-fat yogurt, low-fat frozen yogurt, reduced-fat cheddar cheese, part-skim mozzarella cheese sticks

Meat, fish, and beans: peanuts, almonds, sunflower seeds, hummus, tuna, peanut butter, slices of lean meat or turkey, hard-boiled egg

PART III: COMPONENTS OF THE SAFE WORKOUT

Place students in five groups that represent the five food groups (i.e., place students in the grain group, the fruit group, and so on). Remind students that eating right and keeping the body moving (getting at least 60 minutes of physical activity every day) are equally important and together help keep us healthy and energized.

The following description covers all five areas of the safe workout, including the fitness activity—a movement game that involves choosing healthful snacks.

1. Warm-up (1-2 minutes)

2. Stretch (1-2 minutes)

3. Fitness activity (15-20 minutes)

4. Cool-down (1 minute)

5. Cool-down stretch (1 minute)

6. Stay Healthy Corner (4-5 minutes)

1. Warm-Up: 1 to 2 Minutes

You may use the CD player or radio to play music during the warm-up (optional).

What to Emphasize

▸ Car analogy: Your body is like a cold car—warm it up and then move it!

▸ If you do not warm up, you are more likely to get injured.

▸ You should always warm up before exercising, even when you are at home.

▸ Always do the movements very slowly to warm up.

▸ For example, for a bike ride, warm up by riding slowly at first.

▸ Likewise, when throwing a ball, throw slowly at first.

Semicircle Formation

▸ Students should establish and maintain a safe distance between themselves and others who are in front of, in back of, and on either side of themselves.

▸ There should be enough room between students so that they can do all stretches and exercises without fear of inadvertently hitting or being hit by another student.

▸ Students should stand so they are facing the teacher or group leader. They should be spaced so there is not another student directly in front of them (see figure 8.1).

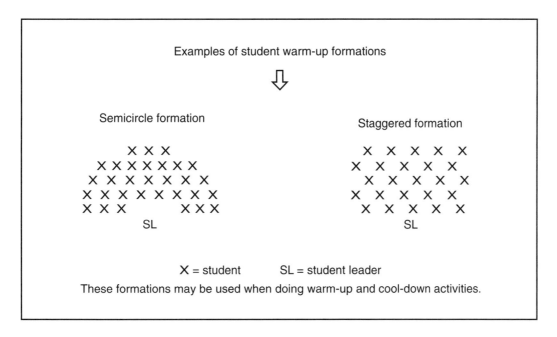

▶ FIGURE 8.1   Examples of student warm-up formations.

Staggered Formation

▶ Have a group of five students form a row with enough space so that they cannot touch each other if their arms are extended at shoulder height. Five more students will form a second row behind row one. Students in the second row should stand behind and between the two students in the row in front of them and, like those in the first row, should make sure that there is enough space between them (and between them and the students in front of them). Continue to put students in rows until all have been placed.

▶ Students should stand so that they are facing (and can see) the teacher or student leader, who will be in the front of the room (see figure 8.1).

2. Stretch: 1 to 2 Minutes

Examples of Student Stretches

Have students perform stretches as they appear in the stretching diagrams in appendix A. One student or a small group of students can help demonstrate the stretches for the class.

What to Emphasize

▶ Stretching improves flexibility fitness.

▶ Activities such as riding a bike or doing push-ups do not improve flexibility.

▶ Even if you aren't going to start a fitness activity, stretch at home while watching TV or when doing nothing in particular.

▶ Hold stretches for 10 or more seconds.

▶ Use slow movements; don't bounce.

3. Endurance Activity: 15 to 20 Minutes

What to Emphasize

▶ Pace, don't race.

▶ Getting fit should be fun.

ENDURANCE ACTIVITY GAME

EAT WELL AND KEEP MOVING: CHOOSING HEALTHFUL SNACKS

a. Equipment needed

1. A variety of pictures of snacks from the different food groups

2. Five hula hoops, boxes, or paper grocery bags (each representing a refrigerator or plate)

3. Music to move to (optional)

b. Introduction

Explain to the students, "The purpose of the game is to determine if each of you knows how to choose healthful snacks. We are also playing this game so that we can become more fit. We will pace ourselves so that we can do the activity for a certain length of time without becoming tired, which will help us build endurance and become stronger. Remember, we need to get at least 1 hour of physical activity every day, and this game will get you on your way to that goal."

c. Procedure

1. Have the class reform into five groups. Each group can be named after a food group (e.g., the grain group).

2. Ask each group to form a line (see figure 8.2 or 8.3).

3. Explain and demonstrate the paths the students will take so that there is no confusion and students can perform their tasks safely.

4. A cone or a distinguishable line on the floor can mark the place where the first person in each line should stand. The second person in the line moves to this place after the first student has left it.

5. Place a hula hoop (or box or paper bag) to the right of each line of students (refer to figure 8.1). This hula hoop can be called a *plate* or a *refrigerator*. Each student will place the food that she has collected in this area and then jog to the back of her food group line.

6. Begin by asking all students who are first in line to take a step forward. You will now walk this group through the course that you would like them to take while pointing out the following:

   a. "The area inside the basketball key (if you are in a gym; if not, your grocery store may be a table or an area in the classroom) has pictures of food all over the floor and is called the *grocery store*. Each student will go shopping for a healthful snack. When you are the first person in line, you will jog in a straight path until you arrive at the grocery store area. Once there, select a snack for your group, pick it up, and jog back to the area we are calling the *refrigerator* (or *plate*) and deposit the food item into it. You will then jog to the back of your line and jog in place until every member of every group has completed this task."

Gym line formation
for shopping fitness activities
[X = one student]

The purpose of the game is to determine if each student in a group knows which food items fit into their food group. We are also playing this game so that we can become fit and learn how to pace ourselves so that we can make our bodies stronger and able to do an activity for a certain length of time without becoming tired.

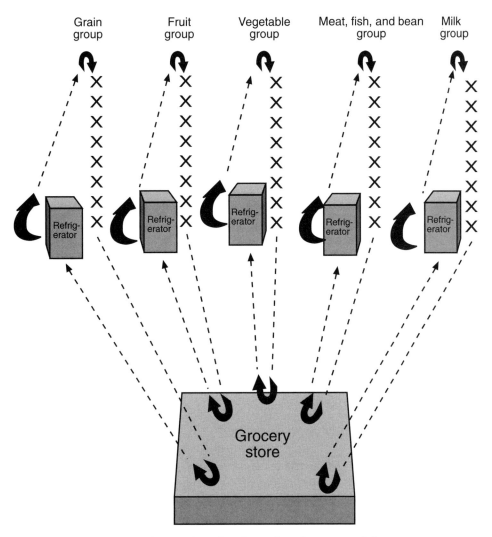

▶ FIGURE 8.2   Gym line formation for shopping fitness activity.

    b. Remind students that this is not a race or a competition between groups. When the first student in each line goes to the grocery store and back, coach them by reminding them to come back on their path so that they can safely jog to their refrigerator (plate).

    c. Tell students to "pace, don't race" so they can continue jogging until each member of their group has gone shopping and brought back a snack item. You may also vary the movement and have students hop in place or skip to the grocery store. Remind the people at the fronts of the lines to wait until the current joggers have reached the end of the line before starting out, so that the activity can be done safely.

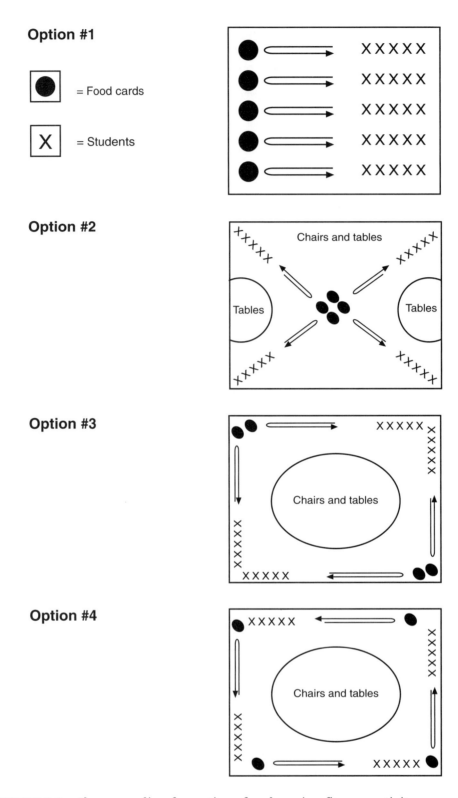

▶ FIGURE 8.3 Classroom line formations for shopping fitness activity.

d. After the first group of students has walked through the course and has moved to the back of the line, ask if there are any questions. If there are no questions, tell the students that they are about to begin with the set of students who are now first in line.

7. This activity will begin with the teacher saying, "Let's go shopping for snacks!" The entire class will jog lightly in place until the last student in each food group has had a turn and has taken a place at the end of the line.

8. Once all have completed the activity, tell the students it is time for the cool-down. Ask students to walk around the gymnasium, cafeteria, or community room three times, with everyone moving in the same direction.

4. Cool-Down: 1 Minute

What to Emphasize

▶ Move slowly.

▶ Remember to cool down after exercising at home too.

5. Cool-Down Stretch: 1 Minute

What to Emphasize

▶ Stretching improves flexibility fitness.

▶ Activities such as riding a bike or doing push-ups do not improve flexibility.

▶ Even if you aren't going to start a fitness activity, stretch at home while watching TV or when doing nothing in particular.

▶ Hold stretches for 10 or more seconds.

▶ Use slow movements; don't bounce.

6. Stay Healthy Corner: 4 to 5 Minutes

Use this time to introduce and reinforce a nutrition concept related to the fitness activity. You can set up a specific area of the classroom for the Stay Healthy Corner and decorate it with pictures or student drawings that represent the Principles of Healthy Living (e.g., healthy foods, children engaged in physical activity, and so on). Or you can simply set aside time for discussion at the end of the lesson.

Choosing Healthier Snacks

1. Tell the students that the class will now look at the snack choices each group made.

2. Ask for volunteers from each group to share 1 or 2 of the snacks that their group chose. Review the students' choices and remind them that a healthful snack is low in saturated and trans fat and high in vitamins and minerals; whole grains, fruits and vegetables, low-fat or fat-free dairy foods, and nuts or seeds are excellent choices. If you like, review some of the foods that were left in the grocery store and ask students why they did not consider them to be healthy snacks.

3. Close the lesson by reminding students to get at least 1 hour of physical activity every day. It is okay to get that activity a little bit at a time—15 minutes of walking to school, 20 minutes of playing tag—just so long as it adds up to an hour per day. Mix it up to keep it fun.

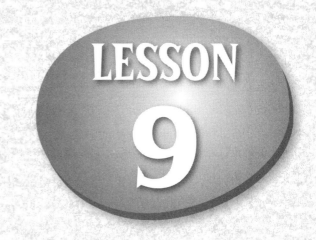

Prime-Time Smartness

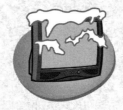

BACKGROUND

In the United States, children watch about 4 hours of TV every day. And this doesn't even count other screen time, like surfing the Web, instant messaging, and playing video games. When added up, TV and other screen time have basically become a full-time job!

And our children are suffering because of it. On average, American youths spend more time watching television each year than they spend in school. This tendency toward an inactive or sedentary lifestyle is a contributing factor to more and more children being overweight. The more television a child watches, the more likely he will be overweight. The increase in television viewing has also been associated with elevated cholesterol levels and poor cardiorespiratory fitness in youths and less time spent on homework.

To combat inactivity, young people should be encouraged to consider healthy alternatives to television viewing and other screen activities, particularly choices that involve more physical activity.

ESTIMATED TEACHING TIME AND RELATED SUBJECT AREAS

Estimated teaching time: 1 hour, 30 minutes
Related subject areas: reading, math

OBJECTIVES

1. Students will identify a television program or programs that they will not view in order to participate in an alternative activity.
2. Students will create a list of alternative activities to consider in place of watching television.

MATERIALS

1. Envelopes containing student letter (page 140) and pledge (page 141)—one per student
2. One teacher-only letter
3. Small white envelopes for signed copy of the pledge—one per student
4. Worksheet 1, My Favorite Prime-Time Shows
5. Packet of Prime-Time Smartness Challenge materials (one for each student who wants to take the challenge):
   - Hello Again
   - The Star Page
   - Prime-Time Smartness Challenge
   - The Questions Page
6. Certificate of Congratulations for students who take the challenge
7. Screen Gem graphic

PROCEDURE

PART I: MOTIVATION

1. Begin by telling the class that the office has delivered special letters addressed to "Student Only." The teacher should also receive a letter marked "Teacher Only." (Pass out an envelope to each child, addressed similarly to the example in figure 9.1; each envelope should contain a student letter and pledge.) If your school can afford the expense (approximately $10.00 U.S. total for postage), you can also have the letters mailed to each student in the class.

2. Provide time for the class to open the letters and read the pages quietly. Encourage students who need assistance to work in pairs. Pretend to open the "Teacher Only" letter, and then tell the students that they have been asked to create a list of things that could be done at home during prime-time hours. (Write the words *prime time* on the board.)

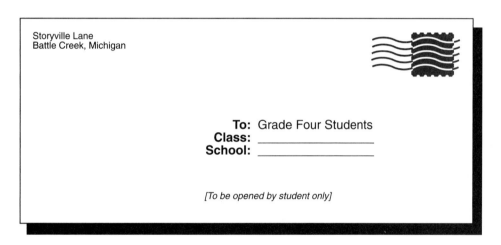

Storyville Lane
Battle Creek, Michigan

To: Grade Four Students
Class: _____
School: _____

[To be opened by student only]

▶ FIGURE 9.1 "Student Only" letter address example.

PART II: DEVELOPMENT

1. Ask the students to define *prime time* as it relates to television viewing.

2. Have students identify some favorite shows that they watch between 4 p.m. and 9 p.m.

3. Conduct a class poll to determine the class's favorite shows: Determine students' first choice, second choice, and third choice (see the example in figure 9.2).

4. Ask the students to study the chart to determine which program would probably be easiest for the class to pass up. For example, if most students picked *SpongeBob SquarePants* as a third choice, it would probably be the easiest show not to watch.

5. Ask students to think of activities in which they could participate when not watching television. As the list is brainstormed, record the suggestions on the board. List 7 to 10 activities.

Prime time refers to the time of the day during which most programs on television record their highest viewing audience.

Program	Show #1	Show #2	Show #3
A. *Jimmy Neutron*	18	15	1
B. *Hannah Montana*	10	14	10
C. *SpongeBob SquarePants*	6	5	23

▶ FIGURE 9.2   A sample poll in which students identify favorite TV shows (first, second, and third choices).

Sample alternatives to TV include reading a book, writing a poem, playing a game with siblings, helping younger siblings, playing basketball, dancing, walking to the store, and helping with chores.

PART III: APPLICATION

1. Have students review and discuss their activities list to determine if the activities are safe.

2. Guide students in reviewing the list again to determine which activities involve the greatest level of physical activity. Code the list as follows:

(+) = some physical activity (e.g., dancing, stretching, playing ball)

(–) = very little physical activity (e.g., reading, playing a board game)

Have students cite the benefits of choosing activities that involve physical activity.

Sample benefits may include the following:

- Exercises the muscles
- Exercises the heart

3. Distribute worksheet 1, My Favorite Prime-Time Shows. Have the students write in their three favorite television programs for each day. Ask them to circle one for each day that they would agree to pass up if they were to take the Prime-Time Smartness Challenge (see part IV).

PART IV: SUMMARY AND EXTENSION

1. Explain the Prime-Time Smartness Challenge to students. Ask students to sign their pledges. Then distribute small white envelopes (one per student) for them to put their pledges into and collect the pledges from the students. Record the names of students who agree to participate. Distribute the packet of materials.

The challenge does not have to be limited to students who watch TV. If a student does not watch any TV, she can still participate in the daily activities of the challenge. Where appropriate, she may substitute physically active time for physically inactive time. For example, instead of sitting and listening to music, the student could dance to the music.

If desired, a different or more challenging comprehension exercise can replace the echidnas paragraph that makes up The Star Page on page 144.

If you substitute for the echidnas paragraph, the exercises on The Questions Page on page 147 will need to reflect the change to The Star Page.

2. Create a bulletin board titled Winner's Circle. Display pictures of students who participate in the Prime-Time Smartness Challenge. Add the Certificates of Congratulations of those students who return their materials to the teacher. Add Screen Gem patches for those who completed the challenge and at least three Screen Time Bonus exercises.

3. Make a bar graph with the class to show the numbers of students who gave up 30 minutes of television each day for the week. Make another bar graph that shows the number of students who gave up 30 minutes of other screen time as part of the Screen Time Bonus exercise.

4. Make a pie chart of an average day (24 hours). Have the students estimate and display the number of hours that they do the following activities during that day:

   Sleep
   Eat
   Spend in school
   Play
   Do homework
   Bathe, dress, brush teeth, and so on
   Watch TV or DVDs
   Play video games
   Surf the Web
   Instant message
   Participate in other activities

5. Explain the Freeze My TV promotion to students (see lesson 27). Tell them it will be another TV and screen activity they will participate in.

Dear Student:

How would you like to be smarter in just 5 days? Yes, that's right! You can be smarter than you are now in just 5 days!

I know you are smart now, but you can become even smarter. I know the secret and I will share it with you, if you promise not to give up after the first or second day. I will prove to you that you can be smarter if you follow my instructions for 5 days.

"WHAT'S THE SECRET?" you ask.

It's so simple, you can easily do it.

Yes . . . you, you, you!

Oh, I almost forgot to tell you. . . . In order to be smarter in 5 days, you *must* believe in yourself. What good is being smarter if you don't believe you are smart already?

What I'm offering you is a chance to be smarter than you are right now. Being smart usually takes a long time, but my method will take only 5 days!

First, I must be honest and tell you that you must sign the pledge on the next page to prove that you are really brave enough to succeed. After signing the pledge, fold the page and put it in an envelope. Then give it to me in exchange for the Prime-Time Smartness Challenge materials.

DO NOT TURN THE PAGE
UNTIL YOU HAVE READ THIS PAGE CAREFULLY!

From L.W.Y. Cheung, H. Dart, S. Kalin, and S.L. Gortmaker, 2007, *Eat Well & Keep Moving*, 2nd ed. (Champaign, IL: Human Kinetics).

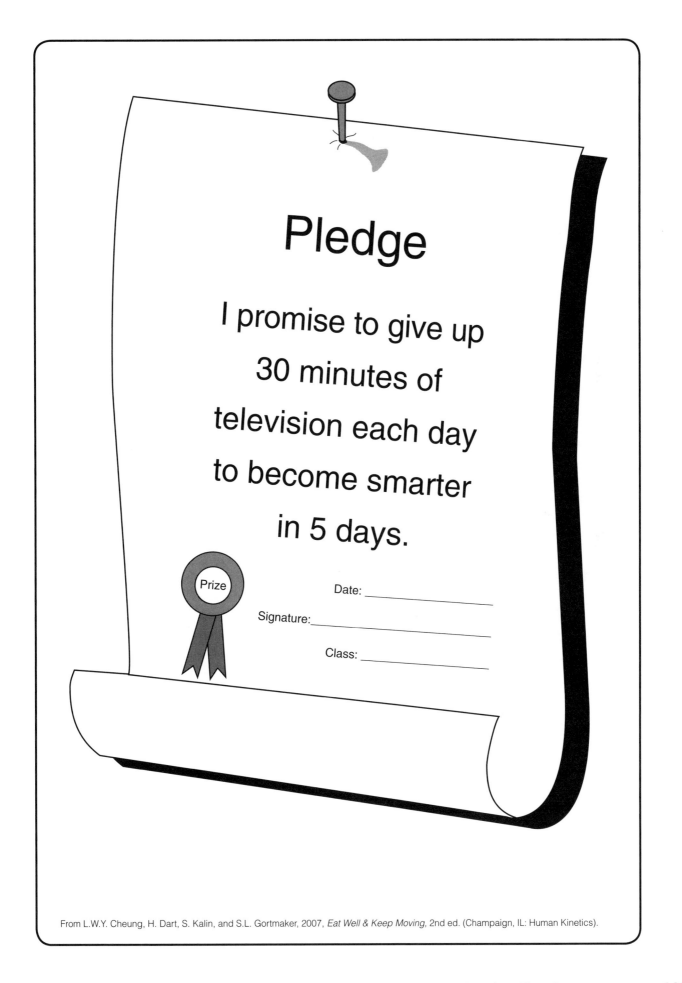

Pledge

I promise to give up
30 minutes of
television each day
to become smarter
in 5 days.

Prize

Date: _____

Signature:_____

Class: _____

From L.W.Y. Cheung, H. Dart, S. Kalin, and S.L. Gortmaker, 2007, *Eat Well & Keep Moving*, 2nd ed. (Champaign, IL: Human Kinetics).

WORKSHEET 1

My Favorite Prime-Time Shows

Directions

Write the names of three of your favorite television shows (in order from most to least favorite) on the lines following each day of the week.

Monday

1._____

2._____

3._____

Tuesday

1._____

2._____

3._____

Wednesday

1._____

2._____

3._____

Thursday

1._____

2._____

3._____

Friday

1._____

2._____

3._____

From L.W.Y. Cheung, H. Dart, S. Kalin, and S.L. Gortmaker, 2007, *Eat Well & Keep Moving,* 2nd ed. (Champaign, IL: Human Kinetics).

Prime-Time Smartness Challenge Materials

Hello Again!

Did you follow the instructions? Great! Now you will begin the real test. Are you ready to follow the steps? Good luck! See you in the winner's circle!

Step 1

List the names of the shows (one each day) that you agree to give up to become smarter. Look at My Favorite Prime-Time Shows if you don't remember which ones you chose.

Step 2

Here comes the real secret. Are you ready? Turn the page to The Star Page. On that page there is a passage for you to read. Please look it over, and then go on to step 3.

Step 3

Now that you have seen The Star Page, here's what you do. . . . Each day, instead of watching one of your favorite television programs, you agree to read The Star Page three times and then do some other activity—but not one that involves screen time, like surfing the Web, instant messaging, or playing computer games. You must read each word of The Star Page. If you skip a word, start over. Remember, read this page instead of watching one of your favorite shows.

Step 4

Keep track of your success on the Prime-Time Smartness Challenge page. Return it and The Questions Page to your teacher after the week is over.

Is giving up 30 minutes of television too much to ask to get smarter?

From L.W.Y. Cheung, H. Dart, S. Kalin, and S.L. Gortmaker, 2007, *Eat Well & Keep Moving*, 2nd ed. (Champaign, IL: Human Kinetics).

The Star Page

Echidnas (e-kid-nas)

Echidnas are egg-laying mammals that are covered with spines. The female deposits a single egg in her pouch while lying on her back. The egg is about the size of a grape. It hatches about 10 days later, but the young echidna (called a "puggle") stays in its mother's pouch and feeds from milk patches until its spines begin to develop.

There are two types of echidnas: short-beaked echidnas and long-beaked echidnas. Both types have long snouts, which they use to find food. Echidnas use their long, sticky tongues to catch their food. Since they do not have teeth, they use their tongues to grind food in their mouths. An echidna's favorite foods are termites and ants. This is why echidnas have the nickname "spiny anteaters."

An echidna's spines are its protection. If threatened, the echidna curls up in a ball, offering a mouthful of sharp spines to other animal attackers. On soft soil, it uses its long fore claws to bury itself and to escape heat and disturbances. The echidna has short but powerful legs, and it can dig a hole rapidly in soft or hard ground. But the echidna does not live in a permanent shelter. Instead, it roams around and finds refuge in hollow logs, in thick brush, or in holes around the roots of trees.

Echidnas are found in Australia and New Guinea. Short-beaked echidnas are common, but scientists believe that long-beaked echidnas are endangered.

From L.W.Y. Cheung, H. Dart, S. Kalin, and S.L. Gortmaker, 2007, *Eat Well & Keep Moving,* 2nd ed. (Champaign, IL: Human Kinetics).

Prime-Time Smartness Challenge

Mark the box next to each day that you succeed in following your pledge:

❏ **Day 1:** I gave up watching _____.
Instead, I read The Star Page three times. For the rest of the 30 minutes I
_____.
(Ideas for possible activities include playing a game, dancing to music, drawing, and helping a family member with a project or chore.)

Screen Time Bonus: I also gave up 30 minutes or more of other screen time (watching DVDs, Web surfing, instant messaging, playing video games).

Yes/No

❏ **Day 2:** I gave up watching _____.
I read The Star Page three times, and then I _____
_____ for the rest of the 30 minutes.

Screen Time Bonus: I also gave up 30 minutes or more of other screen time (watching DVDs, Web surfing, instant messaging, playing video games).

Yes/No

❏ **Day 3:** I'm halfway there—I know I can make it! I gave up watching _____
_____.
After I read The Star Page three times, I _____
_____.

Screen Time Bonus: I also gave up 30 minutes or more of other screen time (watching DVDs, Web surfing, instant messaging, playing video games).

Yes/No

From L.W.Y. Cheung, H. Dart, S. Kalin, and S.L. Gortmaker, 2007, *Eat Well & Keep Moving*, 2nd ed. (Champaign, IL: Human Kinetics).

(continued)

❑ **Day 4:** I'm getting smarter—I can feel it. I gave up watching _____

_____ .

I read The Star Page three times, and then I _____

_____ .

Screen Time Bonus: I also gave up 30 minutes or more of other screen time (watching DVDs, Web surfing, instant messaging, playing video games).

Yes/No

❑ **Day 5:** I gave up watching _____

_____ .

Instead, I did my best to fill out The Questions Page. Now I am finished with the Prime-Time Smartness Challenge!

Screen Time Bonus: I also gave up 30 minutes or more of other screen time (watching DVDs, Web surfing, instant messaging, playing video games).

Yes/No

From L.W.Y. Cheung, H. Dart, S. Kalin, and S.L. Gortmaker, 2007, *Eat Well & Keep Moving*, 2nd ed. (Champaign, IL: Human Kinetics).

? The Questions Page ?

(Save for day 5.)

1. By now, you have learned many facts about echidnas. Please list four of them (or list more than four if you can)! Tonight, go to someone in your home and share one interesting fact that you have learned.

   1. _____

   2. _____

   3. _____

   4. _____

2. If someone said that an echidna would make a great pet, would you agree? Why or why not? Write a short paragraph explaining your answer.

   _____

   _____

   _____

   _____

   _____

   _____

   _____

   _____

   _____

   _____

   _____

From L.W.Y. Cheung, H. Dart, S. Kalin, and S.L. Gortmaker, 2007, *Eat Well & Keep Moving,* 2nd ed. (Champaign, IL: Human Kinetics).

CONGRATULATIONS! YOU'RE A WINNER!

_____

Student's Name

Do you feel smarter?

Did you know about echidnas before you started this assignment?

Think of all you've learned!

You can give up TV for 30 minutes each day!

Keep up the great work!

And remember to be careful with your other screen time.

Screen Gem Patch

Add Screen Gem patches to the Winner's Circle bulletin board for those students who completed the challenge and at least three Screen Time Bonus exercises.

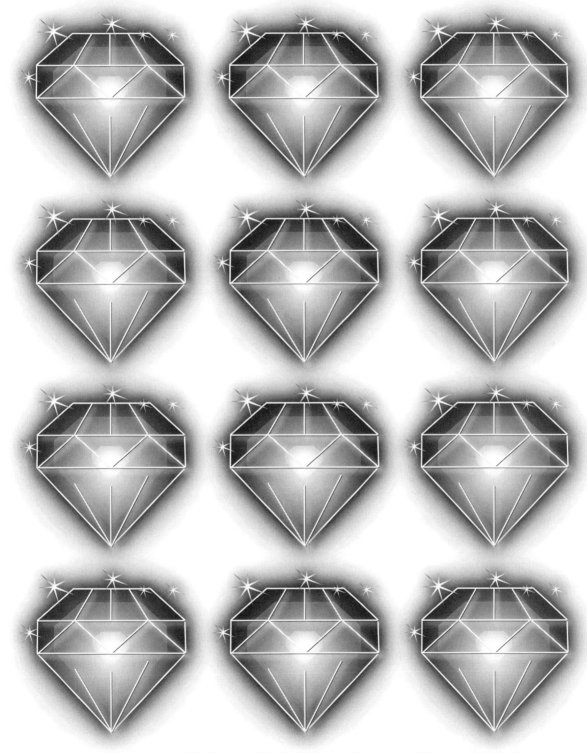

From L.W.Y. Cheung, H. Dart, S. Kalin, and S.L. Gortmaker, 2007, *Eat Well & Keep Moving,* 2nd ed. (Champaign, IL: Human Kinetics).

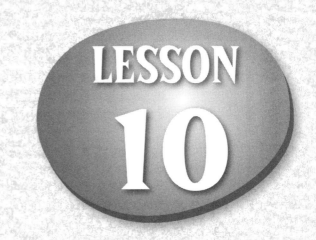

Chain Five

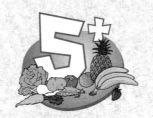

BACKGROUND

Most fruits and vegetables are naturally low in unhealthy fat and provide many essential nutrients and other food components important for health. These foods are excellent sources of vitamin C, vitamin B_6, carotenoids (including those that form vitamin A), folate (folic acid), and fiber. The antioxidants found in plant foods (e.g., vitamin C, carotenoids, vitamin E, and certain minerals) are currently of great interest to scientists because of their potentially beneficial role in reducing the risk of some cancers and other chronic diseases. Scientists are also trying to determine if other substances in plant foods, called *phytochemicals,* protect against some cancers.

The availability of fresh fruits and vegetables varies by season and by region of the country. However, frozen and canned fruits and vegetables are affordable, healthful options that are available throughout the year. The goal is to eat at least 5 servings of fruits and vegetables a day, and more is always better. Choose fruits and vegetables in a rainbow of colors (choose especially dark-green and orange vegetables).

THE GET 3 AT SCHOOL AND 5⁺ A DAY promotion, which encourages students to eat more fruits and vegetables, can be used as an extension to this lesson. See lesson 28 in part III, Promotions for the Classroom, for details.

ESTIMATED TEACHING TIME AND RELATED SUBJECT AREAS

Estimated teaching time: 1 hour, 5 minutes

Related subject areas: science, language arts, art

OBJECTIVES

1. Students will identify the benefits of consuming a variety of fruits and vegetables as well as other foods high in vitamins and minerals.
2. Students will explain how vitamins and minerals obtained from fruits and vegetables contribute to a healthy body.

MATERIALS

1. Blackboard
2. Storage box such as a pencil case or school supply box containing transparent tape, chalk, erasers, a ruler, pencils, pens, and sticky notes
3. Pictures of fruits and vegetables and a picture of low-fat milk
4. Transparency 1, Fruit and Vegetable Labels
5. Transparency 2, Mineral Food Labels
6. Worksheet 1, Chain Five: Vitamins and Minerals
7. Worksheet 2, Vitamins and Minerals Chart
8. Strips of colored paper (use 2 different colors) and paste, tape, or staplers

PROCEDURE

1. Display the contents of the storage box and explain to the class, "This is the box where I get my supplies. These are the things I need to write on the board, to mark papers, to repair papers, and to write notes to identify pages I want to find quickly. My supply box is important to me because it contains things I need. It also works for me by keeping all the things I need together so that they will be ready for use. I must constantly put new things into my storage box. Can anyone tell me why?"

Possible student answers include the following:

- When pencils are used a lot they get shorter and their erasers get smaller.
- All the paper is used up on the sticky pad and you have to get a new pad.
- New supplies must be put in so that they will never run out.

Respond to the students, "All the things in the box have a job to do. They are useful to me and help me do my work. Sometimes they work together. For example, I need my sticky notes and my pen to make notes when reading pages in the teacher's guide. In my red pen there's an ink cartridge that contains the ink I need in order to correct your papers."

2. Explain to the students, "Fruits and vegetables are like the supplies in my container because they are sources of things our bodies need. These things are called *nutrients* (vitamins, minerals, and other nutrients), which are substances our bodies need to be healthy. Just as I need to replace my supplies when they run low, we need to replace the nutrients in our bodies because our bodies use them every day."

3. Ask the students what they think is the most popular breakfast juice. Acknowledge all answers, and ask the following question when orange juice is given as an answer: "What is the primary vitamin found in oranges?" Students should answer, "Vitamin C." Explain that an orange is a citrus fruit and ask if the students can name other fruits that belong in this group (grapefruit, limes, lemons, tangerines, tangelos).

4. Tell the students that other sources of vitamin C include broccoli, cantaloupes, peppers, tomatoes, and sweet potatoes.

5. Write the word *vitamins* on the board. Have students discuss what they know about vitamins.

Students might say the following:

- Vitamins are things your body needs to stay healthy.
- Vitamins are listed on cans, bags, and boxes of food.
- Vitamin pills are purchased and taken by mouth.

6. Display pictures of dark-green, leafy vegetables and yellow-orange

> ### Key Ideas
>
> ▶ Vitamins are important for growth and maintenance of the body.
>
> ▶ Vitamins do not work alone. They work with other nutrients to get a job done.
>
> ▶ When we eat foods containing vitamins, some are broken down, used, and excreted by the body, while others are stored by the body.
>
> ▶ Vitamins reduce the risk of certain chronic diseases such as heart disease and possibly certain cancers.
>
> ▶ Vitamin C helps the body maintain healthy tissue, healthy skin, and healthy blood vessels.
>
> From L.W.Y. Cheung, H. Dart, S. Kalin, and S.L. Gortmaker, 2007, *Eat Well & Keep Moving*, 2nd ed. (Champaign, IL: Human Kinetics).

vegetables. Explain to the students, "These foods contain lots of vitamin A. This vitamin enables us to see at night and gives us healthy skin."

7. Show transparency 1, Fruit and Vegetable Labels, which shows one label for a fruit selection and one for a vegetable selection. Ask the students to identify vitamins listed on each label.

8. Have students suggest reasons why they must eat daily a variety of fruits and vegetables in a rainbow of colors.

   Sample reasons include the following:
   - Foods and nutrients work together to keep the body healthy.
   - There is more than one source of the same nutrient.
   - Many different substances are needed to bring about chemical reactions in the body.
   - Not all nutrients are contained in one food selection.

9. Display a photograph or a container of low-fat or nonfat milk and explain, "It is important to eat a variety of fruits and vegetables so that you get all the vitamins you need. It is also important to eat a variety of foods so that you get all the minerals you need. Like vitamins, minerals are substances that keep your body strong and working well. For example, milk has a lot of calcium, which is a mineral. Calcium builds healthy bones and teeth." Explain that calcium is also found in fortified soy and rice milks and fortified orange juice as well as in foods such as collard greens, tofu, black-eyed peas, and baked beans.

10. Write the word *minerals* on the board and list some important ones. Also explain how each is helpful to the body (see table 10.1).

▶TABLE 10.1 Minerals

Calcium helps keep our bones and teeth strong.	Zinc helps our bodies get energy from the food we eat.
Iron helps blood carry oxygen to all parts of our bodies.	Potassium helps our nerves function and our muscles, especially the heart, work properly.
Iodine helps our bodies get energy from the food we eat.	

11. Explain to the class that we get some minerals from fruits and vegetables, but we also get minerals from other sources such as low-fat and skim milk (and their products, like low-fat cheese and low-fat or nonfat yogurt) and lean meat. We must eat a balanced diet to make sure we get all the vitamins and minerals we need.

12. Show transparency 2, Mineral Food Labels, to the class. Ask the students to identify minerals listed on the label of each food selection. Remember that if the % Daily Value is 5 or less, the food is low in that nutrient.

13. Have the students form pairs or small groups. Distribute worksheet 1, Chain Five: Vitamins and Minerals, and worksheet 2, Vitamins and Minerals Chart. Have pairs or small groups use the chart on worksheet 2 to identify a fruit

or vegetable for each vitamin in the first chain on worksheet 1 and a food source for each mineral in the second chain. Suggest that they select fruits, vegetables, and other foods that they enjoy.

14. As the groups are working, distribute the colored strips of paper (at least five of color 1 and five of color 2 per group) and paste, tape, or staplers. Once the groups have completed the worksheet, have them write one of the vitamins from the worksheet (including the extra vitamin they chose for the fifth box) on each of the strips of color 1 and then have them write the fruit or vegetable source on the backs. On the strips of color 2, have them write each of the minerals, with the food source they chose on the backs.

15. Have each group link their strips together into paper chains, either alternating or grouping colors. You may want to link all of the groups' chains into one to hang up in the classroom or leave them in shorter lengths to decorate various areas of the room.

16. Explain to the students that the chains are a visual reminder to eat a variety of fruits and vegetables (5 or more servings each day) and other foods in order to get all the vitamins and minerals they need for healthy bodies.

Fruit and Vegetable Labels

Plums		
Nutrition Facts		
Serving Size 2 medium		
Amount Per Serving		
Calories 61	Calories from Fat 4	
		% Daily Value*
Total Fat 0.4g		**1%**
Saturated Fat 0g		**0%**
Trans Fat 0g		**0%**
Cholesterol 0mg		**0%**
Sodium 0mg		**0%**
Potassium 207mg		**6%**
Total Carbohydrate 15g		**6%**
Dietary Fiber 2g		**8%**
Sugars 13g		
Protein 1g		
Vitamin A 10% • Vitamin C 20%		
Calcium 0% • Iron 2%		
*Percent Daily Values are based on a 2,000 calorie diet. Your daily values may be higher or lower depending on your calorie needs.		

Sweet Potatoes		
Nutrition Facts		
Serving Size 1 medium		
Amount Per Serving		
Calories 103	Calories from Fat 0	
		% Daily Value*
Total Fat 0g		**0%**
Saturated Fat 0g		**0%**
Trans Fat 0g		**0%**
Cholesterol 0mg		**0%**
Sodium 40mg		**2%**
Potassium 540mg		**15%**
Total Carbohydrate 24g		**8%**
Dietary Fiber 4g		**15%**
Sugars 10g		
Protein 2g		
Vitamin A 440% • Vitamin C 35%		
Calcium 4% • Iron 4%		
*Percent Daily Values are based on a 2,000 calorie diet. Your daily values may be higher or lower depending on your calorie needs.		

Mineral Food Labels

Skim Milk

Nutrition Facts

Serving Size ½ pint (236 ml)
Serving Per Container 1

Amount Per Serving

Calories 90	Calories from Fat 0

	% Daily Value*
Total Fat 0g	**0%**
Saturated Fat 0g	**0%**
Trans Fat 0g	**0%**
Cholesterol <5mg	**1%**
Sodium 130mg	**5%**
Total Carbohydrate 13g	**4%**
Dietary Fiber 0g	**0%**
Sugars 12g	
Protein 8g	

Vitamin A 10%	•	Vitamin C 2%
Calcium 30%	•	Iron 0%

*Percent Daily Values are based on a 2,000 calorie diet. Your daily values may be higher or lower depending on your calorie needs.

Chicken

Nutrition Facts

Serving Size 1 roasted drumstick
(61 g/about 2 oz)
Serving Per Container 6

Amount Per Serving

Calories 110	Calories from Fat 50

	% Daily Value*
Total Fat 6g	**9%**
Saturated Fat 1.5g	**8%**
Trans Fat 0g	**0%**
Cholesterol 85mg	**28%**
Sodium 50mg	**2%**
Total Carbohydrate 0g	**0%**
Protein 14g	**28%**
Iron	**4%**

Not a significant source or dietary fiber, sugars, vitamin A, vitamin C, or calcium

*Percent Daily Values are based on a 2,000 calorie diet. Your daily values may be higher or lower depending on your calorie needs.

From L.W.Y. Cheung, H. Dart, S. Kalin, and S.L. Gortmaker, 2007, *Eat Well & Keep Moving,* 2nd ed. (Champaign, IL: Human Kinetics).

Name _____

Chain Five: Vitamins and Minerals

Part A Directions

Use the Vitamins and Minerals Chart to identify fruits and vegetables for each vitamin in the chain. In the last box of the chain, choose any fruit or vegetable you like and write in a vitamin it provides.

Vitamins

Vitamin C	Vitamin A	Folate	Vitamin K	

Food sources:

_____ + _____ + _____ + _____ + _____

Part B Directions

Use the Vitamins and Minerals Chart to identify a food source for each mineral in the chain. In the last box of the chain, choose any fruit or vegetable you like and write in a mineral it provides.

Minerals

Calcium	Iron	Potassium	Zinc	

Food sources:

_____ + _____ + _____ + _____ + _____

From L.W.Y. Cheung, H. Dart, S. Kalin, and S.L. Gortmaker, 2007, *Eat Well & Keep Moving,* 2nd ed. (Champaign, IL: Human Kinetics).

Vitamins and Minerals Chart

▶ **TABLE 10.2 Vitamins and Minerals Chart**

What's the nutrient?	Where can I get it?
Vitamin A	Carrots, sweet potatoes, greens, kale, spinach, cantaloupes, papayas, mangoes
Vitamin C	Oranges, grapefruits, tangerines, broccoli, bell peppers, tomatoes, sweet potatoes
Vitamin D	Vitamin D fortified low-fat or skim milk, vitamin D fortified soy milk and rice milk, salmon, egg yolks
Vitamin E	Seed oils, corn oil, almonds, sunflower seed kernels
Vitamin K	Green leafy vegetables, broccoli, cabbage, turnip greens, kale, sardines
Folate	Dried beans, green leafy vegetables, kale, spinach, yeast, soybeans, wheat germ, orange juice, most commercial breakfast cereals and breads
B vitamins such as B_1 (thiamine), B_2 (riboflavin), B_3 (niacin)	Liver, whole-grain breads and cereals, whole grains (such as barley, quinoa, whole wheat), lean meat, low-fat or fat-free yogurt, low-fat or skim milk, eggs
Calcium	Low-fat or nonfat milk, low-fat cheese, low-fat or nonfat yogurt, low-fat or nonfat cottage cheese, fortified soy milk and rice milk, fortified orange juice, broccoli, tofu, black-eyed peas, baked beans, collard greens, bok choy, kale
Potassium	Bananas, oranges, apricots, avocados, sweet potatoes, bran, peanuts, dried beans, and lean meat
Iron	Lean meat, whole wheat bread, spinach, lentils, kidney beans, lima beans, tofu, liver
Zinc	Lean meat, seafood, whole wheat bread, eggs, liver, beans, nuts
Iodine	Seafood

From L.W.Y. Cheung, H. Dart, S. Kalin, and S.L. Gortmaker, 2007, *Eat Well & Keep Moving*, 2nd ed. (Champaign, IL: Human Kinetics).

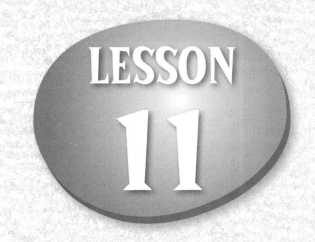

Alphabet Fruit (and Vegetables)

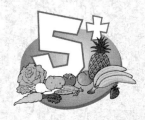 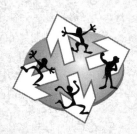

BACKGROUND

This lesson teaches students the importance of eating 5 or more servings of fruits and vegetables each day. Leading health authorities recommend that both adults and children eat at least 5 servings of fruits and vegetables daily, and more is always better. Getting 5 or more each day can help reduce the risk of diabetes, heart disease, obesity, and possibly some cancers. It's especially important to get children excited early on about getting 5 or more each day so that they establish healthy eating patterns that will last a lifetime.

THE GET 3 AT SCHOOL AND 5⁺ A DAY promotion, which encourages students to eat more fruits and vegetables, can be used as an extension of this lesson. See lesson 28 in part III, Promotions for the Classroom, for details.

HELPING YOUR KIDS GET 5⁺ A DAY

Parents and guardians are crucial partners in this task. Photocopying and sharing handout 1, Helping Your Kids Get Their 5⁺ A Day, with parents and guardians will help reinforce the messages of this lesson (as well as other messages in the *Eat Well & Keep Moving* curriculum). Suggest that parents try one tip each week (or each day, if they seem particularly motivated).

Parental involvement is a crucial component of the *Eat Well & Keep Moving* program. For detailed information about potential parent–student activities, see the Parent and Community Involvement Guide (Manual 3) on the CD-ROM.

Here are some tips for parents:

1. **Make more seem like less:** 5⁺ servings each day sounds like a lot unless you divide them up throughout the day and serve 1 at breakfast (a whole orange), 2 at lunch (carrot sticks or bell pepper slices), 1 as a snack (apple, banana, or berries), and 2 at dinner (a salad and a baked sweet potato). That equals 5⁺!

2. **Bring out the cook in you:** Get your child involved with the shopping and preparation of fruits and vegetables for your family. Ask your child to arrange a fruit plate for dessert or a vegetable tray for a party. The more your child helps in the preparation, the more likely he is to eat it.

3. **Dip it, dunk it:** Fruits and vegetables taste better to kids when combined with dips and dressings made with healthy fat (e.g., olive oil, canola oil) or with plain fat-free yogurt.

4. **Serve crunchy munchies:** Raw produce is a great way to help your child get 5 servings. Serve the kids crunchy munchies—apples, pears, carrots, broccoli, celery, and cucumbers, among others.

5. **Explore the unknown:** Most children are afraid to try new fruits and vegetables. Try to offer them a wide variety of fruits and vegetables at an early age. Keep offering those fruits and vegetables to help prevent later dislikes.

6. **Set an example:** Children model what they see their parents and teachers do. If parents and teachers eat plenty of fruits and vegetables, they're more likely to eat them as well.

7. **Gimme more:** Serve up a few different vegetables at dinner—a couple that the kids are familiar with and 1 or 2 that are new.

8. **Proclaim the benefits:** Tell the kids how eating fruits and vegetables will make them look and feel better. Eating 5 or more servings each day helps keep the heart healthy!

9. **Masquerade your mango:** Turn disgust into delicious with a disguise. Smell, color, and texture are three important qualities that can turn kids on or off to fruits and vegetables.

10. **Combine fruits and vegetables with the kids' favorite foods:** For instance, drizzle melted low-fat cheese on top of cauliflower or peanut sauce on top of steamed broccoli.

This lesson will include the five parts of a safe workout and a nutrition concept (eating fruits and vegetables). Students will be moving during the lesson, which will stress how both exercise and eating right help take care of the body. It's a team effort!

ESTIMATED TEACHING TIME AND RELATED SUBJECT AREA

Estimated teaching time: 1 hour
Related subject area: language arts

OBJECTIVES

1. Students will learn about a variety of fruits and vegetables.
2. Students will understand and be able to describe the importance of eating 5 or more fruits and vegetables each day.
3. Students will demonstrate the safe workout and its five parts.

MATERIALS

1. Handout 1, Helping Your Kids Get Their 5+ A Day
2. Five sets of fruit and vegetable cards (1 master set is provided for making copies)
3. Five containers (e.g., bags, boxes) in which to put the cards

PROCEDURE

1. Ask the students if they have eaten any fruits or vegetables today.
2. Ask the students to create a 5+ A Day menu for themselves. Ask them, "What fruit or vegetable could you have for breakfast? For lunch? For a snack? For dinner? Did you eat 5 today? More? Less?"
3. Discuss the reasons why we need to eat 5 or more servings each day. For example, fruits and vegetables help prevent heart disease, they help the

body heal wounds and burns, they prevent and fight infections, and they promote good dental health. Fruits and vegetables are also low in unhealthy fat, sodium, and calories.

4. Lead students through a warm-up and stretch.

> Warm-up—The first part of the safe workout, in which slow movements get the body ready for stretching and the fitness activity.

> Stretch—The part of the safe workout in which you do exercises that improve flexibility fitness and get the body ready for the fitness activity.

5. Explain to the students that they are going to participate in a fitness activity focusing on fruits and vegetables.

> Fitness activity—The part of the safe workout in which strength and endurance fitness exercises are performed.

6. Have the class form five groups.

7. Review the names of the fruits and vegetables on the cards.

8. Place the fruit and vegetable cards in a container in front of each group.

9. Set aside a place on the floor on the opposite side of the classroom where each group can put its fruit and vegetable cards in alphabetical order.

10. The students will be moving nonstop (either walking or jogging in place) behind the card container. On the signal of the teacher, the first person in line will get a card and go to the opposite side of the room, put the card down in the designated space, go back to the group, and high-five the next student in line. The second student will then pick up a card, place it on the floor in alphabetical order, go back to the group, and high-five the next person in line.

11. This will continue until all fruit and vegetable cards are in alphabetical order on the floor.

12. This activity can be completed more than once depending on time.

13. Lead the students in a cool-down and cool-down stretch.

> Cool-down—The part of the safe workout in which your body slows down and recovers from the fitness activity.

> Cool-down stretch—The last part of the safe workout, in which you do exercises that improve flexibility fitness.

14. Begin the Stay Healthy Corner, a time to reinforce a nutrition concept related to the fitness activity. You can set up a specific area of the classroom for the Stay Healthy Corner and decorate it with pictures or student drawings that represent the Principles of Healthy Living (e.g., healthy foods, children engaged in physical activity, and so on). Or you can simply set aside time for discussion at the end of the lesson.

   a. Have each group check to make sure its cards are in alphabetical order. Then have the groups pick five cards and discuss how these five could fit into their daily meals and snacks.

   b. Discuss some tips on how students can get 5 fruits and vegetables each day (see handout 1, Helping Your Kids Get Their 5+ A Day, for ideas) and ask them to offer their own experiences. For example, they might say, "My mom gives me money to pick out any fruits and vegetables I want at the grocery store," "I like crunchy bell pepper slices with hummus," "I like having orange juice for breakfast," and "Sometimes grown-ups don't set the right example—they don't eat fruits and vegetables."

    c. Encourage the students to give advice as to how the class can eat more fruits and vegetables each day.

15. Have students take their Helping Your Kids Get Their 5+ A Day handout home and post it on the refrigerator. Suggest that they work with their parents to try one tip every week (maybe even every day).

Helping Your Kids Get Their 5⁺ A Day

1. **Make more seem like less:** 5⁺ servings each day sounds like a lot unless you divide them up throughout the day and serve 1 at breakfast (orange juice), 2 at lunch (carrot sticks and bell pepper slices), 1 as a snack (apple, banana, or berries), and 2 at dinner (a salad and a baked sweet potato). That equals more than 5!

2. **Bring out the cook in you:** Get your child involved with the shopping and preparation of fruits and vegetables for your family. Ask your child to arrange a fruit plate for dessert or a vegetable tray for a party. The more your child helps in the preparation, the more likely he is to eat it.

3. **Dip it, dunk it:** Fruits and vegetables taste better to kids when combined with dips and dressings made with healthy fat (e.g., olive oil, canola oil) or with plain nonfat yogurt.

4. **Serve crunchy munchies:** Raw produce is a great way to help your child get her 5⁺ servings. Serve the kids crunchy munchies—apples, pears, carrots, broccoli, celery, and cucumbers, among others.

5. **Explore the unknown:** Most children are afraid to try new fruits and vegetables. Try to offer them a wide variety of fruits and vegetables at an early age. Keep offering those fruits and vegetables to help prevent later dislikes.

6. **Set an example:** Children model what they see their parents and teachers do. If parents and teachers eat plenty of fruits and vegetables, they're more likely to eat them as well.

7. **Gimme more:** Serve up a few different vegetables at dinner—a couple that the kids are familiar with and 1 or 2 that are new.

8. **Proclaim the benefits:** Tell the kids how eating fruits and vegetables will make them look and feel better. Eating 5 or more servings each day helps keep the heart healthy!

9. **Masquerade your mango:** Turn disgust into delicious with a disguise. Smell, color, and texture are three important qualities that can turn kids on or off to fruits and vegetables.

10. **Combine fruits and vegetables with the kids' favorite foods:** For instance, drizzle melted low-fat cheese on top of cauliflower or peanut sauce on top of steamed broccoli.

From L.W.Y. Cheung, H. Dart, S. Kalin, and S.L. Gortmaker, 2007, *Eat Well & Keep Moving,* 2nd ed. (Champaign, IL: Human Kinetics).

Fruit and Vegetable Cards

These cards are for use in the fitness activity.

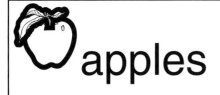 apples

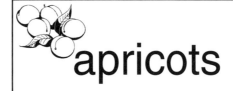 apricots

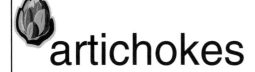 artichokes

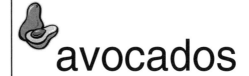 avocados

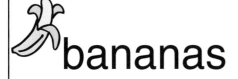 bananas

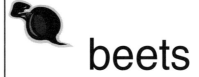 beets

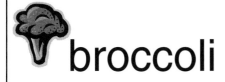 berries

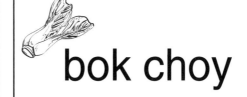 bok choy

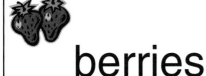 broccoli

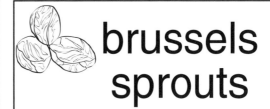 brussels sprouts

From L.W.Y. Cheung, H. Dart, S. Kalin, and S.L. Gortmaker, 2007, *Eat Well & Keep Moving*, 2nd ed. (Champaign, IL: Human Kinetics).

(continued)

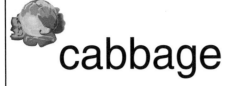 cabbage

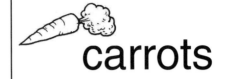 carrots

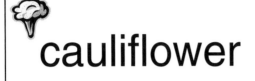 cauliflower

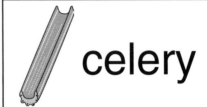 celery

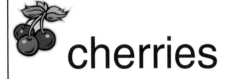 cherries

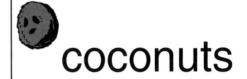 coconuts

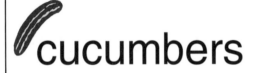 collards

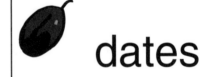 corn

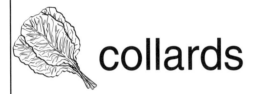 cucumbers

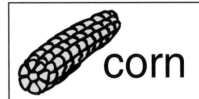 dates

From L.W.Y. Cheung, H. Dart, S. Kalin, and S.L. Gortmaker, 2007, *Eat Well & Keep Moving,* 2nd ed. (Champaign, IL: Human Kinetics).

(continued)

eggplant

 figs

 grapes

 grapefruit

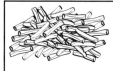 green beans

 green peppers

 kale

 kelp

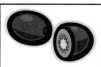 kiwi

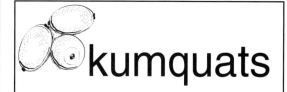 kumquats

From L.W.Y. Cheung, H. Dart, S. Kalin, and S.L. Gortmaker, 2007, *Eat Well & Keep Moving,* 2nd ed. (Champaign, IL: Human Kinetics).

(continued)

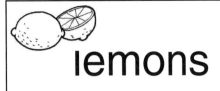 lemons

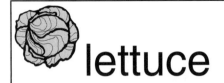 lettuce

 limes

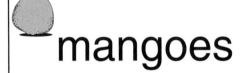 mangoes

 melons

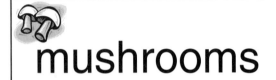 mushrooms

 nectarines

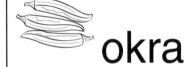 okra

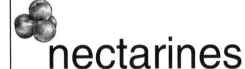 onions

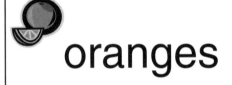 oranges

From L.W.Y. Cheung, H. Dart, S. Kalin, and S.L. Gortmaker, 2007, *Eat Well & Keep Moving,* 2nd ed. (Champaign, IL: Human Kinetics).

(continued)

papayas

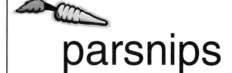 parsnips

 peaches

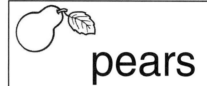 pears

 peas

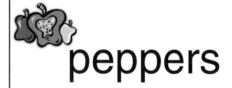 peppers

 persimmons

 pineapples

 plums

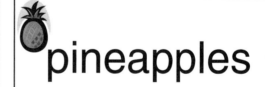 prunes

From L.W.Y. Cheung, H. Dart, S. Kalin, and S.L. Gortmaker, 2007, *Eat Well & Keep Moving,* 2nd ed. (Champaign, IL: Human Kinetics).

(continued)

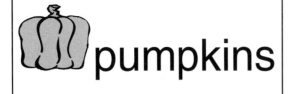 pumpkins

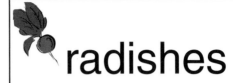 radishes

 raisins

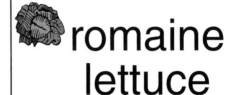 romaine lettuce

 spinach

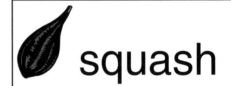 squash

sweet potatoes

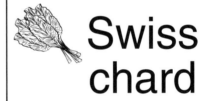 Swiss chard

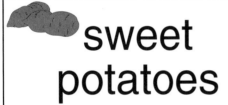 tangerines

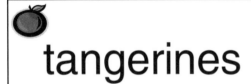 tomatoes

From L.W.Y. Cheung, H. Dart, S. Kalin, and S.L. Gortmaker, 2007, *Eat Well & Keep Moving,* 2nd ed. (Champaign, IL: Human Kinetics).

(continued)

turnips

zucchini

From L.W.Y. Cheung, H. Dart, S. Kalin, and S.L. Gortmaker, 2007, *Eat Well & Keep Moving,* 2nd ed. (Champaign, IL: Human Kinetics).

(continued)

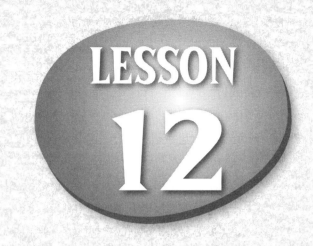

LESSON 12

Brilliant Breakfast*

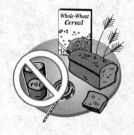
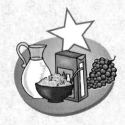

*Lesson adapted from Texas Education Agency Nutrition Education Curriculum Guide Grade 5-8, and a lesson plan developed by Ms. Michele Dorsey.

BACKGROUND**

Breakfast is the most important meal of the day. Eating breakfast gives the body the energy it needs to start the day and perform the morning's tasks, from thinking to doing the dishes to working out. Generally, adults who regularly eat breakfast learned this lifelong good habit when they were children.

Studies show that children who eat breakfast are better prepared for the school day. They perform better in school, are tardy less often, and miss fewer days of school. Students who eat breakfast have also demonstrated that their ability to concentrate is better, their reaction times are faster, their energy levels are higher, and their scores on tests are better.

To help make breakfast a lifelong habit, students (and adults) should be encouraged to start their day by eating breakfast. Any good, nutritious food can be eaten for breakfast. If people don't happen to like typical breakfast foods, such as cereal or toast, they can eat leftovers from dinner, like pizza or a sandwich. The most important thing is to eat a nutritious meal in the morning.

Breakfast is a great time to start the day by eating well. Ideally, breakfast should contain healthy foods such as whole-grain cereal or toast and fresh fruit or a small glass of 100% fruit or vegetable juice—and not foods made with refined grains or added sugars, such as sweetened cereal, doughnuts, pastries, soft drinks, or candy. The carbohydrate in nutritious breakfast foods gives the body energy, and some added protein helps stave off a midmorning drop in blood sugar that can make children lethargic before lunchtime. Protein foods may come from low-fat or nonfat dairy such as 1% milk and low-fat plain yogurt, eggs, nuts (such as peanut butter on whole wheat toast or almonds sprinkled on oatmeal), or even slices of turkey, cubes of tofu, or hummus.

Blood sugar levels indicate how much fuel (in the form of glucose) is immediately available to the body. When blood sugar levels drop, children (and adults) may feel drowsy or less energetic and have trouble concentrating. Breakfast can help keep blood sugar levels up throughout the morning until lunchtime.

Foods such as doughnuts, sweetened cereals, soft drinks, sports drinks, fruit punch, candy bars, and desserts contain a lot of added sugar and are not the best choices for breakfast because they can cause blood sugar levels to drop faster than foods containing a mix of healthy carbohydrate (from fiber-rich whole grains, fruits, and vegetables) and protein.

ESTIMATED TEACHING TIME AND RELATED SUBJECT AREAS

Estimated teaching time: 1 hour
Related subject areas: math, science

**Background information partially from Maryland Food Committee.

OBJECTIVES

1. Students will able to describe why they should eat a healthful breakfast.
2. Students will identify the effects of eating a nutritious breakfast and a less-than-nutritious breakfast.
3. Students will create breakfasts to fit different lifestyles and needs.

MATERIALS

1. Worksheet 1, The Breakfast Club
2. Worksheet 2, International Breakfast Club
3. Transparency 1, Avoiding the Midmorning Slump
4. Solutions to worksheet 1

PROCEDURE

1. Ask the students to raise their hands if they like to eat breakfast.
2. Ask the students if they know what the word *breakfast* means. Tell them that *breakfast* means *breaking the fast* and that a fast is when the body has gone for a long time without food—such as overnight.
3. Tell the students that during a fast, the amount of sugar in the blood decreases (the sugar eventually is transported to muscles and organs to create energy for work). When your blood sugar levels are low, your body is not getting all the energy it needs to work really efficiently whether you are playing or thinking.
4. Tell the students that when they eat breakfast, they are breaking the overnight fast and giving the body what it needs to work until lunchtime. On the other hand, if they skip breakfast in the morning, they may
   - be less alert;
   - feel less energetic;
   - be less efficient at completing tasks;
   - experience headaches, stomach cramps, and irritability; or
   - achieve less.
5. Ask the students what they like to eat for breakfast. Write responses on the board. Tell the students that they should all try to eat breakfast every morning and that eating any type of nutritious food in the morning is better than eating nothing. Some foods, though, are better than others for breakfast.
6. Remind the class of the Principles of Healthy Living (introduced in lesson 1), especially the ones that relate to food choices and breakfast:
   - Eat 5 or more servings of fruits and vegetables each day.
   - Choose whole-grain foods and limit foods and beverages with added sugar.
   - Choose healthy fat, limit saturated fat, and avoid trans fat.
   - Eat a nutritious breakfast every morning.

Look at the list of foods written on the board. Circle the ones that fit the healthy living goals and help students to start the day off in a healthy way. If appropriate, remind students that breakfast is available to them before school in the cafeteria.

7. Tell the students that the ideal breakfast contains carbohydrate (from foods such as whole-grain cereal or toast and fruit or a small glass of 100% fruit or vegetable juice—but not from foods made with refined grains or added sugar, such as soft drinks, candy, sweetened cereal, pastries, or doughnuts) and some protein (from foods such as peanut butter, low-fat or nonfat milk and yogurt, eggs, turkey slices, tofu, hummus). The carbohydrate gives the body energy, and the protein helps stave off a midmorning drop in blood sugar, a drop which can make students feel hungry, drowsy, sluggish, and irritable before lunchtime.

8. Also tell students that foods high in added sugar (such as doughnuts, soft drinks, energy drinks, sports drinks, fruit punches, candy bars, and desserts) are not ideal for breakfast because they can cause blood sugar levels to rise quickly and then drop below fasting levels within a few hours. These types of foods also tend to contain very few other nutrients like vitamins and minerals. If a student does not like typical breakfast foods, grabbing a slice of last night's pizza or making a sandwich on whole-grain bread is better than eating sweets or nothing at all.

9. Distribute and review worksheet 1, The Breakfast Club, with the students. After students have completed the worksheet, use the Avoiding the Midmorning Slump transparency to review their answers and show students what happens to blood sugar levels with each type of breakfast. Discuss the following points for the transparency:
   - Breakfast #1 (the skipped breakfast) did not provide any food, so energy must come from body storage. Blood sugar levels remain at or below fasting levels, which are low and do not provide enough energy for work.
   - Breakfast #2 provides enough protein to keep Tisha alert and to discourage midmorning hunger pangs, and it provides enough healthy carbohydrate and fiber (from whole grains and fruit) and protein for sustained energy, which means that she will be able to concentrate until it is time for lunch.
   - Breakfast #3 contains too much refined sugar and not enough protein to keep blood sugar levels up until lunch. This quick rise in blood sugar makes the body work just as quickly to get the sugar into the cells. The result is a midmorning slump that makes it hard for Omar to concentrate on his work.

10. With the class, write several nutritious breakfast menus that address the specific situations of the people in the following list.
   Breakfasts for people who wake up late:
   - Breakfast shakes with low-fat milk
   - A slice of low-fat cheese and piece of fruit
   - Low-fat yogurt
   - Leftover supper entrees
   - Peanut butter sandwich on whole-grain bread and a juice box of 100% juice

Breakfasts for people who do not like typical breakfast foods:
* Whole wheat crackers with cheese or peanut butter
* English muffin pizzas on a whole wheat English muffin
* Breakfast burritos with a whole wheat tortilla, brown rice, and beans
* Hummus, lettuce, and tomato sandwich on a whole wheat pita

Breakfasts for people who sleep in on the weekend:
* Omelet with tomatoes, reduced-fat cheese, and peppers
* Homemade buckwheat pancakes with low-fat milk
* Turkey sandwich on whole wheat bread and fresh fruit
* Fruit and low-fat yogurt parfait

11. Distribute worksheet 2, International Breakfast Club, and arrange the class in small groups. Have each group review the breakfast foods typically eaten in different parts of the world and create a healthful breakfast that could be served as part of an international breakfast day. Ask students to write how their chosen breakfast affects blood sugar levels and circle the appropiate diagram.

12. Instruct students to create their own nutritious, energizing breakfasts based on their own lifestyles, traditions, and food preferences. Ask some of them to share their breakfast menus with the class.

13. For an optional activity, you may assign students (individually or in pairs) to create a poster depicting a healthful breakfast. This may be a breakfast that they enjoy, a breakfast that fits one of the scenarios discussed previously (for instance, a meal that suits someone who sleeps late or does not like breakfast), or an international breakfast from worksheet 2.

Name _____

The Breakfast Club

Breakfast

Jeremy's Breakfast

Jeremy was late for school, so he left without eating breakfast. By midmorning (around 10 a.m.), he was fidgety and had trouble concentrating. His stomach was grumbling before lunchtime, and he had trouble completing his morning math quiz.

Tisha's Breakfast

Tisha was also running late for school; but when she got there, she went to the cafeteria and ate the school breakfast of a small apple, plain oatmeal, and 1% milk. She felt great all morning and did very well on her math quiz.

Omar's Breakfast

Omar grabbed two doughnuts and a glass of Kool-Aid as he ran out the door for school. He was full of energy and enthusiasm for a while, but then his mind started to wander and, like Jeremy, he had trouble finishing the math quiz.

Why did Jeremy, Tisha, and Omar feel the way they did by lunchtime?

1. _____

_____

_____

2. _____

_____

_____

3. _____

_____

_____

From L.W.Y. Cheung, H. Dart, S. Kalin, and S.L. Gortmaker, 2007, *Eat Well & Keep Moving*, 2nd ed. (Champaign, IL: Human Kinetics).

International Breakfast Club

Your school will have an international breakfast day. You will help plan the meal. Pick two countries and plan a healthy breakfast from each of them. Use table 12.1, Breakfast Foods Around the World.

Circle the graph that shows how each breakfast affects blood sugar levels. Write a sentence describing the effect of each breakfast on blood sugar levels.

Name of students in group:

Country 1:

Breakfast menu:

Effect on blood sugar level:

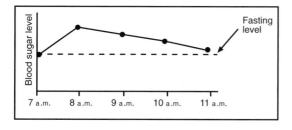

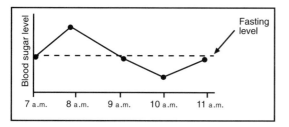

From L.W.Y. Cheung, H. Dart, S. Kalin, and S.L. Gortmaker, 2007, *Eat Well & Keep Moving,* 2nd ed. (Champaign, IL: Human Kinetics).

(continued)

Country 2:

Breakfast menu:

Effect on blood sugar level:

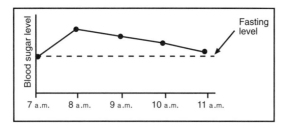

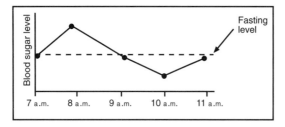

From L.W.Y. Cheung, H. Dart, S. Kalin, and S.L. Gortmaker, 2007, *Eat Well & Keep Moving,* 2nd ed. (Champaign, IL: Human Kinetics).

(continued)

▶TABLE 12.1   Breakfast Foods Around the World

Country	Typical breakfast foods
Mexico	• Fruit (bananas, cactus fruit, mangoes, oranges, pineapple) • Whole-grain tortillas with refried beans and cheese • Eggs with tomato-chili sauce, tortillas, and avocado • Bolillos (wheat rolls) • Chocolate milk or plain milk • Freshly squeezed orange juice
China	• Rice • Congee (rice porridge) • Steamed vegetable dumplings • Soup • Vegetables (bamboo shoots, bok choy, broccoli, eggplant, mushrooms, peppers, snow peas) • Soybeans • Fish
Ghana	• Soup or stew • Fish • Yams • Plantains • Eggs • Millet porridge
India	• Flatbread • Dumplings with coconut chutney • Lentils and rice • Rice noodles with meat curry • Steamed rice cake with bananas • Yogurt

From L.W.Y. Cheung, H. Dart, S. Kalin, and S.L. Gortmaker, 2007, *Eat Well & Keep Moving*, 2nd ed. (Champaign, IL: Human Kinetics).

Avoiding the Midmorning Slump

A good breakfast has healthy carbohydrate (approximately 40 grams) and some protein (12-18 grams). This combination helps the body avoid a midmorning slump in energy.

You can see how many grams of protein or carbohydrate there are in a food by looking at its food label.

When blood sugar drops below the fasting level, a person may have a harder time concentrating on schoolwork, may feel light-headed, and may be less alert.

Jeremy's breakfast:

Breakfast #1

Skips morning meal
Energy must come from body storage

Carbohydrate: 0 grams
Protein: 0 grams

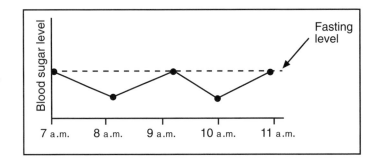

Tisha's breakfast:

Breakfast #2
Optimal morning meal example

1/2 cup plain oatmeal
8 oz. (250ml) 1% milk
1 small apple

Carbohydrate: 44 grams
Protein: 12 grams

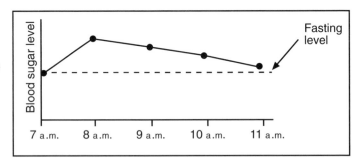

Omar's breakfast:

Breakfast #3
High-carbohydrate morning meal example

2 doughnuts
1/2 cup Kool-Aid

Carbohydrate: 37 grams
Protein: 2 grams

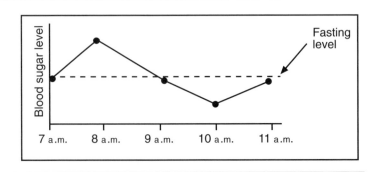

From L.W.Y. Cheung, H. Dart, S. Kalin, and S.L. Gortmaker, 2007, *Eat Well & Keep Moving*, 2nd ed. (Champaign, IL: Human Kinetics).

The Breakfast Club

Breakfast

Jeremy's Breakfast

Jeremy was late for school, so he left without eating breakfast. By midmorning (around 10 a.m.), he was fidgety and had trouble concentrating. His stomach was grumbling before lunchtime, and he had trouble completing his morning math quiz.

Tisha's Breakfast

Tisha was also running late for school; but when she got there, she went to the cafeteria and ate the school breakfast of a small apple, plain oatmeal, and 1% milk. She felt great all morning and did very well on her math quiz.

Omar's Breakfast

Omar grabbed two doughnuts and a glass of Kool-Aid as he ran out the door for school. He was full of energy and enthusiasm for a while, but then his mind started to wander and, like Jeremy, he had trouble finishing the math quiz.

Why did Jeremy, Tisha, and Omar feel the way they did by lunchtime?

1. Jeremy did not eat anything in the morning. He did not break his overnight fast so his energy needed to come from body storage. This kept his blood sugar levels low, making him hungry, lethargic, and distracted.

2. Tisha ate an excellent breakfast with whole grains (oatmeal), a small apple, and some protein (primarily from the 1% milk.) This breakfast held her blood sugar up at normal levels throughout the morning, keeping her alert and energized until lunchtime.

3. It was good that Omar ate a breakfast. However, his breakfast was not ideal. He ate foods that were too high in sugar. With so much sugar (and no milk to provide some protein), Omar felt tired and restless around midmorning because his blood sugar dropped.

From L.W.Y. Cheung, H. Dart, S. Kalin, and S.L. Gortmaker, 2007, *Eat Well & Keep Moving,* 2nd ed. (Champaign, IL: Human Kinetics).

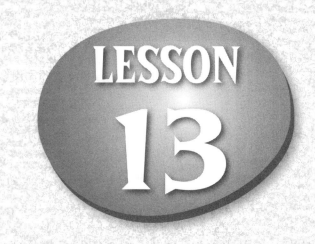

Fitness Walking

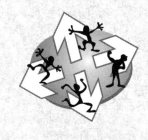

BACKGROUND

Walking is one of the healthiest, safest, and easiest ways to begin a fitness program, and it can be a big step toward improving your health. Fitness or aerobic walking uses all of the major muscle groups in the upper and lower body in a gentle, dynamic, rhythmic action, which is what an ideal exercise should do. Children should get at least 60 minutes of physical activity every day, and walking is a great way for them to reach that goal.

Walking is also free! There are no machines or membership fees, no fancy packaging or expensive clothes. Walking requires only that you pace yourself and do your personal best. What's important is feeling good about yourself and setting your own goals.

Walking can be done with friends or family. It can also be done as an adventure with a school class. An active lifestyle can make you feel better, give you more energy, and enhance your health. We want you and your class to get hooked on walking. It's fun, and it's good for you!

OVERVIEW

This lesson introduces students to the benefits and fun of walking for fitness. The lesson also serves as a kickoff for an ongoing class walking club that can be integrated into geography activities throughout the year.

ESTIMATED TEACHING TIME AND RELATED SUBJECT AREAS

Estimated teaching time: 1 hour

Related subject areas: science, social studies, math, physical education

OBJECTIVES

1. Students will learn the importance of regular exercise and will establish an ongoing class walking club.
2. Students will be exposed to the benefits of walking with family, friends, and classmates.
3. Students will learn walking techniques and learn about the health benefits of raising their heart rate through regular aerobic activity.
4. Students will learn about a particular geographic region of the world.

MATERIALS

1. Comfortable shoes (students and teacher)
2. Worksheet 1, Teacher Classroom Walking Log
3. Worksheet 2, Student Classroom Walking Log (duplicate for students)
4. Worksheet 3, Student Home Walking Log (duplicate for students)

5. Worksheet 4, Bird Behaviors Worksheet (optional Nature Walk extension, duplicate for students)

6. Maps

7. Map pins or thumbtacks

8. Tape recorder, binoculars, and bird identification book (optional, for Nature Walk extension)

9. Pedometers* for each student (optional)

PLANNING A WALKING CLUB

In addition to introducing students to how important and fun walking can be, this lesson focuses on organizing a class walking club.

When planning a walking club, first consider where and when your students can walk. The walks can take place before, during, or after school and can be done in the hallways, gym, playground, or neighborhood—whenever and wherever such a program works best for your school.

An effective way to introduce a walking club into your school is to integrate it with your curriculum. One option is to integrate the club with your social studies curriculum. For example, you can combine walking with lessons on the state in which you live, on the entire United States, or on other countries around the world. If there is an area of the world your students would like to learn about, use the walking club to talk about that area. As a class or individually, design the itinerary of a fitness walk across the region you have chosen to cover, and then pretend you are walking across that region. Students could walk across America together, walk across a specific region of the United States, or walk around the world. The design is completely open.

Give your program a name, such as Walk Across America or Walk Across the World, or let the students choose a name.

Obtain maps of the area you chose to study, and tie in the students' walking progress with movement on the map. Each time the class walks for a certain length of time, equate that time with a particular distance on the map (for example, 5 minutes of walking could equal 50 miles, or 80 kilometers). Each student can have a map to follow, or all of the students can plot their travels on one map. The amount of time the class walks and the distance traveled will depend on the part of the world or country on which you chose to focus. For example, if you decided on a large area of the world, such as Africa, then 5 minutes might equal 200 miles (322 kilometers) traveled. If you chose the state of Maryland, however, 5 minutes might equal 50 miles (80 kilometers).

Keep track of your class walks on the logs provided. There is a log for each class as well as for each student. The class log can be made larger and displayed in the classroom for all to see. A map of the region or country that they are traveling across should be displayed along with the class log. Displaying the map and log will motivate the class and keep everyone more involved.

If it is possible to supply students with pedometers, consider tracking their number of steps instead of tracking walking time. Pedometers can also be a fun way to motivate students to increase their activity. Have students keep track of the number of steps they take each day for a week, and then have them determine

*Low-cost pedometers are available from many sources on the Web. Consult with your school's physical education director to get recommendations for accurate, easy-to-use, low-cost models. In some communities, local health departments, health centers, or health insurers may provide pedometers for free.

their average number of steps per day. Set a goal for students to increase their average number of steps per day by 10%.

Possible extensions for combining geography with the walking program include having students learn the state's or country's capital, natural resources, climate, unique features, major monuments, and historical sites. Students could create posters to illustrate these features or write journal entries or fictionalized accounts of what they "see" along their walk.

Another way to integrate walking with the curriculum is to link an outdoors nature walk with science lessons (see Extension Activity: Taking a Nature Walk, page 193, which gives suggestions and worksheets for taking a bird observation walk). Students can collect samples, describe a habitat, or look for evidence of human effects on the environment. Have students follow up in the classroom with posters or journal entries describing what they saw.

Encourage students to take on the walking program as an after-school, family-and-friend adventure. Have the students keep a log of the dates and times of their after-school walks (see worksheet 3, Student Home Walking Log). They can plot their travels on the maps with pins or thumbtacks. Get the whole school involved in walking—principals, office staff members, custodians, and other teachers and students can join the program. The more the students see others participating, the more they will want to become involved.

PROCEDURE

1. FITNESS WALKING

Explain to the students that fitness walking is walking at a pace (speed) that makes the heart, lungs, and blood vessels work harder than usual. This type of aerobic workout makes the heart muscle pump harder because the body's other muscles—the leg and arm muscles—are working harder and need more blood to keep them going.

Blood delivers energy and oxygen to working muscles. When muscles work hard, such as when you're fitness walking, they need more energy and oxygen. During exercise, the heart works harder to pump blood to these muscles. When the heart works harder, it gets stronger.

Explain to the students that they can check their pulse rate before they begin exercising and again during their fitness workout in order to see firsthand how the heart muscle works harder. (See details on how to do this in the section titled Finding a Pulse on page 191.) Also explain to the students the importance of completing an hour of physical activity on all or most days of the week. It is OK to do that activity a little bit at a time, so a 15-minute or longer walk can help them reach their hour-a-day goal.

2. BENEFITS OF FITNESS WALKING

Ask the students to list the benefits of fitness walking. These can include the following:

a. Walking is an excellent and safe way to improve aerobic fitness. Aerobic exercises like walking strengthen the heart, lungs, and blood vessels. Walking lets you do this with less wear and tear on the body compared to many other types of conditioning.

b. Walking, like other aerobic exercises, can give you more energy and reduce fatigue.

c. Walking can help relieve stress.

d. Walking can improve mood and mental function.

e. Walking can help slow down the progression of osteoporosis (bone loss), which can occur as the body ages.

f. Walking can be performed with friends and family.

3. HOW TO FITNESS WALK

a. Make sure students wear sneakers or comfortable shoes.

b. Review with students the following (and consult figure 13.1):

1. Arm swing: Try to keep the arms swinging faster than they swing when walking normally. The faster the arms swing, the faster the legs will move. Bend the arms 90 degrees at the elbow. Concentrate on moving the arms faster and swinging them from the shoulder. Remember, when you shorten your arms (bending them 90 degrees at the elbow), you can swing them faster and your legs will move faster. Keep your shoulders relaxed. Beginners tend to tense up around the shoulders. Relax!

2. Hands: Form a loose fist. Do not clench your fist and put tension in the arm muscles.

3. Foot placement and toe-off: The power of the step comes from the toe-off. With each step, land the foot on the heel, and then roll forward to the toe and push off.

Tell the students that following these instructions for fitness walking should help them enjoy their walking more. They should do what feels comfortable for them. Do it right, but make it *fun!*

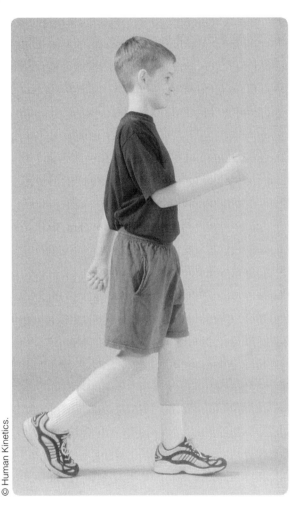

© Human Kinetics.

▶ FIGURE 13.1   Fitness walking.

4. FINDING A PULSE

On the first day of fitness walking (or however often you would like), remind the students that their pulse rate will increase when they exercise and teach them how to find their pulse (refer to figure 13.2).

Explain to the students, "During an aerobic workout, you want your heart, lungs, and blood vessels to work harder than they are used to working. Your pulse can help you know what is going on inside your body. On the side of your neck, just below the jawbone, is a major blood vessel bringing blood to the brain. Put your index and middle fingers together and place them gently on that blood vessel on the side of your neck to feel the pulse. During exercise, the pulse is usually very easy to find." To demonstrate how pulse rate changes from the warm-up to the fitness activity to the cool-down, have the students try to feel their pulse before, during, and after aerobic walking.

Tell the students, "The heart is a muscle that has a huge job to do. It must always be working every second, minute, hour, day, week, month, and year of your lives. Once you understand that this heart muscle of yours has such a huge job, hopefully you will want to take care of it so it can do its job.

"Walking is one way to keep the heart muscle healthy. Likewise, eating right and being active are both a big part of helping the heart stay healthy. If, during the fitness activity, the heart is working harder than it's used to working, then with time the heart will get stronger and stay healthy. The more you include exercise and eating right in your daily lives, the better the body can work and feel!"

5. THE SAFE WORKOUT

Following the steps of the safe workout will help students prevent injuries. The five steps are the following:

Step 1: Warm-up. Start each fitness walk slowly to get the body ready for harder work. Emphasize to the students the importance of warming up and stretching before doing any type of physical activity. During the warm-up, talk about the adventure for the day and review the important facts about the warm-up. (Refer to lesson 3, The Safe Workout: An Introduction.)

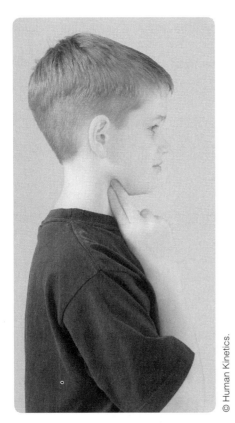

▶ FIGURE 13.2   Finding a pulse.

© Human Kinetics.

Step 2: Stretch. After the warm-up, stretch out and work on flexibility fitness. Review the importance of stretching and the key parts of safe stretching.

Step 3: Fitness activity. Introduce the walking activity you have chosen for your class, such as walking the first leg of a trip across the United States. Have the class set a goal for that particular day. For example, the class goal for the first day may be to walk for 10 minutes without stopping; if students are using pedometers, the goal may be for each student to walk 1,000 steps. Equate the number of minutes walked or number of steps walked to a particular distance on the map. As students get used to the program, the class can set goals to walk longer and more frequently or (if using pedometers) to increase their average number of steps per day by 10%. Remember, the more days that students walk, the greater the opportunity they have to learn and become fit. Take the students on their fitness walk. During the walk, lead a discussion among students about the geographic region they are pretending to walk through on their program. Other topics to discuss include nutrition and physical activity issues.

Step 4: Cool-down. After their fitness walk, have the students walk slowly to let their bodies recover. Review the benefits of the cool-down.

Step 5: Cool-down stretch. After the cool-down, have the students stretch again to prevent soreness, to improve flexibility, and to decrease their chances of injury. While they are stretching, review the benefits of the cool-down stretch and the proper way to cool down.

The Stay Healthy Corner can be an area of the classroom decorated with pictures or student drawings that represent the Principles of Healthy Living (e.g., healthy foods, children engaged in physical activity, and so on). Or it can be simply a time for discussion and reflection on the health messages of the lesson. After the first walk, gather the class together and review the benefits of walking, stressing the enjoyment the students will get from it. Introduce and fill out together the classroom walking logs—worksheet 1, Teacher Classroom Walking Log, and worksheet 2, Student Classroom Walking Log.

Introduce and distribute worksheet 3, Student Home Walking Log, to students. Review with them the four parts of the log sheet—(1) Date, (2) Time or Steps (if you are using pedometers), (3) Miles, and (4) Where—and how to complete the log. You and your students can decide how to use worksheet 3. For example, the students can keep track of their after-school walking program completely on their own and track their progress on separate maps. Or the students can integrate their after-school walking experience with their in-school tracking system. However you approach it, the ultimate goal is to motivate students to exercise at home with family or friends so that they can achieve the goal of being physically active for at least 1 hour every day.

EXTENSION ACTIVITY: TAKING A NATURE WALK

Taking a nature walk is a fun way to introduce additional walking time into the school day, to explore your local surroundings, and to enhance a science, math, or social studies unit. You can walk to a local green space near your school, such as a park, an urban wild, an open field, or a wooded area. You can also take a walk in the neighborhood surrounding your school. Keep track of nature walks on the class walking log. In general, nature walks cover about half the distance of fitness walks for the same amount of time because of the frequent stops to observe and discuss.

LEARNING ABOUT BIRDS

Birds are a fascinating group of animals to study. They have many observable behaviors, their migration patterns are interesting to study and track, and often their physical characteristics provide clues to their natural habitats. You might want to review some of the main characteristics of birds with the class at the start of the walk. Birds have feathers of different colors and sizes and beaks of different sizes and shapes; and they lay eggs, build nests, use their wings to fly, and often follow migration patterns.

Take along a few pairs of binoculars on your walk. Depending on the habitat you walk in, you can look for birds nesting in trees, nesting in tall grass, flying in the sky, flitting in or around bodies of water such as ponds and lakes, and perching on telephone wires and fences.

The changing seasons offer different kinds of explorations and lessons on bird behavior, identification, and observation:

▶ In spring through early summer, when birds are claiming breeding territories and attracting mates, they sing the most. Each species has a recognizable song, with different pitches and tempos. Bring along a tape recorder, binoculars, and a bird identification book (a field guide) and ask your class to match a birdsong to the bird singing it and to match a bird's physical characteristics to the name of its species. Back in the classroom, play your recordings of the birdsong and translate these sounds into writing. Compare the written examples and imitate these sounds using the written versions.

▶ In the fall, some of the birds in any location migrate north or south, while others are year-round residents or merely passing through as transients. The class can observe the migration of birds by looking for large flocks overhead when the temperature turns colder. How birds know when to begin their journey is a fascinating topic to study. As a class you can explore the aspects of nature that trigger migration and how birds absorb this information. You can also research how birds find their way to their new destinations. The science of bird navigation involves studying the roles of the earth's magnetic field, star constellations, geographic land and water features, and much more.

▶ The winter is the best time to search for bird nests abandoned in the spring and summer after the young have learned to fly. They are often revealed when broadleaf (deciduous) trees and shrubs lose their leaves and grasses die off. The nest's size, shape, and materials usually are unique to the bird species. With a field guide, nests are a good way to identify birds that have migrated for the season and those that are wintering over.

You may use the following science extensions of the nature walk to enhance classroom study during any season:

1. Create a field journal

   Field journal entries are a valuable way to capture birding expedition activities, observations, and questions. Observations are usually recorded during the walk. Ask the students to record any distinguishing characteristics such as beak length, size, and shape; bird colors; and bird size (small, medium, or large), and then have the students draw the bird as they see or remember it. Hypotheses, new questions, goals of the expedition, and conclusions are written after the trip.

2. Identify bird behaviors using the Bird Behaviors Worksheet (worksheet 4)

   Birds nest, court, chase each other, fly in all sorts of formations and styles, care for their young, feed, and store food. Introduce and distribute the Bird Behaviors Worksheet before the nature walk and ask the students to complete it as they observe the birds in the neighborhood.

Teacher Classroom Walking Log

▶TABLE 13.1 Teacher Classroom Walking Log

Date	Time or Steps*	Miles	Where

*Log number of steps if your class is using pedometers.

Date: Date of the fitness walk

Time or Steps: Number of minutes walked or number of steps walked

Miles: Number of miles walked (depends on how many minutes or steps your class decided equals 1 mile)

Where: Town, city, state, or country traveled through today

From L.W.Y. Cheung, H. Dart, S. Kalin, and S.L. Gortmaker, 2007, *Eat Well & Keep Moving*, 2nd ed. (Champaign, IL: Human Kinetics).

Name _____

Student Classroom Walking Log

▶TABLE 13.2 Student Classroom Walking Log

Date	Time or Steps*	Miles	Where

*Log number of steps if your class is using pedometers.

Date: Date of the fitness walk

Time or Steps: Number of minutes walked or number of steps walked

Miles: Number of miles walked (depends on how many minutes or steps your class decided equals 1 mile)

Where: Town, city, state, or country traveled through today

From L.W.Y. Cheung, H. Dart, S. Kalin, and S.L. Gortmaker, 2007, *Eat Well & Keep Moving*, 2nd ed. (Champaign, IL: Human Kinetics).

Student Home Walking Log

▶ **TABLE 13.3 Student Home Walking Log**

Date	Time or Steps*	Miles	Where

*Log number of steps if your class is using pedometers.

Date: Date of the fitness walk

Time or Steps: Number of minutes walked or number of steps walked

Miles: Number of miles walked (depends on how many minutes or steps your class decided equals 1 mile)

Where: Town, city, state, or country traveled through today

Name _____

Bird Behaviors Worksheet

For each bird you observe on your walk, mark the box that most closely matches its color and mark the behaviors you see as you watch the bird.

▶TABLE 13.4 Bird Colors

Red	Black and white
Blue	Brown
Yellow	Orange
Black	Green

▶TABLE 13.5 Bird Behaviors

Singing	Drinking	Flocking	Preening
Catching worms	Chasing another bird	Hiding	Soaring in circles
Pecking a tree	Feeding young	Bathing in water	Bathing in dust
Cracking a seed	Calling an alarm	Begging for food	Flying straight
Scratching the ground	Storing food	Taking a roller coaster flight	

If you can name any of the bird species you observe, write them here:

_____

_____

_____

_____

_____

From L.W.Y. Cheung, H. Dart, S. Kalin, and S.L. Gortmaker, 2007, *Eat Well & Keep Moving*, 2nd ed. (Champaign, IL: Human Kinetics).

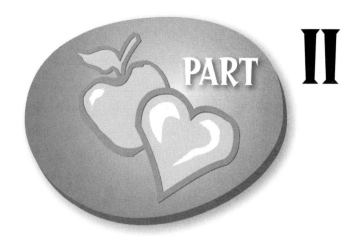

Classroom Lessons for Fifth Graders

Part II includes the fifth-grade classroom lessons. Using the same multidisciplinary approach used in part I, these lessons expand upon the key ideas presented in the fourth-grade lessons while emphasizing skill building and putting knowledge into practice. With activities such as choosing healthy snacks, monitoring food choices, and limiting television and screen time, the fifth-grade lessons provide ample opportunities for students to begin living by the themes of *Eat Well & Keep Moving*. Like the fourth-grade lessons, the fifth-grade lessons and their key messages can be bolstered by the many supporting activities of *Eat Well & Keep Moving* described in parts III through VII and the CD-ROM.

Focusing on the same broad messages taught in the fourth-grade lessons, these fifth-grade lessons teach students to

- eat 5 or more servings of fruits and vegetables each day;
- choose whole-grain foods and limit foods and beverages with added sugar;
- choose healthy fat, limit saturated fat, and avoid trans fat;
- eat a nutritious breakfast every morning;
- be physically active every day for at least an hour per day; and
- limit television and other screen time to no more than 2 hours per day.

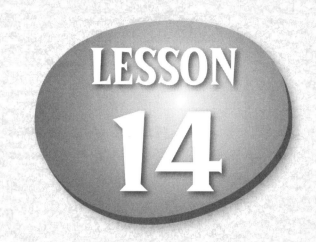

Healthy Living, Healthy Eating

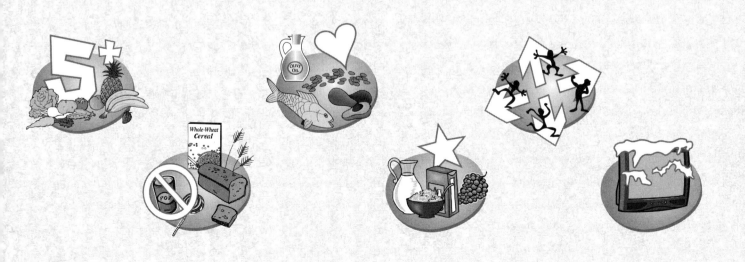

BACKGROUND

HEALTHY LIVING

Healthy living involves making lifestyle choices that maximize our physical and mental well-being. Healthy living encompasses more than just eating a balanced diet. It also involves getting the exercise and rest our bodies need, staying away from harmful substances (such as tobacco and drugs), and engaging in activities that we enjoy and that enhance our mental well-being.

It is important to recognize that our physical health and our mental health are interrelated. For example, eating a balanced diet and exercising not only helps maintain good physical health but also boosts mental health by increasing energy levels and improving our ability to cope with stress. Spending time with friends can provide support for the many challenges in life as well as provide companions for physical activity. The key to healthy living is a balance of all aspects of life, including the physical, intellectual, social, and emotional.

Again, eating a balanced diet and exercising are the cornerstones of a healthy lifestyle. Eating the right foods (plenty of fruits, vegetables, and whole grains without excess saturated and trans fat) provides us with the energy and nutrients our bodies need to stay healthy and helps us fight and prevent infections and diseases. Similarly, regular physical activity helps prevent heart disease, diabetes, osteoporosis, and a host of other disorders. What we eat and how much activity we get not only affect how our bodies perform and feel today but also affect our health for the next 10, 20, and 30 years and beyond.

Healthy living means being aware of and making an effort to enhance those aspects of our lives that keep us healthy, make us feel good, and help us lead active, full lives.

BUILD A HEALTHY FOUNDATION

The following guidelines can help you eat well and can keep you moving toward a lifetime of healthy living:

Principles of Healthy Living

- **Eat 5 or more servings of fruits and vegetables each day.** Fruits and vegetables are packed with vitamins, minerals, antioxidants, and fiber, and they provide healthy carbohydrate that gives us energy. Choose fruits and vegetables in a rainbow of colors (choose especially dark-green and orange vegetables). For more on fruits and vegetables, refer to lessons 10, 11, and 23 and to the school-wide promotion Get 3 At School and 5+ A Day (lesson 28).

- **Choose whole-grain foods and limit foods and beverages with added sugar.** Minimally processed whole grains make better choices than refined grains do. Whole grains contain fiber, vitamins, and minerals, and the refining process strips away many of these beneficial nutrients. Even though some refined grains are fortified with vitamins and minerals, fortification does not replace all of the lost nutrients. In addition, the body absorbs refined grains very quickly, which causes sugar levels in the blood to spike. In response, the body quickly takes up sugar from the blood to bring blood sugar levels down to normal; but it can overshoot things a bit, making blood sugar levels a bit low, and this can cause feelings of false hunger even after a big meal. Choose whole grains whenever possible, making sure that at least half of the grain servings you eat each day are made with whole grains. For more on whole grains and healthy carbohydrate, refer to lessons 2 and 12.

In addition to selecting whole-grain foods, limit your intake of sugary beverages such as soft drinks and limit foods with added sugar. Sweetened drinks are said to be filled with empty calories because they provide many calories but few of the nutrients the body needs to stay healthy and grow strong. A growing body of research suggests that consuming sugar-sweetened beverages is associated with excess weight gain in children and adults. For more on sugar-sweetened beverages, refer to lesson 18.

• **Choose healthy fat, limit saturated fat, and avoid trans fat.** Plant-based foods, including plant oils (such as olive, canola, soybean, corn, sunflower, and peanut oils), nuts, and seeds, are natural sources of healthy fat, as are fish and shellfish. Healthy fat can lower the risk of heart disease, stroke, and possibly diabetes. Unhealthy fat—namely, saturated fat and trans fat—increases the risk of heart disease, stroke, and possibly diabetes. Much of the fat that comes from animals, including dairy fat, the fat in meat or poultry skin, and lard, is saturated. Saturated fat should make up no more than 10% of your total calorie intake. Trans fat is formed when healthy vegetable oils are partially hydrogenated (a process that makes the oil solid or semisolid and makes the fat more stable for use in packaged foods). This is the worst type of fat because it raises the risk of heart disease in a number of different ways, and it may possibly raise the risk of diabetes. For more on choosing healthy fat, refer to lessons 5, 6, and 17.

• **Eat a nutritious breakfast every morning.** Breakfast is a critical meal since it gives the body the energy it needs to perform at school, work, or home. Studies have shown that breakfast can improve learning, and it helps boost overall nutrition. Many common breakfast foods are rich in whole grains; breakfast is also a great time to get started toward the daily goal of consuming 5 or more servings of fruits and vegetables. For more on eating breakfast, refer to lesson 24.

• **Be physically active every day for at least an hour per day.** Regular physical activity not only improves our physical health (it helps maintain a healthy weight and prevents several chronic diseases) but also benefits our emotional well-being. Children should get at least 60 minutes of physical activity every day. This should include moderate- and vigorous-intensity activities, and it can be accumulated throughout the day in sessions of 15 minutes or longer. For more on physical activity, refer to lessons 16 and 26, as well as the physical education lessons and microunits in parts IV through VII.

• **Limit TV and other screen time to no more than 2 hours per day.** The more television you watch, the less time you have to engage in physical activity or other healthy pursuits; the same goes for surfing the Web, text messaging, and playing video games. Watching more television means watching more ads for unhealthy foods, and evidence suggests that this leads to eating extra calories. Such sedentary behavior combined with poor diet can lead to excess weight gain. Children should watch no more than 2 hours of quality television or videos each day; watching less is better. Children should limit total screen time, including watching television, playing computer games, watching DVDs, and

Web surfing, to no more than 2 hours each day. For more on reducing TV viewing and screen time, refer to lesson 21 and the school-wide promotion Freeze My TV (lesson 27).

FOOD GROUPS AT A GLANCE

There are five basic food groups: grains; vegetables; fruit; meat, fish, and beans (meat, poultry, fish, nuts, dry beans, and meat alternatives); and milk. Each food group provides nutritional benefits, and so foods from each group should be consumed each day. The key to a balanced diet is to recognize that whole grains, vegetables, and fruits are needed in greater proportion than are the foods from the meat, fish, and beans and milk groups. This concept is illustrated by the Balanced Plate for Health (see figure 14.1). A healthy and balanced diet also contains a variety of foods from each food group, since each food offers different nutrients (see table 14.1). Note

▶TABLE 14.1 Food Items From Each Food Group

Food group	Food items	Best choices*
Grains	Whole grains (barley, brown rice, buckwheat, bulgur, millet, quinoa, wheat), breads (whole wheat or rye bread, whole-grain rolls, stone-ground corn or whole wheat tortillas, whole wheat pitas), cereals (oatmeal, seven-grain hot cereal, ready-to-eat cereals made with whole oats, whole wheat, or other whole grains), pasta (whole wheat noodles, soba noodles), crackers (whole wheat crackers, whole rye crispbread), pancakes (whole wheat or buckwheat)	• Whole grains or foods made with minimally processed whole grains • Choose foods that list a whole grain as the first ingredient.
Vegetables	Collard greens, mustard greens, spinach, kale, chard, bok choy, green cabbage, red cabbage, winter squash, summer squash, zucchini, sweet potatoes, broccoli, carrots, tomatoes, corn, turnips, string beans, lettuce, onions, okra, beets, cauliflower, brussels sprouts, dry beans and peas (kidney beans, black beans, soybeans, chickpeas, lentils, black-eyed peas)	• Choose a rainbow of colors, especially dark green and orange. • Choose dry beans and peas.**
Fruits	Peaches, nectarines, cantaloupe, watermelon, grapefruit, raisins, apples, pears, oranges, bananas, strawberries, tangerines, grapes, pineapple, mangoes, blueberries, cherries, figs, kiwi fruits, avocados	• Choose a rainbow of colors. • Choose whole fruits or sliced fruits (rather than fruit juices).
Meat, fish, and beans	Fish (salmon, trout, cod, shrimp, crab, scallops, light tuna, sardines), nuts (almonds, hazelnuts, walnuts), nut butters (peanut butter, almond butter), seeds (sunflower, pumpkin), dry beans and peas (kidney beans, black beans, soybeans, chickpeas, lentils, black-eyed peas), chicken, turkey, meat (beef, pork, ham), eggs, tofu and other high-protein vegetarian alternatives (tempeh, falafel, veggie burgers)	• Choose dry beans and peas,** fish, poultry, nuts, and high-protein vegetarian alternatives more often than meat. • When eating meat, choose lean cuts.
Milk	Plain milk (nonfat or 1%), low-fat flavored milk, string cheese (reduced-fat mozzarella sticks), low-fat or nonfat cottage cheese, low-fat cheddar cheese, plain low-fat or nonfat yogurt, low-fat frozen yogurt	• Choose plain low-fat (1%) or nonfat milk, yogurt, and other dairy foods.***

*Best-choice foods contain the most nutrients and contribute to overall health.

**Dry beans and peas can be considered part of the vegetable group or part of the healthy protein group.

***Students who cannot drink milk can choose lactose-free milk or calcium-fortified nondairy alternatives such as unflavored and unsweetened rice milk or soy milk.

that the Balanced Plate for Health does not contain sweets, foods that are high in saturated or trans fats, or foods that are low in nutrients. These are "sometimes" foods, not everyday foods. "Sometimes" foods should be eaten in moderation, and they are depicted on a small side plate. For more information on food groups and the serving sizes of foods in each food group, visit the MyPyramid Web site, www.mypyramid.gov.

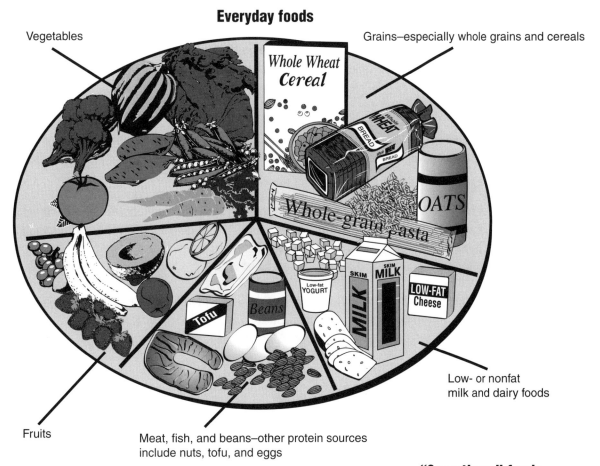

Everyday foods

Vegetables

Grains–especially whole grains and cereals

Low- or nonfat milk and dairy foods

Fruits

Meat, fish, and beans–other protein sources include nuts, tofu, and eggs

The key to a balanced diet is to recognize that grains (especially whole grains),vegetables, and fruits are needed in greater proportion than are the foods from the meat, fish, and beans and milk groups.

"Sometimes" foods

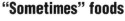
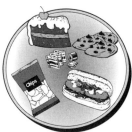

▶ Figure 14.1   The Balanced Plate for Health.

ENERGY NUTRIENTS: CARBOHYDRATE, PROTEIN, AND FAT

The foods that we eat contain many kinds of nutrients. Nutrients are the chemical substances in food that the body uses to maintain health. Macronutrients (carbohydrate, fat, and protein) are the major food components, and they all provide the body with energy. Micronutrients (vitamins and minerals) are the nutrients that we need in very small amounts and that are present in many foods. Both groups of nutrients are important for a healthy body.

All foods contain 1, 2, or all 3 of the macronutrients. Protein provides the body with the building blocks for making and repairing tissue (like muscle and skin). Foods from animals, such as fish, lean meats, poultry, eggs, and low-fat or nonfat dairy foods, are good sources of protein, as are nuts, seeds, and dry beans or legumes. Fat helps the body transport certain vitamins. Healthy unsaturated fat is found in plant foods like vegetables and vegetable oils (olive, canola, and soybean oils), nuts, seeds, and whole grains, as well as in fish. Carbohydrate (starches and sugars) provides the body with the quickest source of energy, and this energy can be readily used in every single cell in the body. But not all types of carbohydrate are healthy choices. Some are better than others.

Whole grains are preferable over refined grains since they contain more vitamins, minerals, and fiber. Fruits and vegetables also contain vitamins, minerals, and fiber, and they provide antioxidants. Other good sources of carbohydrate include dried beans (legumes) and low-fat (1%) or nonfat milk and yogurt. Foods and beverages with added sugar (such as soft drinks, energy drinks, punches, cookies, and candy) also provide carbohydrate. But unfortunately, these foods typically have sugar as one of their main ingredients (and may also be high in saturated and trans fat), and these drinks basically contain just sugar and water. Sugary foods and beverages also usually contain very few micronutrients (vitamins and minerals). These foods should be eaten only in small amounts or once in a while. The Harvard Prevention Resource Center recommends that children consume no more than 2 8-ounce servings of sugar-sweetened beverages per week; less is better.

VITAMINS AND MINERALS

Vitamins and minerals are nutrients (micronutrients, specifically) needed to keep the body healthy. There are many vitamins and minerals in the foods that we eat. Table 14.2 lists some of the vitamins and minerals many Americans do not get enough of. It is important to eat a variety of food every day so that we get all the vitamins and minerals we need.

ESTIMATED TEACHING TIME AND RELATED SUBJECT AREA

Estimated teaching time: 1 hour, 45 minutes
Related subject area: science

▶TABLE 14.2 Selected Vitamins and Minerals

Nutrients	Healthy sources	Role
VITAMINS		
Vitamin A	Dark-green, yellow, and orange vegetables and fruits (such as kale, spinach, broccoli, romaine lettuce, carrots, cantaloupe, apricots)	Helps with night vision, bone growth, and tissue maintenance
Vitamin C	Oranges, grapefruit, tangerines, cantaloupe, mangoes, papaya, strawberries, broccoli, tomatoes, bell peppers	Keeps skin and tissue healthy
Vitamin E	Almonds, sunflower seeds, sunflower oil, safflower oil, peanut butter, corn oil, soybean oil, canola oil, spinach, broccoli, dandelion greens, tomato sauce	Helps protect cells from damage (antioxidant)
MINERALS		
Calcium	Low-fat or nonfat milk, low-fat cheese, low-fat or nonfat yogurt, low-fat or nonfat cottage cheese, kale, broccoli, greens, tofu (bean curd), calcium-fortified 100% juice, calcium-fortified nondairy milks	Helps keep bones and teeth strong
Potassium	Sweet potatoes, tomatoes, winter squash, peaches, cantaloupe, bananas, greens, spinach, dried beans (white beans, lentils, kidney beans), low-fat or nonfat yogurt	Helps the body maintain fluid balance, electrolyte balance, and acid–base balance

OBJECTIVES

1. Students will review the concepts of wellness, balanced lifestyle, and the role of carbohydrate in the diet.
2. Students will gain a further understanding of the food groups and the healthy eating guidelines.
3. Students will learn the roles of vitamin A and calcium in the diet.

MATERIALS

1. Worksheet 1, Building Block for Healthy Living (tip: copy onto cardstock)
2. Worksheet 2, Help! You're the Doctor
3. Worksheet 3, Menu Planning
4. Food picture cards (the National Dairy Council produces cutout models of approximately 200 foods and beverages that can be ordered by calling 800-426-8271 or by contacting your local Dairy Council) or pictures of food cut out from magazines (be sure to include vegetables, fruit, whole-grain breads, whole-grain cereals, and dairy products that are high in carbohydrate)
5. Solutions to worksheet 2
6. Solutions to worksheet 3

7. Teacher resource page 1, Carbohydrate Foods
8. Teacher resource page 2, Low-Carbohydrate Foods
9. Transparency 1, Principles of Healthy Living
10. Transparency 2, The Balanced Plate for Health (copy and distribute to students)

PROCEDURE

1. Provide each student with worksheet 1, Building Block for Healthy Living, and have students assemble the cube. Use transparency 1 to discuss the details of the six healthy living messages. Explain how a balanced diet and balanced lifestyle keep individuals healthy.

2. Discuss the role of carbohydrate and how some carbohydrate foods are healthier than others (see background information and teacher resource pages 1 and 2).

3. Explain that to stay healthy, our bodies need special nutrients called *vitamins* and *minerals.* Small amounts of these nutrients are found in healthy foods from all of the food groups. Discuss the roles of vitamin A and calcium in the diet and list foods that are good sources of these nutrients (see background information).

If you like you may also discuss other vitamins and minerals, such as vitamin E or potassium.

4. From the food picture cards (or foods cut out of magazines), select several foods that contain carbohydrate, vitamin A, and calcium (see background information for examples of such foods). Place these cards on the board and select students to identify a food and then explain the benefits of eating that particular food. The students should also name a nutrient that is found in that food and describe its role in the body.

5. Distribute worksheet 2, Help! You're the Doctor. Have students read the three cases about people who have health concerns and answer the questions in the spaces provided on the worksheet.

6. Explain to students that healthy living involves a lifestyle that is balanced and varied. It is important to eat a balanced and varied diet and to engage in a variety of activities in all aspects of life, including the social, intellectual, physical, and emotional. Possible activities include spending time with friends, talking with family members, walking, dancing, running, playing sports, and even spending quiet time reading or listening to music.

7. Distribute worksheet 3, Menu Planning. Review the healthy living concepts and the Balanced Plate for Health (transparency 2) with students, distributing a copy of transparency 2.

8. Have students complete worksheet 3 as instructed. Invite the students to share and discuss their menu ideas.

Building Block
for Healthy Living

Directions

1. Using scissors, cut out the entire cube on page 210 by cutting along the outside lines.

2. Fold the paper so that it forms the cube and tape the round tabs on the inside of the cube to hold it together.

(continued)

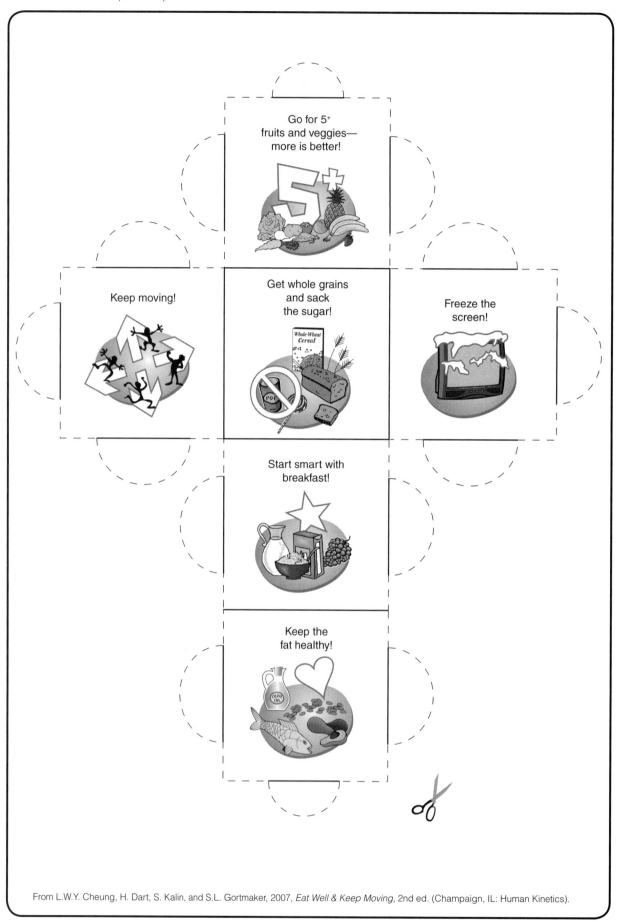

Go for 5⁺ fruits and veggies— more is better!

Keep moving!

Get whole grains and sack the sugar!

Freeze the screen!

Start smart with breakfast!

Keep the fat healthy!

Help! You're the Doctor

Directions

Read the following paragraphs and complete the exercises.

1. Members of the Lee family have been told by a doctor that they should eat more foods that contain lots of vitamins and minerals. The family eats a lot of foods from the grain, milk, and protein food groups. Popular family dinners include spaghetti with meatballs, Italian bread, and 2% milk and steak, mashed potatoes, and white rolls. The family members need a greater variety of foods in their daily diet.

    List some foods that would help the Lee family improve its diet. List five foods that contain lots of vitamins and minerals.

    _____

    _____

    _____

    _____

    _____

2. James, a fifth-grade student, eats toast for breakfast and a meat sandwich for lunch. He eats an apple or orange each day, and he always has one type of vegetable for his evening meal along with meat, chicken, or fish. He goes to the park or beach with his family on weekends, but during the week his only exercise is walking 150 yards (137 meters) from his home to his school.

    Which food group (or groups) is missing from James's diet? Why is this food group important? What else could James do to improve his health? (Use the Building Block for Healthy Living for ideas.)

    _____

    _____

    _____

    _____

    _____

From L.W.Y. Cheung, H. Dart, S. Kalin, and S.L. Gortmaker, 2007, *Eat Well & Keep Moving*, 2nd ed. (Champaign, IL: Human Kinetics).

(continued)

WORKSHEET 2

3. Maria plays basketball for 2 hours each afternoon at the school gym. Recently she noticed that she has no energy after the first hour, which is something that never used to happen. She has been watching a lot of television and staying up late at night, and she wakes up at 6 a.m. each morning to go to school. Sometimes she skips breakfast because she slept through her alarm.

List two reasons why Maria may not have enough energy. How can she improve her energy level?

_____

_____

_____

_____

_____

Name the food groups that give us energy for action sports.

_____

_____

_____

_____

_____

From L.W.Y. Cheung, H. Dart, S. Kalin, and S.L. Gortmaker, 2007, *Eat Well & Keep Moving,* 2nd ed. (Champaign, IL: Human Kinetics).

Name _____

Menu Planning

Directions

Complete the following exercises, providing suggestions for improving the diets of the Lee family, James, and Maria (discussed in worksheet 2, Help! You're the Doctor). Remember to choose a variety of foods from each of the food groups. Keep in mind the tips offered on the Building Block for Healthy Living and the Balanced Plate for Health when you plan meals and snacks for our friends.

1. Create an afternoon snack menu for the Lee family for the next school week. Refer to worksheet 2 to see what they need.

   Monday _____

   Tuesday _____

   Wednesday _____

   Thursday _____

   Friday _____

2. Suggest two healthy dinners that the Lee family can enjoy in place of their usual selections.

   _____

   _____

   _____

   _____

3. Suggest drinks and snacks that would help James eat from the one food group he is missing (remember, this group provides him with calcium, which is good for his bones and teeth).

   _____

   _____

   _____

   _____

From L.W.Y. Cheung, H. Dart, S. Kalin, and S.L. Gortmaker, 2007, *Eat Well & Keep Moving,* 2nd ed. (Champaign, IL: Human Kinetics).

(continued)

4. List fun activities that James could do during the week to keep him active. Pick a different activity for each day of the week:

Sunday _____

Monday _____

Tuesday _____

Wednesday _____

Thursday _____

Friday _____

Saturday _____

5. Suggest some high-carbohydrate foods (including whole grains) that are low in added sugar that Maria should consider eating before playing basketball.

_____

_____

_____

_____

Help! You're the Doctor

1. Members of the Lee family have been told by a doctor that they should eat more foods that contain lots of vitamins and minerals. The family eats a lot of foods from the grain, milk, and protein food groups. Popular family dinners include spaghetti with meatballs, Italian bread, and 2% milk and steak, mashed potatoes, and white rolls. The family members need a greater variety of foods in their daily diet.

   List some foods that would help the Lee family improve its diet. List five foods that contain lots of vitamins and minerals.

   Answer: The Lee family needs to eat more fruits and vegetables. Fruits and vegetables are a wonderful source of vitamins and minerals, and so eating at least 5 servings of these each day would be a great improvement to the Lee family diet. Eating even more servings would be better. Lee family members should include dark-green and orange vegetables for vitamin A, and citrus fruits are a great way to get vitamin C. They should also include more whole-grain breads and whole-grain side dishes (brown rice, barley, bulgur, millet, quinoa) in place of white rolls or pasta to add nutrients as well as fiber. They like milk, but they should switch to a lower-fat type (1% or nonfat). Finally, they could replace foods that provide unhealthy fat (such as butter and steak) with foods that provide healthy fat (such as olive oil for dipping bread into or sautéed vegetables and fish instead of steak).

2. James, a fifth-grade student, eats toast for breakfast and a meat sandwich for lunch. He eats an apple or orange each day, and he always has one type of vegetable for his evening meal along with meat, chicken, or fish. He goes to the park or beach with his family on weekends, but during the week his only exercise is walking 150 yards (137 meters) from his home to his school.

   Which food group (or groups) is missing from James's diet? Why is this food group important? What else could James do to improve his health? (Use the Building Block for Healthy Living for ideas.)

From L.W.Y. Cheung, H. Dart, S. Kalin, and S.L. Gortmaker, 2007, *Eat Well & Keep Moving*, 2nd ed. (Champaign, IL: Human Kinetics).

(continued)

Answer: James is missing foods from the milk group. He should add low-fat or fat-free foods from the milk group along with 1% or skim milk to his diet. Dairy products provide the calcium his body needs to build and maintain strong bones and teeth, and he needs 3 servings each day. If James cannot drink milk, nondairy calcium-fortified milks (such as unflavored rice milk or soy milk) are a good substitute; calcium is also available in fortified 100% orange juice (limit juice to no more than 8 ounces, or 250 milliliters, a day). James would also benefit from more fruit (especially different types of fruit) and vegetables. He also needs to find ways to exercise during the week.

3. Maria plays basketball for 2 hours each afternoon at the school gym. Recently she noticed that she has no energy after the first hour, which is something that never used to happen. She has been watching a lot of television and staying up late at night, and she wakes up at 6 a.m. each morning to go to school. Sometimes she skips breakfast because she slept through her alarm.

List two reasons why Maria may not have enough energy. How can she improve her energy level?

Answer: The reason why Maria doesn't have enough energy to play basketball for more than an hour is likely a combination of factors. By staying up late and waking early, Maria is not getting enough sleep, which makes her feel tired and less energetic throughout the day. This may be especially true on the days that she skips breakfast. In addition, she may not be eating foods that provide her body with energy, such as high-carbohydrate foods. Carbohydrate is the fuel for the muscles. Foods that are excellent sources of carbohydrate can be found in all food groups, but Maria should focus on foods that pack many vitamins and minerals such as whole grains, fruits, vegetables, low-fat or fat-free dairy, and legumes. Turning off the TV at night to get more sleep and start the day refreshed, eating a balanced breakfast, and choosing some healthy carbohydrate snacks can all give her the energy she needs to play basketball all afternoon. Grabbing a candy bar, sweet, or soft drink may give her a quick shot of sugar, but it won't keep her energy levels high for an entire afternoon of play.

From L.W.Y. Cheung, H. Dart, S. Kalin, and S.L. Gortmaker, 2007, *Eat Well & Keep Moving,* 2nd ed. (Champaign, IL: Human Kinetics).

Menu Planning

Improving the Diets of the Lee Family, James, and Maria

1. Following is a sample snack menu for the Lee family:

   Monday: raw carrots and whole wheat crackers (made with healthy fat, not with partially hydrogenated oils) with spinach dip

   Tuesday: fruit smoothie (blend fresh or frozen berries and bananas with 1% milk and ice)

   Wednesday: melon with low-fat plain yogurt

   Thursday: whole wheat pita chips and broccoli dipped in hummus

   Friday: ants on a log (celery sticks spread with peanut butter and topped with raisins) and apple slices

2. Two healthy dinner menus for the Lee family may include the following:

   a. Whole wheat spaghetti with garden tomato sauce, whole wheat rolls dipped in olive oil, tossed green salad drizzled with an olive-oil vinaigrette, low-fat (1%) milk, strawberries

   b. Grilled salmon, barley pilaf, green beans, cucumber salad, low-fat (1%) milk, mandarin orange slices

3. Drink and snack suggestions for James include the following:

   Glass of low-fat (1%) milk or plain calcium-fortified nondairy milk and grapes

   Low-fat cheese (such as string cheese or reduced-fat cheddar)

   Broccoli with low-fat yogurt dip

   Whole-grain cereal with low-fat milk, a banana, and strawberries

   Plain low-fat yogurt with canned peaches

   Fruit smoothie made with plain low-fat yogurt and 1% or nonfat milk

From L.W.Y. Cheung, H. Dart, S. Kalin, and S.L. Gortmaker, 2007, *Eat Well & Keep Moving*, 2nd ed. (Champaign, IL: Human Kinetics).

(continued)

4. Fun activities for James might include the following:

   Sunday: playing Frisbee at the beach

   Monday: roller skating

   Tuesday: bike riding

   Wednesday: playing baseball

   Thursday: playing basketball

   Friday: tossing a football

   Saturday: playing soccer at the park

5. Examples of snacks that are high in carbohydrate, low in unhealthy saturated or trans fat, and convenient to eat include the following: oranges, pears, plums, grapes, apples, bananas, whole wheat bread sticks, whole wheat bagels with low-fat cheese, whole-grain cereal, low-fat milk, whole-grain crackers and fig bars (check the label to make sure that these do not include partially hydrogenated oils), trail mix (almonds, raisins, and whole-grain pretzel sticks), low-fat yogurt, and whole wheat pitas with hummus.

From L.W.Y. Cheung, H. Dart, S. Kalin, and S.L. Gortmaker, 2007, *Eat Well & Keep Moving,* 2nd ed. (Champaign, IL: Human Kinetics).

Carbohydrate Foods

Best-Choice Carbohydrate Foods

Best-choice carbohydrate foods are filled with vitamins, minerals, and often fiber; they have little or no added sugar, little or no saturated fat, and no trans fat. Making healthy carbohydrate choices helps avoid spikes in blood sugar. Examples of these nutritious carbohydrate sources include the following:

Grains: Whole grains (the less processed the better) such as barley, brown rice, buckwheat, bulgur, millet, whole oats, quinoa, or whole wheat; whole wheat (or other whole-grain) breads, bagels, rolls, English muffins, pitas, or tortillas; hot whole-grain cereals such as steel-cut oatmeal and kasha; whole-grain ready-to-eat cereals* such as shredded wheat or oat squares; whole wheat spaghetti or pasta; home-popped or air-popped popcorn; whole-grain crackers;** whole-grain pancakes or waffles (without syrup)

Fruits: Fresh fruit, frozen fruit, or fruit canned in its own juice, including oranges, grapefruit, pineapple, blackberries, raspberries, blueberries, cantaloupe, honeydew, kiwi, mango, papaya, raisins and other dried fruit (e.g., prunes), peaches, nectarines, bananas, apples, pears

Vegetables: Fresh, frozen, or canned vegetables without added saturated or trans fat, including sweet potatoes, winter squash, corn, and parsnips (other vegetables that are healthy choices but have smaller amounts of carbohydrate are beets, turnips, green beans, kale, spinach, carrots, tomatoes)

Meat, fish, and beans: Dry beans without added unhealthy saturated or trans fat, such as black beans, kidney beans, chickpeas, pinto beans, lentils, black-eyed peas

Milk: Low-fat (1%) or nonfat milk, plain low-fat or nonfat yogurt

---

Refined grains (e.g., white bread, white rice, white pasta, other products made with white flour) may be fortified with vitamins and minerals, but they are still not as healthy as whole-grain foods. Potatoes are high in carbohydrate, but they are digested quickly and are similar to refined grains in their effect on blood sugar. These foods are not best choices; they should only be eaten, at most, a few times a week.

---

*Make sure that sugar is not one of the first three ingredients.

**Make sure to choose products that contain no trans fat and are low in saturated fat; for more information on choosing healthy fat, see lessons 5 and 6.

From L.W.Y. Cheung, H. Dart, S. Kalin, and S.L. Gortmaker, 2007, *Eat Well & Keep Moving*, 2nd ed. (Champaign, IL: Human Kinetics). Adapted from National Heart, Lung, and Blood Institute, We Can! (n.d.). Go, Slow, and Whoa Foods. Retrieved March 14, 2007, from www. nhlbi.nih.gov/health/public/heart/obesity/wecan/downloads/gswtips.pdf.

(continued)

"Sometimes" Carbohydrate Foods

Some carbohydrate-containing foods have few vitamins and minerals, are low in fiber, and contain large amounts of added sugar or added saturated and trans fat. While sweetened breakfast cereals and milk products do contain vitamins and minerals, they often have large amounts of added sugar or contain unhealthy fat. These foods should only be eaten once in a while, if at all. Examples of these less nutritious carbohydrate sources include the following:

Grains: Doughnuts, pastries, fruit and cereal bars, sugar-sweetened cereals

Fruits: Fruit canned in heavy syrup, fruit punches or -ades (lemonade), fruit leather, dried sweetened fruit

Milk: Chocolate milk, ice cream, frozen yogurt, pudding

Sweets: Candy, cookies, cakes, soft drinks, sports drinks, energy drinks, fruit punches, other sweetened beverages

From L.W.Y. Cheung, H. Dart, S. Kalin, and S.L. Gortmaker, 2007, *Eat Well & Keep Moving,* 2nd ed. (Champaign, IL: Human Kinetics). Adapted from National Heart, Lung, and Blood Institute, We Can! (n.d.). Go, Slow, and Whoa Foods. Retrieved March 14, 2007, from www. nhlbi.nih.gov/health/public/heart/obesity/wecan/downloads/gswtips.pdf.

Low-Carbohydrate Foods

Many protein foods such as meat, poultry, fish, and cheese do not contain carbohydrate, while some vegetables contain only minimal amounts. Examples of foods that are low in carbohydrate include the following:

▶ Meat

▶ Fish

▶ Hamburgers (without bun)

▶ Eggs

▶ Hot dogs (without bun)

▶ Cheese

▶ Chicken or turkey

▶ Nuts

▶ Sunflower seeds

▶ Greens

▶ Lettuce

▶ Cucumbers

▶ Mushrooms

▶ Celery

From L.W.Y. Cheung, H. Dart, S. Kalin, and S.L. Gortmaker, 2007, *Eat Well & Keep Moving,* 2nd ed. (Champaign, IL: Human Kinetics).

Principles of Healthy Living

Go for 5 Fruits and Veggies—More Is Better!

Eat 5 or more servings of fruits and vegetables each day! Eat a variety of colors—try red, orange, yellow, green, blue, and purple.

Get Whole Grains and Sack the Sugar!

Choose healthy whole grains for flavor, fiber, and vitamins. Limit sweets. Candy, soft drinks, and other sugary drinks have almost nothing in them that is good for you—no vitamins or minerals or other healthy things. They contain just sugar.

Keep the Fat Healthy!

We need fat in our diets, but not all types of fat are good for us. Our bodies like the healthy fat that tends to come from plants and is liquid at room temperature. Examples are olive oil, canola oil, vegetable oil, and peanut oil. Our bodies do not like unhealthy fat, which is solid at room temperature. Examples include saturated fat (usually found in animal products, such as meat and whole milk) and trans fat (found in fast-food fries and store-bought cookies). Of the unhealthy fats, trans fat is the worst and should rarely, if ever, be eaten.

Start Smart With Breakfast!

Eating breakfast helps you focus on schoolwork and gives you energy to play. Breakfast is a great meal for adding whole grains, fruit, and low-fat or nonfat milk to your day!

Keep Moving!

Being active is a very important part of healthy living. Do what you like most, and keep your body moving for at least an hour a day!

Freeze the Screen!

Watching TV, playing video games, or playing on the computer keeps your body still. Keep screen time as low as it can go and never let it add up to more than 2 hours per day.

From L.W.Y. Cheung, H. Dart, S. Kalin, and S.L. Gortmaker, 2007, *Eat Well & Keep Moving*, 2nd ed. (Champaign, IL: Human Kinetics).

The Balanced Plate for Health

Everyday foods

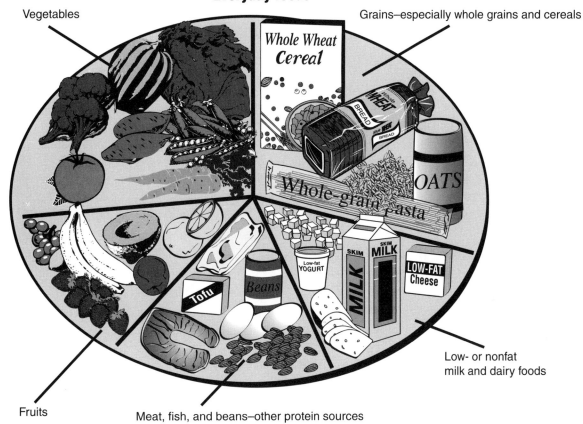

Vegetables

Grains—especially whole grains and cereals

Whole Wheat Cereal

WHEAT BREAD

Whole-grain Pasta

OATS

Low-fat YOGURT

SKIM MILK

SKIM MILK

LOW-FAT Cheese

Tofu

Beans

Low- or nonfat milk and dairy foods

Fruits

Meat, fish, and beans—other protein sources include nuts, tofu, and eggs

"Sometimes" foods

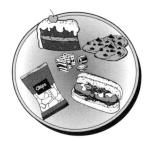

Chips

The key to a balanced diet is to recognize that grains (especially whole grains), vegetables, and fruits are needed in greater proportion than are the foods from the meat, fish, and beans and milk groups.

From L.W.Y. Cheung, H. Dart, S. Kalin, and S.L. Gortmaker, 2007, *Eat Well & Keep Moving,* 2nd ed. (Champaign, IL: Human Kinetics).

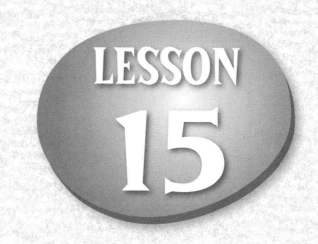

Keeping the Balance

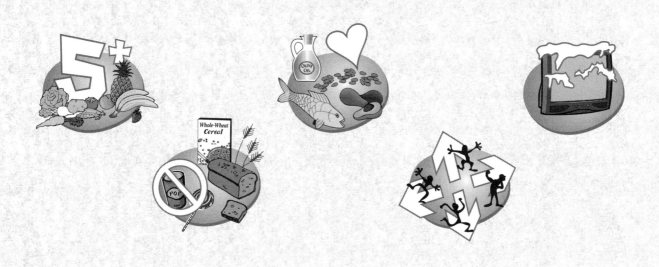

BACKGROUND*

A balanced diet is important because different foods contain different combinations of nutrients. No single food can supply all the nutrients the body needs to maintain good health. This is why balance and variety go hand in hand. For example, oranges provide vitamin C but not vitamin B_{12}, while cheese provides vitamin B12 but not vitamin C. Remember that foods in one food group cannot replace those in another. Choosing a variety of foods among groups and within groups will make your diet more interesting as well as balanced.

The carbohydrate, fat, and protein in food supply energy, which is measured in calories. Carbohydrate and protein provide 4 calories per gram. Fat provides 9 calories per gram. People must balance the amount of energy in food eaten with the amount of energy the body uses. Achieving this balance does not need to occur absolutely every day, but it should be achieved generally, such as over a few days.

Physical activity is an important way to use up food energy. Most Americans spend much of their working day in activities that require little energy. In addition, many Americans of all ages now spend a lot of daily leisure time being inactive —watching television, surfing the Web, or playing computer or video games. To use up dietary energy, people must spend less time doing sedentary activities like sitting and spend more time doing activities, such as walking to the store or around the block and climbing stairs rather than using elevators. Less sedentary activity and more moderate and vigorous activity help reduce body fat and the risk of disease.

The kinds and amounts of food people eat affect their ability to maintain a healthy weight. Soft drinks, energy drinks, fruit punch, cookies, candy, and other foods with lots of added sugar are said to be filled with empty calories because they provide many calories but few of the nutrients the body needs to stay healthy and grow strong. Eating too much of these foods makes it difficult to meet other nutrient needs without eating excessive calories, and this can contribute to excess weight gain. However, even when people eat nutrient-filled foods, they can gain weight from eating too much of them. One key way to avoid eating too much is to choose sensible portion sizes at meals, but choosing the right sizes can be a big challenge these days given the dramatic growth in portion sizes over the past 20 years.

The pattern of eating is also important. Snacks provide a large percentage of daily calories for many Americans. Unless nutritious snacks are part of the daily meal plan, snacking may lead to the intake of lots of unhealthy foods.

Children need enough food for proper growth. To promote growth, development, and good health and to prevent kids from becoming overweight, teach children to choose whole grains, vegetables, fruits, and healthy fat as well as low-fat dairy and other protein-rich foods. Also teach them to participate in at least an hour of physical activity every day. Limiting television and other screen time and encouraging children to play actively in a safe environment are helpful steps.

---

*Background material from U.S. Department of Health and Human Services and U.S. Department of Agriculture. (2005). Dietary Guidelines for Americans, 2005. Retrieved March 14, 2007, from www.health.gov/dietaryguidelines/dga2005/document/pdf/DGA2005.pdf.

ESTIMATED TEACHING TIME AND RELATED SUBJECT AREAS

Estimated teaching time: 1 hour

Related subject areas: math, science

OBJECTIVES

1. Students will discuss the importance of a balanced diet containing all six types of nutrients.
2. Students will learn ways to balance the food they eat with physical activity.

MATERIALS

1. Transparency 1, Food, Nutrients, and You
2. Transparency 2, Energy Balance
3. Worksheet 1, Keeping the Balance
4. Worksheet 2, How Is My Balance?
5. Solutions to worksheet 1
6. Clear drinking glass
7. Pitcher of water (add food coloring for visibility)
8. Low-sided baking dish

PROCEDURE

PART I

1. Set up the following demonstration so that all students can see it. Place the drinking glass in the baking dish (the dish is for catching any overflow of water) and fill the glass to the top with colored water. Explain that this full glass represents a person who is full of the nutrients needed to remain healthy and active.
2. Ask the students what happens to the level of nutrients in the person's body throughout the day. (The level goes down.) Pour some of the water back into the pitcher to show a partially empty glass.
3. Ask the students what the person needs to do to get back to the right level of nutrients. (Eat nutritious foods.) Fill the glass up to the top again.
4. Ask the students what happens when a person regularly eats more than he needs for his daily energy requirements for body growth and maintenance. (He will put on excess weight.) Pour extra water into the already full glass, allowing it to overflow. Explain that the overflowing water represents extra energy that the body will need to store, usually in the form of extra fat.
5. Explain that in today's lesson the students will take a closer look at how they can get nutrients their bodies need without getting too many calories beyond their requirements for growth and maintenance.

PART II

1. Ask the students, "What are nutrients and why are they important?" The answer is nutrients are the parts of foods that give you energy and allow your body to grow and repair itself.

2. Project transparency 1, Food, Nutrients, and You, and discuss the six types of nutrients, their functions, and their food sources. Explain that we must eat a variety of foods in order to get all the nutrients the body needs.

   You may want to make an extra laminated copy of the Food, Nutrients, and You transparency (for increased durability) and create a game that allows students to review the contents of the transparency with each other.

3. Write the word *calorie* on the board. Explain that a calorie is a measure of how much energy a food provides. Some foods, such as fruits and vegetables, are full of nutrients and are also low in calories. Other foods, such as junk foods, can have many calories and very few nutrients.

   Tell the students, "If a food contains 100 calories, it gives you 100 units of energy. Most women need 1,800 to 2,000 calories a day and most men need 2,200 to 2,400 calories a day. Active men and women need more calories than average men and women need. Girls probably need about 1,600 calories a day and boys need 1,800 calories a day; girls and boys who are very physically active may need more than that, up to 2,000 calories a day for girls and 2,200 calories per day for boys."

4. Project transparency 2, Energy Balance, and explain that if the nutrients and calories taken into the body do not equal the nutrients and energy used by the body, the body can have problems. Point to the box at the top of the transparency and review how teeter-totters work (the lighter side goes up and the heavier side goes down). Point to the picture labeled "not enough nutrients and calories" and ask, "What can happen if the nutrients and energy used are greater than the nutrients and calories taken in?" (Answer: The body gets tired, can't grow or repair tissue, begins to break down lean body tissue and fat stores, and loses weight.) Ask, "What can a person do to fix the imbalance?" (Answer: Eat more nutrients and calories.)

5. Point to the picture labeled "too many nutrients and calories" and ask, "What might happen if the amount of calories taken in is consistently greater than the amount of energy used?" (Answer: Excess energy will be stored as fat, and the body will put on weight.) Ask, "What can this person do to fix the imbalance?" (Answer: Eat fewer calories; exercise more.)

6. Point to the picture labeled "nutrient and calorie balance" and explain that eating the right amount of nutrients and calories for body size and activity level means that the body creates an energy and nutrient balance. This is the way to maintain a healthy body.

7. Have the students form pairs, and then distribute worksheet 1, Keeping the Balance. Explain that everything a person does, even sleeping, requires the body to use calories for energy. Some activities require a lot more units of energy than others do. The chart shows approximately how many calories

a 100-pound (45-kilogram) person requires to do various activities. Instruct each pair of students to use the chart and their combined knowledge to answer the questions on the worksheet.

8. Once the students have completed the worksheet, discuss their answers. Encourage them to think about how they might use this information to improve their own energy balance.

9. For an optional activity, distribute worksheet 2, How Is My Balance?, and have students fill it out for a day. You may want to repeat this activity more than once.

Food, Nutrients, and You

▶TABLE 15.1 Food, Nutrients, and You

Nutrients and their functions	Food sources
Water • Helps cool your body when it is working hard • Helps you digest your food • Helps nutrients get to different parts of the body	• Water, other beverages,* fruits, soup
Carbohydrate • Gives you energy quickly • Can be stored as energy for later use • Gives sweetness and texture to foods • Provides a good source of vitamins, minerals, and fiber	• Whole grains, fruits, starchy and root vegetables (like yams and sweet potatoes), legumes and dry beans (like kidney beans or black eyed peas), low-fat or nonfat milk, low-fat or nonfat yogurt
Protein • Builds and repairs muscles • Helps your body grow • Gives you energy	• Lean meat, poultry, fish, dry beans, nuts, low-fat and nonfat milk and milk products, eggs, tofu
Fat • Gives you energy, especially for long-term use • Makes you feel less hungry • Makes food taste good • Helps keep your skin smooth	• Vegetable oil, olive oil, canola oil, peanut oil, nuts, seeds, and fish are rich in healthy fat • Fatty meats and dairy products are high in unhealthy fat; choose lean meats and low-fat or nonfat dairy products instead
Minerals • Help your blood carry oxygen and nutrients to your muscles and other body parts (iron) • Help build strong bones and teeth (calcium)	• Lean meat, some vegetables (spinach), whole grains and fortified cereals, legumes (navy or black beans) (iron) • Low-fat or nonfat milk, low-fat cheese, low-fat or nonfat yogurt, dark-green vegetables (broccoli, kale), tofu, fortified 100% orange juice, fortified nondairy milk (calcium)
Vitamins • Help you see better at night (vitamin A) • Help your body get energy from the food you eat (B vitamins) • Help your body heal cuts and bruises (vitamin C) • Help you fight off infections (vitamin C)	• Vegetables (especially dark green and orange), fruits, low-fat or nonfat milk (vitamin A) • Whole grains, fish, poultry, lean meat, low-fat or skim milk (B vitamins) • Fruits (especially citrus), vegetables (vitamin C)

*Best choices do not have caffeine or sugar.

From L.W.Y. Cheung, H. Dart, S. Kalin, and S.L. Gortmaker, 2007, *Eat Well & Keep Moving,* 2nd ed. (Champaign, IL: Human Kinetics).

Energy Balance

On teeter-totters, the lighter side goes up and the heavier side goes down. When both sides are equal, the board is level.

Lighter   Heavier   Heavier   Lighter   Same weight   Same weight

Not enough nutrients and calories

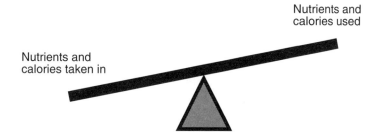

Nutrients and calories taken in

Nutrients and calories used

Too many nutrients and calories

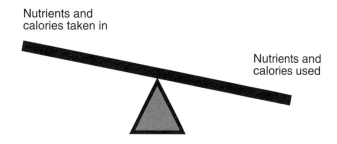

Nutrients and calories used

Nutrients and calories taken in

Nutrient and calorie balance

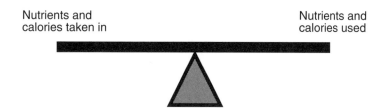

Nutrients and calories taken in

Nutrients and calories used

Name _____

Keeping the Balance

| Everything you do, even sleeping and growing, requires your body to use calories. | Almost everything you eat or drink, except water, contains calories. |

Activity	Calories used in 1/2 hour by a 100 lb.(45 kg) person
bike riding	93
running	183
swimming	150
resting/sitting	40
walking	81

Answer the following questions, assuming that you weigh 100 pounds (45 kilograms).

1. How many calories would you use watching television from 4:00 to 6:30 p.m.?

_____

_____

2a. How many more calories would you use if you rode your bike for an hour compared to watching TV for an hour?

_____

_____

2b. How many extra calories would you use over a week if you substituted an hour of bike riding for an hour of TV watching each day?

_____

_____

From L.W.Y. Cheung, H. Dart, S. Kalin, and S.L. Gortmaker, 2007, *Eat Well & Keep Moving,* 2nd ed. (Champaign, IL: Human Kinetics).

(continued)

2c. How about for a month (30 days)?

_____

_____

3. Jason spends the day in school and then takes the bus home. He fixes himself a snack (usually chips and a soft drink) and then does his homework. After dinner, Jason is allowed 1 1/2 hours of television or computer games. He sometimes reads a book or talks with friends on the phone. Jason is a little overweight. What can he do to improve his weight and overall health?

_____

_____

_____

_____

4. How many calories would you use if you ran laps around the playground for 10 minutes and then rode your bicycle home for 10 minutes?

_____

_____

5. Extra credit: Assume you weigh 100 pounds (45 kilograms). How many calories would you use walking 20 minutes to your friend's house and 20 minutes back home each day?

_____

_____

Name _____

How Is My Balance?

Draw a picture of the scale to show how you think you balanced your nutrients and calories with the energy you used today. (Remember that growing takes energy too, probably less than 100 calories a day.) Then think of ways you can improve your balance.

Here are the changes I want to make tomorrow to create a better nutrition and energy balance:

_____

_____

_____

_____

_____

_____

Keeping the Balance

1. How many calories would you use watching television from 4:00 to 6:30 p.m.?

Answer:

Step 1: resting or sitting = 40 calories per 30 minutes

Step 2: 4:00 to 6:30 p.m. = 2.5 hours or 5 30-minute periods

Step 3: 5 30-minute periods × 40 calories per 30 minutes = 200 calories

2a. How many more calories would you use if you rode your bike for an hour compared to watching TV for an hour?

Answer:

Step 1: 186 calories – 80 calories = 106 calories

2b. How many extra calories would you use over a week if you substituted an hour of bike riding for an hour of TV watching each day?

Answer:

Step 1: 106 calories per day × 7 days = 742 calories

2c. How about for a month (30 days)?

Answer:

Step 1: 106 calories per day × 30 days = 3,180 calories

3. Jason spends the day in school and then takes the bus home. He fixes himself a snack (usually chips and a soft drink) and then does his homework. After dinner, Jason is allowed 1 1/2 hours of television or computer games. He sometimes reads a book or talks with friends on the phone. Jason is a little overweight. What can he do to improve his weight and overall health?

Possible answers:

Jason could walk or ride his bike to school.

Jason could do something active in the evening.

Jason could eat fruit instead of chips and a soft drink.

From L.W.Y. Cheung, H. Dart, S. Kalin, and S.L. Gortmaker, 2007, *Eat Well & Keep Moving,* 2nd ed. (Champaign, IL: Human Kinetics).

(continued)

4. How many calories would you use if you ran laps around the playground for 10 minutes and then rode your bicycle home for 10 minutes?

Answer:

Step 1: (183 calories per half hour of running) ÷ (3 10-minute periods in a half hour) = 61 calories for each 10-minute period of running

Step 2: (93 calories per half hour of bike riding) ÷ (3 10-minute periods in a half hour) = 31 calories for each 10-minute period of bike riding

Step 3: 61 calories for 10 minutes of running + 31 calories for 10 minutes of riding bike = 92 calories

5. Extra credit: Assume you weigh 100 pounds (45 kilograms). How many calories would you use walking 20 minutes to your friend's house and 20 minutes back home each day?

Answer:

Step 1: Walking 20 minutes to friend's house + 20 minutes walking home = 40 minutes of walking, or 4 10-minute periods

Step 2: (81 calories per half hour of walking) ÷ (3 10-minute periods in a half hour) = 27 calories for every 10 minutes of walking

Step 3: (27 calories for every 10 minutes of walking) × (4 10-minute periods of walking) = 108 calories

From L.W.Y. Cheung, H. Dart, S. Kalin, and S.L. Gortmaker, 2007, *Eat Well & Keep Moving,* 2nd ed. (Champaign, IL: Human Kinetics).

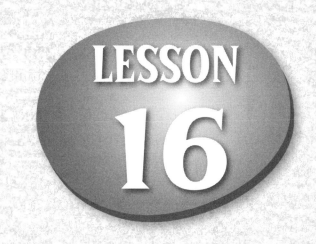

The
Safe Workout:
A Review

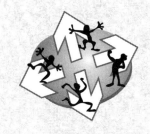

BACKGROUND

The human body can do amazing things. However, in order for the body to perform well, it must be taken care of. To keep our bodies healthy, we must choose good foods, exercise regularly, stay away from harmful substances (such as tobacco and other drugs), and get plenty of sleep. We must also give our bodies good food for energy, growth, and repair. Exercising regularly helps keep the body healthy. Some exercises make the heart, lungs, and blood vessels stronger, while others help with flexibility and the body's ability to bend. The body needs all kinds of exercise. This lesson teaches students the safe way to exercise and at the same time review the five basic food groups.

This lesson reviews the five parts of a safe workout. The concept of the safe workout is introduced in lesson 3, which includes a detailed description of the different workout components. The amount of time spent reviewing the components in this lesson will depend on how much your students were exposed to the safe workout when they were working on lesson 3 in fourth grade.

The five parts of a safe workout help prevent injuries from exercising. These parts are (1) the warm-up, (2) the stretch, (3) the fitness activity, (4) the cool-down, and (5) the cool-down stretch. Each part will be introduced with a statement on why it is important and an explanation of how to do it correctly. Because of time constraints, the parts of the workout practiced during the lesson are shorter than what they normally are in an actual workout. For example, the lesson warm-up lasts only 2 minutes, when ideally the warm-up should last at least 5 minutes. What's important is that the students learn that a warm-up is the first part of a safe workout and that it should be done whenever they get ready for active sports or play. For instance, they should warm up at home before they ride their bike or play basketball.

Children should get at least 60 minutes of physical activity every day; this should include moderate- and vigorous-intensity activities and can be accumulated throughout the day in sessions of 15 minutes or longer. But exercising and doing the five parts of a safe workout is only half of the story! In addition to being physically active, eating right is the other half of the winning combination that keeps our bodies healthy. In this lesson the students will be learning about the food groups and how to choose foods wisely while moving!

This activity can be used as a practice lesson for the other physical activity lessons, which will be taught in the gymnasium, community room, or cafeteria.

ESTIMATED TEACHING TIME AND RELATED SUBJECT AREA

Estimated teaching time: 1 hour, 20 minutes

Related subject area: physical education

OBJECTIVES

1. Students will be able to identify and sequence the components of a safe and healthy workout.
2. Students will discuss and demonstrate each component of a safe workout.

3. Students will be able to identify the five food groups and how to make daily food choices based on the Principles of Healthy Living (for a review of the principles, see pages 202-204 in lesson 14).

4. Students will be able to choose positive health practices based on their knowledge about the safe workout and healthy food selections.

MATERIALS

1. Pictures of various foods (the National Dairy Council produces cutout models of approximately 200 foods and beverages that can be ordered by calling 800-426-8271 or by contacting your local Dairy Council)

2. Stretch and Strength Fitness Diagrams (see appendix A, pages 565-569)

3. Portable CD player or radio (optional)

4. Five hula hoops or large paper bags

PROCEDURE

1. Go over the pertinent vocabulary for this lesson:

   Warm-up—The first part of the safe workout, in which slow movements get the body ready for stretching and the fitness activity.

   Stretch—The part of the safe workout in which you do exercises that improve flexibility fitness and get the body ready for fitness activity.

   Fitness activity—The part of the safe workout in which strength and endurance fitness exercises are performed.

   Cool-down—The part of the safe workout in which your body slows down and recovers from the fitness activity.

   Cool-down stretch—The last part of the safe workout, in which you do exercises that improve flexibility fitness.

   Pacing—Maintaining a comfortable speed so that you can perform your exercise for an extended time.

   Flexibility fitness—The ability to bend; the part of fitness that stretches the muscles and areas around the muscles to get your body ready for action.

   Strength fitness—The part of fitness that makes your muscles (except the heart muscle) stronger and healthier.

   Endurance fitness—The part of fitness that improves the heart muscle, lungs, and blood vessels.

2. Provide motivation for the lesson. Ask students to raise their hands if they would like to

   • grow up to be as healthy as they can be;

   • be able to play, dance, and run longer; and

   • feel good about themselves.

   Tell students that if they raised their hands in response to any of the questions, then this lesson is an important one for them. It's their chance to learn the benefits of eating right and exercising.

3. Briefly introduce the lesson. Tell the students, "A healthy lifestyle involves getting the right amounts and kinds of food daily and moving our bodies and participating in regular physical activity. We have learned that we should eat a variety of foods from each of the food groups and that we should choose carefully to make sure we get all of the nutrients that we need, without eating unnecessary sugar or unhealthy fat. Making the right choices about the food we eat affects the health of our bodies. Eating balanced meals helps our bodies stay healthy, grow, and perform physical activities like playing and dancing.

   "Participating in regular, moderate to vigorous physical activity is also important to our body's health. We need to get at least an hour of physical activity every day. The safe workout steers us in the right direction so that we can exercise and participate in physical activities in ways that are good for our bodies. Today we will learn about the components of a safe workout."

4. Have the class form five groups and assign each group the name of one of the five food groups: Group 1 is the grain group; group 2 is the vegetable group; group 3 is the fruit group; group 4 is the meat, fish, and beans group, and group 5 is the milk group.

5. Review with the class the foods that belong to each group (see transparency 2, The Balanced Plate for Health, in lesson 14, and student handout 1, Best-Choice Foods in Each Food Group, in lesson 1). Have the students in each group work together to list as many foods as they can that belong to their food group. Have each group share its list with the class, and see if the other groups can add any other foods.

6. Keep the students in their food groups. Stress that to be healthy and energized, moving the body (through exercise) is just as important as eating right. The following sections describe all five areas of the safe workout, including the shopping fitness activity, which is a movement game that reviews the food groups. The Stay Healthy Corner at the end of the safe workout is a review of what was learned in the activity and how to apply it to daily life. You can set up a specific area of the classroom for the Stay Healthy Corner and decorate it with pictures or student drawings that represent the Principles of Healthy Living (e.g., healthy foods, children engaged in physical activity, and so on). Or you can simply set aside time for discussion at the end of the lesson.

   You will be guiding the class through the safe workout and Stay Healthy Corner. Have groups of students move into the warm-up formation. Pick the formation that best suits the classroom; see examples in figure 16.1.

   1. Warm-up (1-2 minutes)
   2. Stretch (1-2 minutes)
   3. Fitness activity (15-20 minutes)
   4. Cool-down (1 minute)
   5. Cool-down stretch (1 minute)
   6. Stay Healthy Corner (4-5 minutes)

WARM-UP: 1 TO 2 MINUTES

Why Warm Up?

- ▶ Helps prevent injuries
- ▶ Increases body temperature; gets body warmer before you make it work hard
- ▶ Gets body ready for the rest of the workout, including the stretching and fitness activity

How to Warm Up

- ▶ Perform a series of slow movements such as slow jogging in place or slow jumping jacks.

What to Emphasize

- ▶ Car analogy: Your body is like a cold car—warm it up and then move it!
- ▶ If you do not warm up, you are more likely to get injured.
- ▶ You should always warm up before exercising, even when you are at home.
- ▶ Always do the movements very slowly to warm up.
- ▶ For example, when beginning a bike ride, warm up by riding slowly at first.
- ▶ Likewise, when throwing a ball, throw slowly at first.

Examples of Student Warm-Up Formations

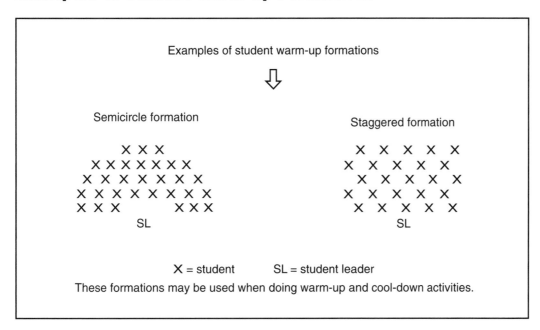

▶ FIGURE 16.1   Examples of student warm-up formations.

Semicircle Formation

1. Students should establish and maintain a safe distance between themselves and the students who are in front of, in back of, and on either side of themselves.

2. There should be enough room between students so that they will be able to do all the stretches and exercises without inadvertently hitting or being hit by another student.

3. Students should stand so that they are facing you or a group leader. Likewise, they should be spaced so that there is not another student directly in front of them (see figure 16.1).

Staggered Formation

1. Have a group of five students form a row with enough space between each of them so that they cannot touch each other if their arms are extended at shoulder height. Five more students will form a second row behind the first. Students in the second row should stand behind and between the two students in the row in front of them and, like those in the first row, should make sure that there is enough space between them. Continue to put students in rows until all have been placed.

2. Students should stand so that they are facing (and can see) you or the student leader who will be in front of the room (see figure 16.1).

STRETCH: 1 TO 2 MINUTES

Why Stretch?

▶ Improves flexibility fitness, or the ability to bend, twist, and stretch and the ability of muscles and joints to move through their complete range of motion

▶ Muscles work better when they are long and bendable.

▶ Body moves better; makes you better at sport skills

▶ Helps prevent injuries

How to Stretch

▶ Hold stretch for 10 or more seconds (count out loud: 1 Mississippi, 2 Mississippi . . . 10 Mississippi).

▶ Don't bounce; hold the stretch gently.

▶ Stretch slowly.

▶ Use proper form to avoid injuries.

▶ Examples of stretches are the neck stretch, butterfly, and quadriceps burner (thigh stretch).

Examples of Student Stretches

Have students perform the stretches as they appear in the diagrams in appendix A (pages 565-567). One student or a small group of students can help demonstrate the stretches for the class.

What to Emphasize

▶ Stretching improves flexibility fitness.

▶ Activities such as riding a bike or doing push-ups do not improve flexibility.

▶ Even if you aren't going to start a fitness activity, stretch at home while watching TV or when doing nothing in particular.

▶ Hold stretches for 10 or more seconds.

▶ Use slow movements; don't bounce.

FITNESS ACTIVITY: 15 TO 20 MINUTES

Benefits of Endurance Fitness

▶ Improves your heart, lungs, and blood vessels (builds cardiorespiratory fitness)

▶ Gives you energy

How to Improve Endurance Fitness

▶ Do activities that involve nonstop, continuous movement, such as bike riding, walking, or rope jumping (students may jog or walk in place to demonstrate endurance activities in class).

▶ Find a pace (speed) you can do for a long time—"Pace, don't race!"

▶ Find endurance activities that you like so you will want to do them.

What to Emphasize

▶ Pace, don't race.

▶ Getting fit should be fun.

ENDURANCE ACTIVITY GAME

EAT WELL AND KEEP MOVING: MAKING A HEALTHFUL MENU GAME

a. Equipment needed

    1. Food models for general audiences (a variety of food pictures from the different food groups)

    2. Five hula hoops or large paper bags

    3. Music to move to (optional)

b. Introduction

Explain to the students, "The purpose of the game is to determine if each of you knows how to use the Principles of Healthy Living to make healthy meal choices. We are also playing this game so that we can improve our fitness and learn how to pace ourselves to make our bodies stronger. Making our bodies stronger will enable us to do an activity for longer durations without becoming tired."

c. Instructions

    1. Keep the class in the five food groups and ask each group to form a line (see figures 16.2 and 16.3). The formation used will depend on the layout and space of the room.

2. Using a cone or distinguishable line, designate a place where the first person in each line can stand. The second person in line will move to this place after the first student has left it.

3. Point out to the students an area in the room where numerous and various pictures of foods from the different food groups are scattered. This is the grocery store. (You can put pictures into place before class begins.)

4. Place a hula hoop or large paper bag to the right of each line of students. This hula hoop can be called a *plate* or a *refrigerator* (as noted in figure 16.2).

Gym line formation
for shopping fitness activities
[**X** = one student]

The purpose of the game is to determine if each student in a group knows which food items fit into their food group. We are also playing this game so that we can become fit and learn how to pace ourselves so that we can make our bodies stronger and able to do an activity for a certain length of time without becoming tired.

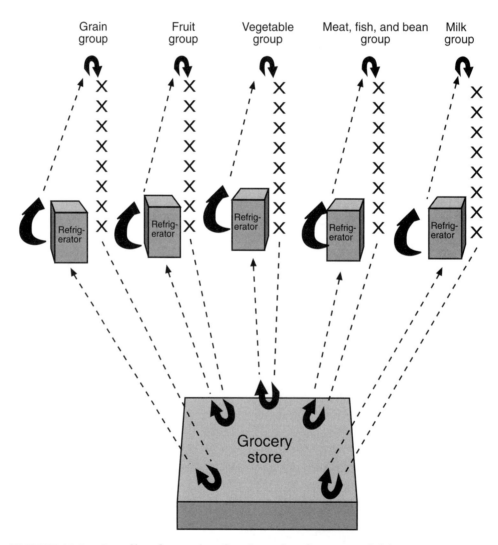

▶ FIGURE 16.2 Gym line formation for shopping fitness activities.

Option #1

Option #2

Option #3

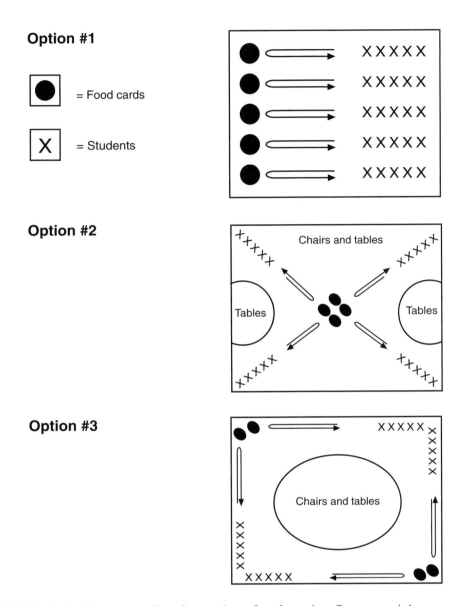

▶ FIGURE 16.3 Classroom line formations for shopping fitness activity.

5. Explain to the students, "Each of you will go to the grocery store to shop for a food that is part of a healthy, well-balanced meal. Remember the Principles of Healthy Living and the Balanced Plate for Health, which call for a variety of foods from each food group, whole grains, fruits and vegetables, healthy fat, and few if any added sugars." Students should collect enough food to create at least two meals per group (meals may be breakfast, lunch, dinner, or snacks). Give the groups a minute to decide which meals they will shop for.

6. Explain the path the students will take so that there is no confusion and students can perform the tasks safely. Tell the students, "When you reach the front of the line and it is your turn, jog in a straight path until you get to the grocery store. Once there, select a food for your chosen meal, pick it up, and jog back to the refrigerator (or plate) and deposit the food picture in it. Then jog to the back of your line and jog in place until every member of every group has taken at least two trips to the grocery store."

7. Each member of the group will be responsible for finding a food or drink from any food group, making sure the item helps to create a balanced meal. If necessary, review the Principles of Healthy Living, the Balanced Plate for Health, and the importance of gathering more foods from the grains, fruits, and vegetables groups and fewer foods from the milk and meat, fish, and beans groups; students may choose healthy sources of fat but should avoid or limit sweets and unhealthy fat.

8. This activity will begin when you say, "Let's go shopping for food!" The entire class will jog lightly in place until the last student in each food group has had a turn and has taken a place at the end of the line. You may also modify the movement by having the students skip to the store or hop in place. Tell the students to "pace, don't race," so they can continue jogging until each member of their group has gone shopping and brought back a food item.

9. When the first students in each line perform this activity, coach them by reminding them to come back on their path so that they can safely jog to their refrigerator (plate). Remind the people at the fronts of the lines to wait until the current joggers have reached the end of the line before starting out, so that the activity can be done safely.

10. Once students have each had the opportunity to collect at least two foods from the store, tell the students it is time for the cool-down. Ask the students to walk around the gymnasium, cafeteria, or community room three times, with everyone moving in the same direction.

COOL-DOWN: 1 MINUTE

What to Emphasize

▶ Move slowly.

▶ Remember to cool down after exercising at home.

After the cool-down, instruct students to get into a staggered or semicircle formation for the cool-down stretch.

COOL-DOWN STRETCH: 1 MINUTE

Why the Cool-Down Stretch?

▶ Helps prevent soreness

▶ Improves flexibility fitness

How to Do the Cool-Down Stretch

▶ Hold stretch for 10 or more seconds (count out loud: 1 Mississippi, 2 Mississippi . . . 10 Mississippi).

▶ Examples include the neck stretch, butterfly, and quadriceps burner (thigh stretch).

What to Emphasize

▶ Stretching improves flexibility fitness.

▶ Activities such as riding a bike or doing push-ups do not improve flexibility.

▶ Even if you aren't going to start a fitness activity, stretch at home while watching TV or when doing nothing in particular.

▶ Hold stretches for 10 or more seconds.

▶ Use slow movements; don't bounce.

STAY HEALTHY CORNER: 4 TO 5 MINUTES

1. When the cool-down stretch has been completed, have all the groups re-assemble and have each group share with the class its healthy meal selections.

2. Explain to the students, "Eating right and exercising are best friends! Healthy living means that we eat well and exercise too!" Talk about how the students can use this healthy living information at home. Ask them what kind of physical activities they can do at home with their family and friends so that they can achieve the goal of being physically active for at least an hour every day. Encourage them to trade screen time for active time. Stress that having the family involved is very helpful for achieving healthy living. Ask the students what they can do to involve their family with healthy lifestyles. Remind students that this involvement begins at the grocery store. Either in groups or as a class, students can create a healthy shopping list for their families.

3. Have the students complete an individual writing assignment about two things that they can do to create a healthier lifestyle.

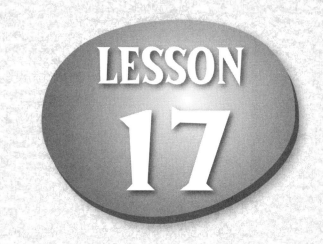
Hunting for Hidden Fat

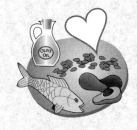

BACKGROUND

Fat is a necessary part of our diets. Fat makes food taste good, and it helps in the absorption and transportation of fat-soluble vitamins, such as vitamins A, D, E, and K. Fat is the primary way energy is stored in the body, and body fat cushions and protects our internal organs. In addition, components of fat are involved in other important body functions such as maintaining healthy skin and hair.

The problem is that most Americans consume too much of the wrong type of fat (namely, saturated fat and trans fat). This is one of the main reasons why so many people die of or are disabled by heart attacks in the United States. Every year, over half a million people die from heart disease in this country; heart disease is the leading cause of early death and disability in the United States. Research suggests that the type of fat consumed rather than the total amount of fat consumed is more indicative of disease risk. High intakes of saturated and trans fat increase the risk of heart disease. The good news is that both decreasing the intake of unhealthy fat and including healthy fat in the diet can reduce the risk of heart disease.

FAT FACTS*

Healthy fat, meaning monounsaturated and polyunsaturated fat, can decrease the risk of heart disease. It is liquid at room temperature. Examples of foods high in monounsaturated fat include olive, canola, and peanut oils; almonds; and avocados. Nuts (such as walnuts) and soybean, corn, and cottonseed oils are rich in polyunsaturated fat. Fatty ocean fish contain a special type of polyunsaturated fat (omega-3 fat) that is also very healthy.

Unhealthy fat, meaning saturated and trans fat, can increase the risk of heart disease. Saturated fat is solid at room temperature and comes mainly from animal-based foods. Examples include full-fat dairy products (such as whole milk, cream, butter, and full-fat ice cream), fatty cuts of meat, poultry skin, and lard, as well as palm oil and coconut oil. One way to minimize intake of unhealthy fat is to choose lean meats, remove poultry skin, select low-fat or nonfat dairy products, and replace saturated fat with unsaturated fat in food preparation (for instance, sautéing vegetables in olive oil instead of butter).

Trans fat is formed when polyunsaturated vegetable oils are partially hydrogenated. This process turns the normally liquid oils into solid or semisolid fat. Trans fat is found in hard stick margarines, commercial baked goods and crackers, and many processed and fast foods (especially fried foods). The consumption of trans fat is strongly associated with an increased risk of coronary heart disease, sudden death, and possibly diabetes.

The *Dietary Guidelines for Americans* recognizes the importance of reducing saturated fat intake and sets a daily limit of 10% of total daily calories from saturated fat. The American Heart Association recommends an even lower limit for saturated fat—7% of total calories. The *Dietary Guidelines for Americans* also advises keeping trans fat consumption as low as possible. Research suggests it may be prudent to limit trans fat consumption from partially hydrogenated oils to no more than 0.5%

*Information in part from President and Fellows of Harvard College.

of total energy intake per day. For a diet based on 2,000 calories per day, that means limiting trans fat intake from partially hydrogenated oils to roughly 1 gram per day. For practical purposes, that means avoiding trans fat.

While the milk and meat, fish, and beans food groups contain some foods that are high in saturated fat, there are many healthy options in these groups from which to choose. Low-fat or nonfat milk, yogurt, and cheeses are available in many schools and supermarkets; fish, skinless poultry, and dried beans provide protein without a lot of saturated fat.

The same goes for grain-based foods. While there are many healthy options, some grain-based foods contain high amounts of saturated or trans fat. Examples include muffins and pastries (these foods are often high in sugar as well). Food preparation is another way unhealthy fat can sneak into food. Frying fish in partially hydrogenated oil or sautéing vegetables in butter, for example, can add unhealthy fat to a dish. Choosing healthy fat sources (like olive, vegetable, or canola oil) for frying and sautéing is an easy way to avoid adding unhealthy fat.

Reading food labels is an effective way to compare the fat and nutrient content of various foods. The place to find out whether a food is relatively high or low in a nutrient is the % Daily Value (% DV) column on the Nutrition Facts label. The % DV for saturated fat is particularly important when making food decisions. If the % DV for saturated fat in an individual food is 5 or less, the food is considered low in saturated fat. Foods that have a % DV of 20 or more for saturated fat are considered high in saturated fat. The more foods chosen that have a % DV of 5 or less for saturated fat, the easier it is to stay within the saturated fat limit. The overall daily goal is to select foods that together have less than 100% of the DV for saturated fat. The % DV is based on a diet of 2,000 calories per day. A person's actual daily caloric needs vary depending on age, gender, and level of activity; for more information on caloric needs, see lesson 15, Keeping the Balance, page 228.

There is no % DV for trans fat because it is unclear if there is any safe level of intake. But food labels do list the number of grams of trans fat per serving. Keep in mind that products made with partially hydrogenated oils can still claim "0 grams trans fat" if the product contains less than 0.5 grams of trans fat per serving. These small amounts of trans fat can add up over the day. So make sure to watch out for the words *partially hydrogenated vegetable oil* in the ingredients list. Switch to an alternative product that does not contain partially hydrogenated oil, especially if it is a product you consume regularly.

Teacher Information: How Is % Daily Value Calculated?

Although all food labels provide % DV for nutrients, it is good to know how to calculate these values. The following describes how the % DV for one specific nutrient (saturated fat) is calculated:

To calculate % DV for a particular food, divide the number of grams of saturated fat per serving by 22 and multiply by 100 to get a percentage (22 is used because it is recommended that a person eating a 2,000-calorie daily diet consume no more than 22 grams of saturated fat each day).

For example, a cup of whole milk has 5 grams of saturated fat: $(5 \div 22) \times 100 = 23\%$. While 5 grams may not sound like much, just 1 cup of whole milk contains 23% of the DV for saturated fat for a person who eats 2,000 calories a day.

ESTIMATED TEACHING TIME AND RELATED SUBJECT AREAS

Estimated teaching time: 1 hour, 15 minutes

Related subject areas: math, science, art

OBJECTIVES

1. Students will explain why fat is an important part of the diet.
2. Students will be able to examine food labels to identify foods that contain unhealthy saturated and trans fat.
3. Students will discriminate between solid and liquid fat.

MATERIALS

1. Chalkboard
2. Food wrappers (including nutrition labels) from canned fruits and vegetables, soups, candy bars, desserts, and baked goods (collect some on your own and ask students to bring some from home; you may want to assign foods from different food groups to ensure a variety of food labels)
3. Small opaque container and a small object (such as a cotton ball, a piece of paper, or a feather) to place in the container
4. Transparency 1, Reading the Food Label
5. Handout 1, Food Labels (select a sample from the food labels provided to copy to round out the collection of labels brought in by students)
6. Handout 2, Reading the Food Label
7. Worksheet 1, Can You Find It?
8. Worksheet 2, Graphing Fat

PROCEDURE

PART I

1. Before class, place a cotton ball, a piece of paper, a feather, or another small object in a small, covered, opaque container.
2. During class, ask the students to guess the contents of the container (provide a few clues). Have them give reasons for their answers.
3. After several guesses have been given, say to the students, "Some of the foods we eat are like this container. They contain hidden ingredients that cannot be seen. Today, we're going to go on a hunt for foods that contain saturated and trans fat."

PART II

1. Ask the students to tell you where they might find fat in foods. Write the names of each food group (grains; fruits; vegetables; meat, fish, and beans; and

milk) on the board and have the students name some foods from each group that contain fat. List fats such as butter, margarine, oil, and salad dressing separately.

2. Discuss with students the reasons fat is an important part of their diets (see background material).

3. Stress the fact that there are different types of fat (saturated, unsaturated, and trans) that not only look differently but also behave differently in the body:

   • Healthy fat—monounsaturated and polyunsaturated fat—is liquid at room temperature; it comes primarily from plant sources, such as olive oil, canola oil, peanut oil, corn oil, and safflower oil. Healthy fat is also found in nuts, peanut butter, avocados, and fish. Healthy fat can help reduce the risk of heart disease.

   • Unhealthy fat—saturated fat and trans fat—is solid at room temperature; it often comes from animal sources or from oils that have been partially hydrogenated, a chemical process that turns liquid oil into a solid. Unhealthy fat increases the risk of heart disease.

   • Discuss why a person should pay attention to the types of fat eaten.

4. Tell students that they will investigate all of the food groups to find foods that contain healthy fat as well as foods that contain unhealthy fat.

PART III

1. Distribute handout 1, Food Labels, and actual food labels or food containers or copies of food labels to students. If possible, hand out a wide variety of labels, including labels from canned and frozen fruits and vegetables, desserts, and frozen dinners.

2. Explain to students that food labels contain information that can help a person make smart decisions about whether a particular food fits into the healthful and balanced diet she is trying to eat.

3. Display transparency 1 and distribute handout 2 (both are entitled Reading the Food Label) to the students. Explain that one specific thing food labels address is the amount and type of unhealthy fat (saturated or trans fat) contained in a food. Food labels also present other information, such as the number of calories a food provides, certain vitamins and minerals a food contains, and a list of ingredients in the food (with the most abundant ingredient listed first).

4. Name one of the foods for which there is a label, and before examining the label, have students decide if they think the food contains fat and, if so, what type of fat it contains. Record students' answers on the board before investigations begin.

5. Have students find the following information on one of the food labels:

   Food name _____

   Serving size _____

   Saturated fat per serving (grams) _____

   Trans fat per serving (grams) _____

   % Daily Value (% DV) of saturated fat _____

Explain that the % Daily Value of saturated fat can help the students figure out how much 1 serving of food contributes to their daily maximum allowance of saturated fat. If they add together the % DVs of saturated fat of all the foods they eat in a day, it should total to no more than 100%. Ask for volunteers to stand and state the % DV of saturated fat found on their food labels. As each student stands, record the food on the board and add the percentages until the total reaches 100%. Try different combinations of foods to see how quickly it can take to reach 100% or how long it can take when eating foods with little saturated fat. From this information, ask students to identify foods and food groups that contain foods that are low in saturated fat.

Also explain that there is no % DV for trans fat; trans fat should be avoided.

6. Write on the board the following words: *bacon, steak, chicken, fish, butter, muffins, olive oil, canola oil, shortening, stick margarine, avocado, peanut butter, almonds, peanuts, cashews, guacamole, salad dressing made with vegetable oil, lunch meats, candy bars, hot dogs, pies, cheese, cakes, doughnuts, Twinkies, puddings, ice creams,* and *cookies.* Discuss foods that contain visible fat (fat that can be seen before, during, and after preparation). Have the students identify the foods with visible, unhealthy fat (bacon, steak, butter, shortening, and stick margarine) and the foods with visible, healthy fat (olive oil, canola oil, salad dressing made with vegetable oil). Point out that some foods may not appear to have fat in them but actually do have fat hidden inside (chicken, fish, and muffins). Have students identify the foods with hidden unhealthy fat (chicken with skin, lunch meats, candy bars, hot dogs, pies, cheese, cakes, doughnuts, Twinkies, puddings, ice creams, cookies) and the foods with hidden healthy fat (almonds, peanuts, cashews, avocado, guacamole).

7. Ask the students, "What are some foods that you know are prepared with fat or oils?"

Responses may include French fries, doughnuts, pies, cakes, fried fish, fried chicken, stir-fries, sautéed dishes, and so on.

8. Have students describe food preparation processes involving fat. As each type of fat (butter, oil, lard, margarine, etc.) is mentioned, list it on the board (see sample in table 17.1).

►TABLE 17.1 Food Preparation Processes

What?	How prepared?	Using what?
French fries	Deep-fried	Partially hydrogenated vegetable oil, lard
Cake	Baked	Butter, vegetable oil
Fish	Fried	Vegetable oil (in restaurants, partially hydrogenated oil), lard
Chicken	Stir-fried	Canola oil, peanut oil
Broccoli	Sautéed	Butter, olive oil, peanut oil

9. Have students distinguish between fat sources that are solid at room temperature and fat sources that are liquid at room temperature. (Butter, lard, shortening, and partially hydrogenated vegetable oil are solid at room temperature; most vegetable oils, including olive oil and squeeze margarine, are liquid at room temperature.)

10. Have students tell what happens to solid fat when it is heated. (It becomes liquid.)

11. Explain to students that most of the time they should choose fat (and foods prepared with fat) that is liquid at room temperature over fat that is solid at room temperature. Liquid fat is unsaturated and is better for the body.

12. Distribute worksheet 1, Can You Find It? Have students (in pairs or small groups) examine various food labels and ingredient lists (using the labels they brought from home) and record the amount of saturated and trans fat in each food selection on the worksheet. Have students make bar graphs to compare the amounts of saturated and trans fat in various foods (use worksheet 2, Graphing Fat, as a guide).

PART IV

1. Have the students identify foods low in saturated fat and that have 0 grams of trans fat—foods they should choose to reduce the amount of saturated and trans fat in their diet. Use the results from the activity on worksheet 1 as a basis for this discussion.

2. Stress that students should not be fearful of fat. Remind the students to enjoy foods with healthy fat, such as olive, canola, and other plant oils; nuts and peanut butter; avocados; and fish. It is okay to occasionally eat a small serving of a food that is high in saturated fat (also known as a "*sometimes*" *food*). But on a regular basis, students should choose foods that are low in saturated fat and avoid trans fat.

PART V

1. Have students look in their refrigerators and pantries at home and make a list of the foods they find that contain less than 5% of the DV for saturated fat per serving (they can use worksheet 2 for this assignment), contain 0 grams of trans fat, and contain no partially hydrogenated oils or shortening in the ingredients list. A food with less than 5% of the DV for saturated fat per serving is considered to be low in saturated fat by the FDA.

2. Have students collect and make a collage of labels from foods with less than 5% of the DV for saturated fat, 0 grams of trans fat, and no partially hydrogenated oils. Encourage them to be creative in designing their collage and to add a message about nutrition and foods low in saturated fat appropriate for other students in their class or school. Display the collages for others to view.

SUMMARY ACTIVITY (OPTIONAL)

Play a game of 20 questions by taping a food label on each player's back. Instruct the students to walk around the room and ask yes or no questions to determine which foods are posted on their backs. Students should only ask one question at a time and then move to another player. Sample questions may include the following:

Does my food contain fat?

Is the fat visible?

Does the food contain saturated fat?

Does the food contain a high amount of saturated fat?

Is the food from the milk group?

Is the food fried?

Reading the Food Label

Nutrition Facts

Serving Size ①cup (228g) —————————— | Serving size |

Servings Per Container② ——————————— | Servings per container |

Amount Per Serving

Calories 250   Calories from Fat 120

                     % Daily Value*

Total Fat 13g	**20%**
Saturated Fat ③g	**15%**
Trans Fat ③g	
Cholesterol 31mg	**10%**
Sodium 470mg	**20%**
Total Carbohydrate 31g	**10%**
Dietary Fiber 0g	**0%**
Sugars 5g	
Protein 5g	

Vitamin A 4%	•	Vitamin C 2%
Calcium 15%	•	Iron 4%

*Percent Daily Values are based on a 2,000 calorie diet. Your daily values may be higher or lower depending on your calorie needs:

	Calories	2,000	2,500
Total Fat	Less than	65g	80g
Sat. Fat	Less than	20g	25g
Cholesterol	Less than	300mg	300mg
Sodium	Less than	2,400mg	2,400mg
Total Carbohydrate		300g	375g
Dietary Fiber		25g	30g

Calories per gram:
Fat 9 • Carbohydrate 4 • Protein 4

| Saturated fat per serving |

| *Trans* fat per serving: Choose foods that have 0g of *trans* fat |

| % DV of saturated fat: Foods with a DV for saturated fat of 5 or less are low in saturated fat. Foods with a % DV for saturated fat of 20 or more are high in saturated fat. The daily goal is to choose foods that together contain less than 100% of the DV for saturated fat. |

From L.W.Y. Cheung, H. Dart, S. Kalin, and S.L. Gortmaker, 2007, *Eat Well & Keep Moving,* 2nd ed. (Champaign, IL: Human Kinetics).
http://cfsan.fda.gov/~dms.labtr.html.

Food Labels

Glazed Cake Doughnut

Nutrition Facts

Serving Size 1 doughnut
Servings Per Container 1

Amount Per Serving

Calories 350   Calories from Fat 170

	% Daily Value*
Total Fat 19g	**30%**
Saturated Fat 5g	**27%**
Trans Fat 4g	
Cholesterol 25mg	**8%**
Sodium 340mg	**14%**
Total Carbohydrate 41g	**14%**
Dietary Fiber 1g	**4%**
Sugars 21g	
Protein 4g	

Vitamin A 0%	•	Vitamin C 0%
Calcium 2%	•	Iron 8%

*Percent Daily Values are based on a 2,000 calorie diet. Your daily values may be higher or lower depending on your calorie needs.

Plums

Nutrition Facts

Serving Size 2 medium

Amount Per Serving

Calories 61   Calories from Fat 4

	% Daily Value*
Total Fat 0.4g	**1%**
Saturated Fat 0g	**0%**
Trans Fat 0g	**0%**
Cholesterol 0mg	**0%**
Sodium 0mg	**0%**
Potassium 207mg	**6%**
Total Carbohydrate 15g	**6%**
Dietary Fiber 2g	**8%**
Sugars 13g	
Protein 1g	

Vitamin A 10%	•	Vitamin C 20%
Calcium 0%	•	Iron 2%

*Percent Daily Values are based on a 2,000 calorie diet. Your daily values may be higher or lower depending on your calorie needs.

From L.W.Y. Cheung, H. Dart, S. Kalin, and S.L. Gortmaker, 2007, *Eat Well & Keep Moving*, 2nd ed. (Champaign, IL: Human Kinetics).

(continued)

Sweet Potatoes

Nutrition Facts

Serving Size 1 medium

Amount Per Serving

Calories 103 · Calories from Fat 0

	% Daily Value*
Total Fat 0g	0%
Saturated Fat 0g	0%
Trans Fat 0g	0%
Cholesterol 0mg	0%
Sodium 40mg	2%
Potassium 540mg	15%
Total Carbohydrate 24g	8%
Dietary Fiber 4g	15%
Sugars 10g	
Protein 2g	

Vitamin A 440%	•	Vitamin C 35%
Calcium 4%	•	Iron 4%

*Percent Daily Values are based on a 2,000 calorie diet. Your daily values may be higher or lower depending on your calorie needs.

Skim Milk

Nutrition Facts

Serving Size ½ pint (236 ml)
Serving Per Container 1

Amount Per Serving

Calories 90 · Calories from Fat 0

	% Daily Value*
Total Fat 0g	0%
Saturated Fat 0g	0%
Trans Fat 0g	0%
Cholesterol <5mg	1%
Sodium 130mg	5%
Total Carbohydrate 13g	4%
Dietary Fiber 0g	0%
Sugars 12g	
Protein 8g	

Vitamin A 10%	•	Vitamin C 2%
Calcium 30%	•	Iron 0%

*Percent Daily Values are based on a 2,000 calorie diet. Your daily values may be higher or lower depending on your calorie needs.

Chicken

Nutrition Facts

Serving Size 1 roasted drumstick
(61 g/about 2 oz)
Serving Per Container 6

Amount Per Serving

Calories 110 · Calories from Fat 50

	% Daily Value*
Total Fat 6g	9%
Saturated Fat 1.5g	8%
Trans Fat 0g	0%
Cholesterol 85mg	28%
Sodium 50mg	2%
Total Carbohydrate 0g	0%
Protein 14g	28%
Iron	4%

Not a significant source or dietary fiber, sugars, vitamin A, vitamin C, or calcium

*Percent Daily Values are based on a 2,000 calorie diet. Your daily values may be higher or lower depending on your calorie needs.

From L.W.Y. Cheung, H. Dart, S. Kalin, and S.L. Gortmaker, 2007, *Eat Well & Keep Moving,* 2nd ed. (Champaign, IL: Human Kinetics).

Reading the Food Label

Nutrition Facts

Serving Size (1 cup) (228g) ——————— | Serving size |

Servings Per Container ② ——————— | Servings per container |

Amount Per Serving

Calories 250   Calories from Fat 120

	% Daily Value*
Total Fat 13g	**20%**
Saturated Fat (3g)	(15%)
Trans Fat (3g)	
Cholesterol 31mg	**10%**
Sodium 470mg	**20%**
Total Carbohydrate 31g	**10%**
Dietary Fiber 0g	**0%**
Sugars 5g	
Protein 5g	

Vitamin A 4%	•	Vitamin C 2%
Calcium 15%	•	Iron 4%

*Percent Daily Values are based on a 2,000 calorie diet. Your daily values may be higher or lower depending on your calorie needs:

	Calories	2,000	2,500
Total Fat	Less than	65g	80g
Sat. Fat	Less than	20g	25g
Cholesterol	Less than	300mg	300mg
Sodium	Less than	2,400mg	2,400mg
Total Carbohydrate		300g	375g
Dietary Fiber		25g	30g

Calories per gram:
Fat 9 • Carbohydrate 4 • Protein 4

| Saturated fat per serving |

| *Trans* fat per serving: Choose foods that have 0g of *trans* fat |

| % DV of saturated fat: Foods with a DV for saturated fat of 5 or less are low in saturated fat. Foods with a % DV for saturated fat of 20 or more are high in saturated fat. The daily goal is to choose foods that together contain less than 100% of the DV for saturated fat. |

From L.W.Y. Cheung, H. Dart, S. Kalin, and S.L. Gortmaker, 2007, *Eat Well & Keep Moving,* 2nd ed. (Champaign, IL: Human Kinetics). http://cfsan.fda.gov/~dms.labtr.html.

Name _____

Can You Find It?

Nutrition facts	**Nutrition facts**
Name of product _____	Name of product _____
Serving size_____	Serving size_____
Saturated fat per serving _____	Saturated fat per serving _____
Trans fat per serving _____	Trans fat per serving _____
% DV of saturated fat_____	% DV of saturated fat_____
Nutrition facts	**Nutrition facts**
Name of product _____	Name of product _____
Serving size_____	Serving size_____
Saturated fat per serving _____	Saturated fat per serving _____
Trans fat per serving _____	Trans fat per serving _____
% DV of saturated fat_____	% DV of saturated fat_____
Nutrition facts	**Nutrition facts**
Name of product _____	Name of product _____
Serving size_____	Serving size_____
Saturated fat per serving _____	Saturated fat per serving _____
Trans fat per serving _____	Trans fat per serving _____
% DV of saturated fat_____	% DV of saturated fat_____

▶ FIGURE 17.1 Nutrition facts.

Name _____

Graphing Fat

Instructions

Use different colored pencils to graph the saturated fat and the trans fat in your food.

15		
14		
13		
12		
11		
10		
9		
8		
7		
6		
5		
4		
3		
2		
1		
	Grams saturated fat	Grams trans fat

15		
14		
13		
12		
11		
10		
9		
8		
7		
6		
5		
4		
3		
2		
1		
	Grams saturated fat	Grams trans fat

From L.W.Y. Cheung, H. Dart, S. Kalin, and S.L. Gortmaker, 2007, *Eat Well & Keep Moving,* 2nd ed. (Champaign, IL: Human Kinetics).

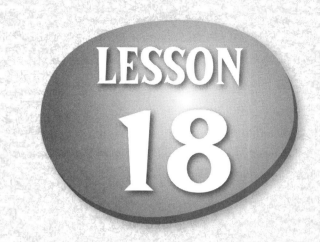

Beverage Buzz: Sack the Sugar

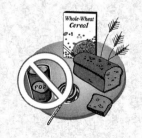

BACKGROUND

A major source of sugar in the American diet is sugar-sweetened beverages such as soft drinks, fruit punches, energy drinks, sweetened iced teas, and sports drinks. Children's consumption of soft drinks is rising. Teenage girls and boys drink an average of 20 ounces (600 milliliters) of soft drink per day, compared to just 9 ounces (270 milliliters) of milk per day.

The steady climb in children's intake of sugar-sweetened beverages is troubling for many reasons. As children's soft drink consumption has increased, their milk consumption has decreased. That is a worrisome trend, given that adolescence is a time of rapid bone development and increased calcium needs. Teenagers who do not maximize bone development during these crucial years (by getting enough calcium and regular physical activity) may increase their risk of osteoporosis in late adulthood.

Sugar-sweetened beverages are considered a source of empty calories because they basically contain just sugar and water, and they do not provide vitamins, minerals, or other key nutrients. A growing body of research strongly suggests that sugar-sweetened beverage consumption is associated with excess weight gain in children and adults. One study found that middle school students who increased their sugar-sweetened beverage consumption gained excess weight; for each additional 12-ounce (375-milliliter) serving of sugar-sweetened beverage consumed per day, the odds of becoming obese increased by 60%. Reducing or avoiding empty calories from sugar-sweetened beverages may help with weight control: Another study found that when overweight teenagers reduced their consumption of sugar-sweetened beverages by replacing these beverages with calorie-free ones, they lost about 1 pound (0.5 kilogram) per month. Other research connects the consumption of sugar-sweetened beverages with a risk for type 2 diabetes.

Over the years, little by little, beverage packaging sizes have increased. In the 1950s, a typical bottle of soft drink held 6.5 ounces (195 milliliters); in 2005, the typical bottle held 20 or 24 ounces (600 or 720 milliliters). Restaurants and convenience stores offer supersized drink cups that hold up to 64 ounces (1.9 liters) of soft drink. Some experts believe that the supersizing of sugar-sweetened beverages, combined with creative marketing, has increased the likelihood that children and adults will consume even greater amounts of soft drink. This lesson helps make children informed consumers by teaching them to assess their own beverage consumption and to consider the nutritional consequences of their choices. Children will also discuss popular ads for sweetened drinks and will be encouraged to select healthier beverages such as water for quenching thirst or low-fat and skim milk for calcium; calcium-fortified soy drinks* and calcium-fortified 100% orange juice are also good sources of calcium.

A healthy eating plan includes few if any beverages with added sugar. The Harvard Prevention Research Center recommends that children consume no more than 2 8-ounce glasses of sugar-sweetened beverages per week. This includes soft drinks, fruit punches, sweetened iced teas, and sports drinks.** Children should also avoid consuming artificially-sweetened beverages, since the long-term effects of artificial sweetener consumption are unknown and since artificial sweeteners may encourage a taste for sweetness. The consumption of 100% fruit juice should be limited to no more than 8 ounces (250 milliliters) per day. Juice

*Choose soy or other nondairy drinks that have no more than 12 grams of sugar per 8-ounce (250-milliliter) serving.

**During most types of physical activity, children can get adequate hydration and energy by drinking water and having a healthy snack (such as orange slices). Most sports drinks are designed for endurance athletes who compete for more than an hour at high intensity. Save sports drinks for when children are participating in high-intensity, long-duration sports competitions (greater than 1 hour) or for when children are vigorously active for a long time in the heat.

contains vitamins and minerals, but it naturally contains a large amount of fruit sugar (fructose) and it lacks the fiber found in fresh whole fruit. To make it easier to stay within the 8-ounce fruit juice limit, dilute a small amount of 100% fruit juice (4 ounces) with sparkling water.

Source of background material in part from Center for Science in the Public Interest. (2005). *Liquid Candy: How Soft Drinks are Harming America's Health*. Washington, DC: Center for Science in the Public Interest.

ESTIMATED TEACHING TIME AND RELATED SUBJECT AREAS

Estimated teaching time: 1 hour, 15 minutes

Related subject areas: math, health, language arts (vocabulary)

OBJECTIVES

1. Students will measure the amount of sugar they consume from soft drinks and other sugar-sweetened beverages and evaluate the results.
2. Students will recognize how the media entices people to consume sweetened beverages.
3. Students will learn about the body's response to sugar.
4. Students will identify the health benefits of different beverages.
5. Students will learn to replace soft drinks and other sugar-sweetened beverages with healthy drinks.

MATERIALS

1. Sugar (2-5 pounds, or 1-2 kilograms)
2. Measuring teaspoons
3. Plain paper cups or clear plastic cups
4. Worksheet 1, Where's the Sugar?
5. Worksheet 2, What's Up With This Ad?
6. Worksheet 3, Beverage Buzz
7. Worksheet 4, Your Top Three (optional)
8. Student resource 1, Beverage Facts
9. Solutions to worksheet 3
10. Teacher resource page 1, Evaluating Media Advertising
11. Transparency 1, Supersized Soft Drinks

PROCEDURE

PART I: EVALUATION OF SUGAR INTAKE

1. Ask students to name the drink they had last night at supper. Create a histogram on the board (combine similar drinks such as juice cocktails, fruit

You may need to assist students in estimating the amount of soft drinks and other sugary beverages they consumed if they consumed something other than the listed beverage sizes. This exercise is not meant to be an exact record but rather a rough estimate of the amount of sugar consumed from beverages.

Students who did not drink soft drinks or other sweetened beverages over the past 2 days may fill out the sheet based on what they drink on a typical day; if several students did not drink soft drinks over the past 2 days or some students rarely drink soft drinks because of household rules, it may be more effective to conduct this activity in groups.

punches, and lemonade). Calculate the percentage of students consuming the various drinks. What percentage had milk? What percentage had soft drinks or other sugary drinks? Explain that children aged 6 to 11 years derive almost 20% of their total energy intake from soft drinks, sugary beverages, and other types of sweets.

2. Explain to the students that they will be analyzing their beverage intake from the past 2 days. Distribute worksheet 1 (Where's the Sugar?) to the students and instruct them to complete the table by recording the cans of soft drink, bottles of sports drink, and pouches of fruit punch that they consumed over the previous 2 days. Then ask the students to calculate the number of teaspoons of sugar consumed from soft drinks, sports drinks, and fruit punches and to sum these amounts to determine the total amount of sugar they consumed from sugar-sweetened beverages over the past 2 days.

3. Have the students evaluate their total intake of sugar. Distribute the cups and instruct the students to measure out the teaspoons of sugar they consumed over the past 2 days. Have them pour their sugar into the cups to visualize the amount. Discuss student observations—were the students surprised at the amount of sugar they consumed?

4. For a homework assignment, have students complete parts II and III of worksheet 1 at home.

   a. In part II (How Much Sugar Is This?), students will assess their sugar intake by converting teaspoons to cups, calculating their average intake of sugar and projecting their intake of sugar over time. A child who consumes just 1 can of soft drink and 1 juice-box size of a sweetened drink per day (a total of 16 teaspoons, or 80 milliliters, of sugar) may consume 112 teaspoons (560 milliliters) of sugar over 1 week, which translates to more than 4.5 pounds (2 kilograms) of sugar each month (using the simple calculation of 4 weeks in 1 month) and 56 pounds (25 kilograms) of sugar each year.

   b. In part III (Calcium Switch), students will calculate the amount of calcium they would consume if they drank low-fat or nonfat milk instead of soft drinks. Students will first calculate the amount of soft drinks they consumed in ounces, and they will then use that number to determine the amount of calcium contained in the same amount of low-fat or nonfat milk.

   c. In part IV (What Can You Say About Your Drinks?), students will write a paragraph that describes their current beverage intake and make recommendations for improvement.

PART II: SUGAR AND THE MEDIA

1. Display transparency 1, Supersized Soft Drinks, to show how soft drink packaging has changed over time. Explain how the change in serving size has made it more likely for people to drink more soft drinks when they eat out or when they buy a bottle from a vending machine or a convenience store.

2. Discuss other ways that companies encourage the consumption of their products. Instruct students to think about the advertisements that they see on television. Can they recall any ads for healthy beverages? Ask them to name some of the advertisements for sugar-sweetened beverages.

3. Divide the class into small groups and give each group one copy of worksheet 2 (What's Up With This Ad?). Instruct the groups to select one beverage

advertisement to consider. Read the five questions and have each group answer the questions about its selected advertisement. Discuss the group responses as a class (see teacher resource page 1 for ideas).

PART III: IDENTIFICATION OF SUGAR

1. Distribute worksheet 3 (Beverage Buzz) and student resource 1 (Beverage Facts) to help students identify alternate words for sugar and sources of healthy nutrients. Students may work on the crossword individually or in groups. Display the solutions as an overhead and discuss the answers with the class.

2. Invite students to create a list of healthy drink options, and discuss the best choices according to their health benefits. For example, the students might list

   * plain or sparkling water (alleviates thirst and promotes hydration),
   * nonfat or low-fat milk (provides calcium for strong bones and teeth), and
   * 100% fruit juice (offers vitamins and minerals); note that consumption of 100% fruit juice should be limited to no more than 8 ounces per day.

> In addition to containing large amounts of sugar, energy drinks often contain caffeine, herbs, and other additives that may not be healthy for children.

PART IV: APPLICATION AND EXTENSION OF INFORMATION

1. Ask students to describe why we might want or need sugar (it tastes good; it gives us energy). In what foods and beverages do we find sugar? We find sugar naturally in fruits and vegetables; these foods are healthy because they provide fiber and many vitamins and minerals. Low-fat and nonfat milk and some dairy foods also contain sugar. Other foods and drinks have sugar added to them.

2. Remind students that soft drinks and other sweet drinks contain high amounts of sugar and usually nothing else that is good for us—they basically contain just sugar and water. And the energy boost from sugary drinks does not last.

3. Have the class stand up and do the wave (raising and lowering the arms as you might do at a sporting event). Explain that this is what happens in our bodies when we drink a whole can of sugary drink all at once (or eat sugary foods, like a pack of jelly beans): There is a quick rise in blood sugar, giving us energy, but our bodies work quickly to pull that sugar out of the blood and into storage (in our muscles). That is why the quick boost of energy we feel after drinking a sugary drink does not last.

4. Read the following scenario to the class.

   Michael is playing chess as part of the chess club at school. During a break, the chess club coach gives Michael and other club members fruit punch to drink. Michael starts playing chess again, and at first he is feeling great, but he starts to feel sluggish before the end of the afternoon and has a hard time concentrating on his final match.

   a. Ask the students to discuss (in small groups or as a class) what happened. How could Michael and his coach have prevented the late-afternoon slump?

   b. Possible solutions may include the following: The coach can provide water to quench the players' thirst and fruit such as orange wedges, bananas, or unsweetened dried fruit to provide energy (without causing the quick rise and fall in blood sugar that occurs with a sugary fruit punch).

EXTENSION ACTIVITIES

1. Create posters discouraging the consumption of soft drinks and other sugary drinks and post them near the cafeteria.

2. Create television ads that send the message that sugary drinks do not make healthy choices or that promote consumption of a healthy beverage, such as water. Have students work in groups; each group can determine the audience for its ad (for instance, children or parents) and then perform its skit for the class.

3. Evaluate top beverage choices using optional worksheet 4 (Your Top Three). Instruct students to pretend that they just got back from recess or gym class and to choose their top three drink choices from the list provided. Students can use student resource 1 (Beverage Facts) to determine the grams of sugar in each drink, whether the drink contains vitamins or minerals, and whether the drink contains added sugars. Then the students can determine which one is the healthiest choice.

Where's the Sugar?

Part I: What Did You Drink?

Fill in the Beverage Count table (table 18.1) with the number of cans of soft drinks, bottles of sports drink, and pouches of fruit punch you had yesterday and the day before yesterday.

You may need to estimate the amounts that you drank and round to a whole number. For instance, if you opened a 20-ounce (600-milliliter) bottle of soft drink but only drank half of it, you consumed approximately one 12-ounce (375-milliliter) can of soft drink.

▶TABLE 18.1 Beverage Count

	Soft drink—12 oz. (375 ml) can (10 tsp. of sugar)	Sports drink—16 oz. (500 ml) bottle (7 tsp. of sugar)	Fruit punch—7 oz. (210 ml) pouch (7 tsp. of sugar)
How many did you drink yesterday?			
How many did you drink the day before yesterday?			
Total drinks			

Calculate the total teaspoons of sugar you consumed from drinks over the past 2 days.

1. How many teaspoons of sugar did you consume from soft drinks over the past 2 days?

   For example, if you drank 2 cans, then 2 cans × 10 teaspoons = 20 teaspoons of sugar.

From L.W.Y. Cheung, H. Dart, S. Kalin, and S.L. Gortmaker, 2007, *Eat Well & Keep Moving*, 2nd ed. (Champaign, IL: Human Kinetics). Adapted, by permission, from J. Carter et al., 2007, *Planet Health*, 2nd ed. (Champaign, IL: Human Kinetics), lesson 19.

(continued)

2. How many teaspoons of sugar did you consume from sports drinks over the past 2 days?

For example, if you drank 1 bottle, then 1 bottle × 7 teaspoons = 7 teaspoons of sugar.

3. How many teaspoons of sugar did you consume from fruit punch over the past 2 days?

For example, if you drank 2 juice pouches, then 2 juice pouches × 7 teaspoons = 14 teaspoons of sugar.

4. Add it all up: How many teaspoons of sugar did you consume from soft drinks, sports drinks, and fruit punches over the past 2 days?

Teaspoons of sugar from soft drinks: _____

+ teaspoons of sugar from sports drinks: _____

+ teaspoons of sugar from fruit punch: _____

= total teaspoons of sugar: _____

Part II: How Much Sugar Is This?

1. There are 24 teaspoons in 1/2 cup. How many cups of sugar did you consume in the past 2 days by drinking sugary beverages?

2. What is your average intake of sugar per day from soft drinks and other sweet drinks? (Hint: Divide the total number of teaspoons from the past 2 days by 2.)

3. If you continue drinking the same amount of soft drinks and other sweet drinks, how many teaspoons of sugar will you consume over 1 week? (Hint: Use the average teaspoons of sugar consumed each day to calculate the teaspoons of sugar consumed over 1 week.)

4. If 108 teaspoons of sugar equals 1 pound (0.5 kilogram), then how many pounds of sugar might you consume from soft drinks and other sweet drinks over a month (use the average of 4 weeks in a month)? Over a year?

From L.W.Y. Cheung, H. Dart, S. Kalin, and S.L. Gortmaker, 2007, *Eat Well & Keep Moving*, 2nd ed. (Champaign, IL: Human Kinetics). Adapted, by permission, from J. Carter et al., 2007, *Planet Health*, 2nd ed. (Champaign, IL: Human Kinetics), lesson 19.

(continued)

Part III: Calcium Switch

Soft drinks and other sweet drinks contain high amounts of sugar and usually nothing else that is good for us—they basically contain just sugar and water. That's why we say that sugar-sweetened drinks give us empty calories. Determine how much calcium you could consume if you drank low-fat or nonfat milk in place of the soft drinks you drank over the past 2 days.

   1. How much soft drink did you drink?

   Number of cans of soft drink _____ × 12 ounces (375 milliliters) per can = _____ ounces of soft drink.

   2. Each ounce (30 milliliters) of milk provides 38 milligrams of calcium. How much calcium would you have consumed by drinking milk instead of soft drinks?

Note that children need 1,300 milligrams of calcium each day.

Part IV: What Can You Say About Your Drinks?

Write a statement that describes your drinks over the past 2 days. Describe at least one health effect of your drinks. Do you need to make healthier choices? What could you do to improve your drink choices?

Name _____

What's Up With This Ad?

As a group, select one beverage product for which you can recall a television advertisement. Use the ad for that product to answer the following questions. If you need more space, write on the back of this worksheet. Remember, members of your group may have different opinions, and that is okay.

Names of group members:

Name of product:

What is going on in the advertisement?

1. Which company is sending the message?

2. What do you like about the ad? Think about how the ad catches your attention. What do you dislike about the ad?

3. Who is this ad for? Consider how you feel about the ad and how others (maybe someone older or younger or of a different gender) might feel about the ad.

4. What does this ad tell you about how people live? Can you relate to the ideas or lifestyles depicted in the message? Is anything left out?

5. What is the message trying to tell you or sell you?

From L.W.Y. Cheung, H. Dart, S. Kalin, and S.L. Gortmaker, 2007, *Eat Well & Keep Moving*, 2nd ed. (Champaign, IL: Human Kinetics). Adapted, by permission, from Center for Media Literacy, 2005. Available www.medialit.org.

Beverage Buzz

Complete the crossword puzzle using the words in the following list. For help with answering the clues, look at the Nutrition Facts labels on the Beverage Facts sheet that your teacher gives you.

Calcium	Corn syrup	Fruit	Fruit punch	Soft
Sports	Sucrose	Sugar	Vitamin C	Water

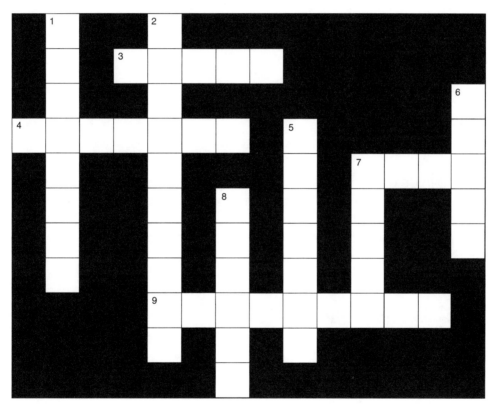

Down

1. A nutrient in orange juice (2 words)
2. Sounds healthy but has a lot of sugar (2 words)
5. Scientific name for table sugar
6. The best thirst quencher
7. 10 teaspoons of this are found in a 12-ounce soft drink
8. Sodium can be found in this type of drink

Across

3. Fructose is the natural sugar in this food
4. A mineral in milk
7. This drink provides empty calories
9. Sounds like a vegetable but is really a sugar (2 words)

From L.W.Y. Cheung, H. Dart, S. Kalin, and S.L. Gortmaker, 2007, *Eat Well & Keep Moving*, 2nd ed. (Champaign, IL: Human Kinetics).

WORKSHEET

NName _____

Your Top Three

Pretend that you just got back from gym class or recess and you are thirsty. Out of the beverages in the following list, what would you want to drink?

▶ Water

▶ Gatorade

▶ Capri Sun Fruit Punch

▶ Soft drink

▶ Skim milk

▶ Chocolate milk

▶ Orange juice

▶ Lemonade

Pick your top three choices and list them in table 18.2. For each drink, use the Beverage Facts sheet to fill in the number of grams of sugar, the names of the vitamins and minerals (if any), and the names of the added sugars (if any). Remember that there are many names for added sugar: corn syrup, dextrose, fructose, glucose, high fructose corn syrup, honey, maltose, molasses, sucrose, and sugar.

▶TABLE 18.2 Your Top Three

What are your three favorite drinks?	Sugar (grams)	Vitamins and minerals	Added sugars
1.			
2.			
3.			

Which one do you think is the healthiest drink and why?

From L.W.Y. Cheung, H. Dart, S. Kalin, and S.L. Gortmaker, 2007, *Eat Well & Keep Moving,* 2nd ed. (Champaign, IL: Human Kinetics).

Beverage Facts

Capri Sun Fruit Punch Ingredients

Water, high fructose corn syrup, pear and grape juice from concentrate, citric acid, water extracted orange and pineapple juice concentrates, ascorbic acid, vitamin E acetate, natural flavor

Orange Juice (Minute Maid) Ingredients

100% pure squeezed orange juice from concentrate (pure filtered water, premium concentrate orange juice)

Nutrition Facts

Serving Size 6.75 fl oz (200 ml)

Amount Per Serving	% DV*
Calories 100	
Total Fat 0g	0%
Sodium 15mg	1%
Total Carbohydrate 27g	8%
Sugars (27g)	
Protein 0g	

Vitamin C 0%

Not a significant source of calories from fat, saturated fat, trans fat, cholesterol, dietary fiber, vitamin A, calcium, or iron.
*Percent Daily Values are based on a 2,000 calorie diet. Your daily values may be higher or lower depending on your calorie needs.

Nutrition Facts

Serving Size 8 fl oz (250 ml)

Amount Per Serving		% DV*
Calories 110		
Total Fat 0g		0%
Sodium 15mg		1%
Potassium 450 mg		13%
Total Carbohydrate 27g		15%
Sugars (24g)		
Protein 2g		
Vitamin C 120%	B$_6$	4%
Thiamin 10%	Niacin	2%
Folate 15%	Calcium	2%

Magnesium 6%

Not a significant source of calories from fat, saturated fat, trans fat, cholesterol, dietary fiber, vitamin A, calcium, or iron.
*Percent Daily Values are based on a 2,000 calorie diet. Your daily values may be higher or lower depending on your calorie needs.

- -

Note: This drink may be sold in bottles that contain more than one serving. A 10-ounce bottle contains 30 grams of sugar.

From L.W.Y. Cheung, H. Dart, S. Kalin, and S.L. Gortmaker, 2007, *Eat Well & Keep Moving,* 2nd ed. (Champaign, IL: Human Kinetics). Nutrition information retrieved from company Web sites on July 6, 2007: Capri Sun Fruit Punch, www.kraftfoods.com/CapriSun/1_1_CS_Base. html; Minute Maid Orange Juice, www.minutemaid.com/productsMain.jsp?group=Variety_Juices_and_Drinks.

(continued)

Gatorade Thirst Quencher Ingredients

Water, sucrose syrup, glucose–fructose syrup, citric acid, natural and artificial flavors, salt, sodium citrate, monopotassium phosphate, vegetable juice (for color), ester gum

---

Note: This drink may be sold in bottles that contain more than one serving. A 24-ounce bottle contains 42 grams of sugar.

Nutrition Facts
Serving Size 8 fl oz (250 ml)

Amount Per Serving	% DV*
Calories 50	
Total Fat 0g	0%
Sodium 110mg	5%
Potassium 30 mg	1%
Total Carbohydrate 14g	5%
Sugars (14g)	
Protein 0g	

Not a significant source of calories from fat, saturated fat, trans fat, cholesterol, dietary fiber, vitamin A, vitamin C, calcium, or iron.
*Percent Daily Values are based on a 2,000 calorie diet. Your daily values may be higher or lower depending on your calorie needs.

Low-Fat Milk Ingredients

Low-fat milk (pasteurized and homogenized), vitamin A palmitate, vitamin D_3

Nutrition Facts
Serving Size 8 fl oz (250 ml)

Amount Per Serving	% DV*
Calories 110	
Total Fat 2.5g	4%
Saturated Fat 1.5g	8%
Trans Fat 0g	0%
Cholesterol 15mg	4%
Sodium 130mg	5%
Total Carbohydrate 13g	4%
Sugars 12g	
Protein 8g	

Vitamin A 10%	•	Vitamin C 2%
Calcium 30%	•	Vitamin D 25%

Not a significant source of dietary fiber or iron.
*Percent Daily Values are based on a 2,000 calorie diet. Your daily values may be higher or lower depending on your calorie needs.

Water Ingredients

Natural spring water

Nutrition Facts
Serving Size 8 fl oz (250 ml)

Amount Per Serving	% DV*
Calories 0	
Total Fat 0g	0%
Sodium 0mg	0%
Total Carbohydrate 0g	0%
Sugars 0g	
Protein 0g	

*Percent Daily Values are based on a 2,000 calorie diet. Your daily values may be higher or lower depending on your calorie needs.

From L.W.Y. Cheung, H. Dart, S. Kalin, and S.L. Gortmaker, 2007, *Eat Well & Keep Moving,* 2nd ed. (Champaign, IL: Human Kinetics). Nutrition information retrieved from company Web sites on July 6, 2007: Gatorade, www.gatorade.com/products/gatorade_thirst_quencher/.

(continued)

Coca-Cola Ingredients

Carbonated water, high fructose corn syrup and/or sucrose, caramel color, phosphoric acid, natural flavors, caffeine

Note: This drink may be sold in bottles that contain more than one serving. A 24-ounce bottle contains 78 grams of sugar.

Nutrition Facts
Serving Size 12 fl oz (375 ml)

Amount Per Serving	% DV*
Calories 110	
Total Fat 0g	0%
Sodium 5mg	1%
Total Carbohydrate 29g	10%
Sugars 29g	
Protein 0g	

*Percent Daily Values are based on a 2,000 calorie diet. Your daily values may be higher or lower depending on your calorie needs.

McDonald's Low-Fat Chocolate Milk Ingredients

Low-fat milk, high fructose corn syrup, sugar, cocoa, cocoa processed with alkali, skim milk, carrageenan, salt, artificial flavor, vitamin A palmitate, vitamin D_3

Minute Maid Lemonade Ingredients

Pure filtered water, sweeteners (high fructose corn syrup, sugar), lemon juice from concentrate, lemon pulp, natural flavors

Nutrition Facts
Serving Size 8 fl oz (250 ml)

Amount Per Serving	
Calories 170	
	% DV*
Total Fat 3g	4%
Saturated Fat 1.5g	9%
Trans Fat 0g	0%
Cholesterol 15mg	0%
Sodium 15mg	6%
Total Carbohydrate 26g	9%
Dietary Fiber 1g	3%
Sugars 25g	
Protein 8g	
Vitamin A 10% • Vitamin C 6%	
Calcium 30% • Iron 2%	
Vitamin D 25% • Phosphorus 25%	

*Percent Daily Values are based on a 2,000 calorie diet. Your daily values may be higher or lower depending on your calorie needs.

Nutrition Facts
Serving Size 8 fl oz (250 ml)

Amount Per Serving	
Calories 100	
	% Daily Value*
Total Fat 0g	0%
Sodium 15mg	1%
Total Carbohydrate 28g	19%
Sugars 27g	
Protein 0g	

*Percent Daily Values are based on a 2,000 calorie diet. Your daily values may be higher or lower depending on your calorie needs.

Note: This drink may be sold in bottles that contain more than one serving. A 20-ounce bottle contains 68 grams of sugar.

From L.W.Y. Cheung, H. Dart, S. Kalin, and S.L. Gortmaker, 2007, *Eat Well & Keep Moving*, 2nd ed. (Champaign, IL: Human Kinetics). Nutrition information retrieved from company Web sites on July 6, 2007: Coca Cola, www.thecoca-colacompany.com/us_nutrition.html; McDonald's low-fat chocolate milk, www.mcdonalds.com/usa/eat/nutrition_info.html; Minute Maid Lemonade, www.minutemaid.com/productsMain. jsp?group=Variety_Juices_and_Drinks.

3 WORKSHEET

SOLUTIONS

Beverage Buzz

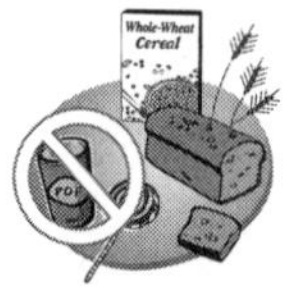
Whole-Wheat Cereal

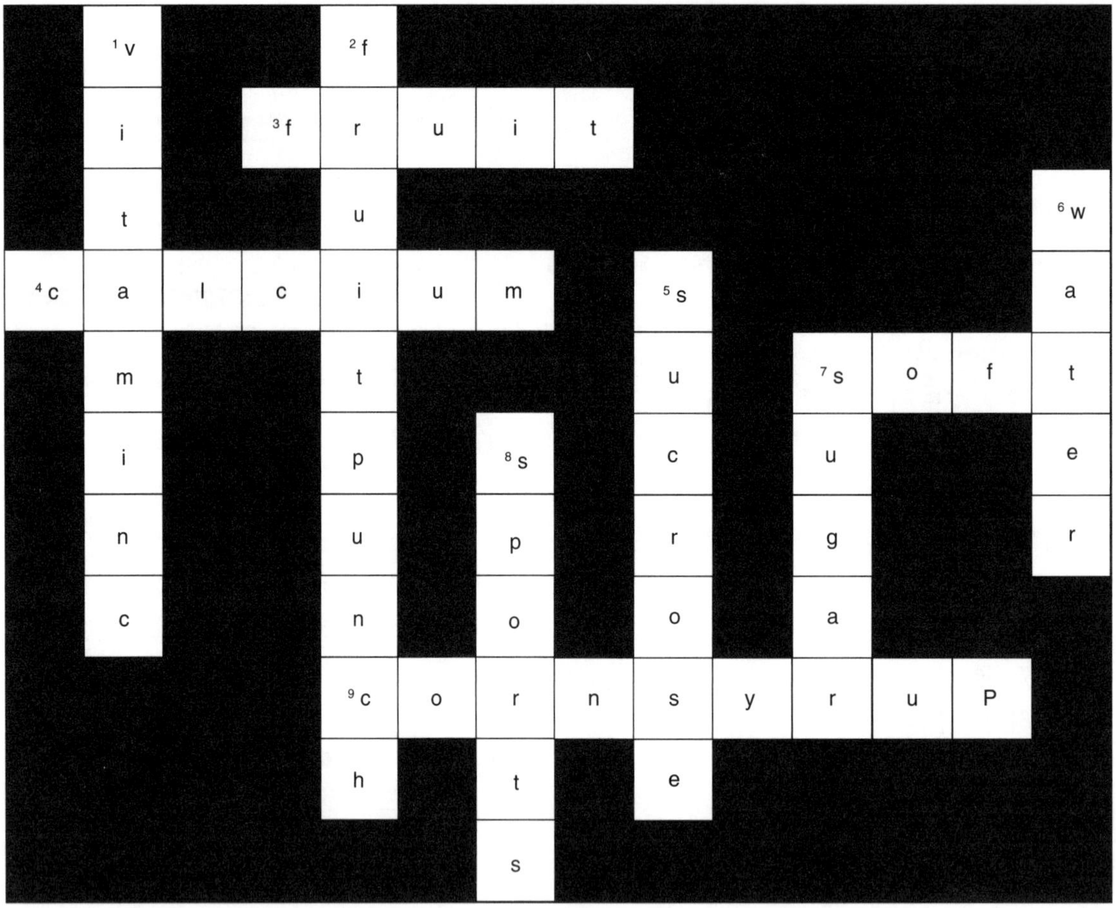
1 vitaminc
2 fruitpunch
3 fruit
4 calcium
5 sucrose
6 water
7 soft
7 sugar
8 sports
9 cornsyruP

From L.W.Y. Cheung, H. Dart, S. Kalin, and S.L. Gortmaker, 2007, *Eat Well & Keep Moving,* 2nd ed. (Champaign, IL: Human Kinetics).

Evaluating Media Advertising

Media messages can be evaluated by considering five key questions and five core concepts.

Five Key Questions

1. Who created this message?

2. What creative techniques are used to attract my attention?

3. How might different people understand this message differently from me?

4. What values, lifestyles, and points of view are represented in, or omitted from, this message?

5. Why is this message being sent?

Five Core Concepts

1. All media messages are constructed.

2. Media messages are constructed using a creative language with its own rules.

3. Different people experience the same media message differently.

4. Media messages have embedded values and points of view.

5. Most media messages are organized to gain profit or power (or both).

From L.W.Y. Cheung, H. Dart, S. Kalin, and S.L. Gortmaker, 2007, *Eat Well & Keep Moving*, 2nd ed. (Champaign, IL: Human Kinetics). Adapted, by permission, from Center for Media Literacy, 2005. Available at www.medialit.org.

Supersized Soft Drinks

Growth in soft drink container size

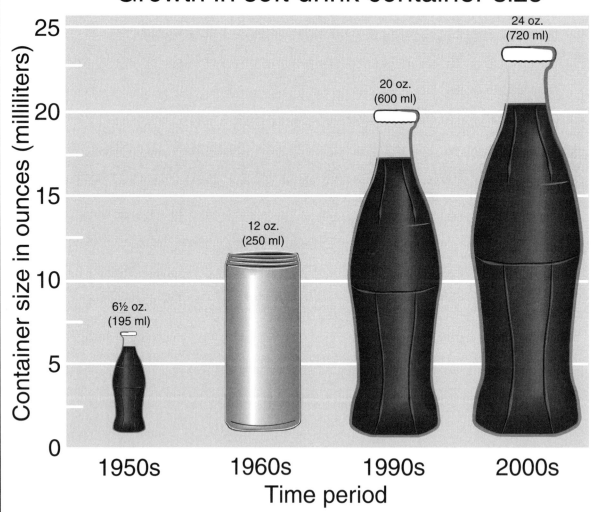

Container size in ounces (milliliters)

24 oz.
(720 ml)

20 oz.
(600 ml)

12 oz.
(250 ml)

6½ oz.
(195 ml)

25

20

15

10

5

0

1950s   1960s   1990s   2000s

Time period

From L.W.Y. Cheung, H. Dart, S. Kalin, and S.L. Gortmaker, 2007, *Eat Well & Keep Moving*, 2nd ed. (Champaign, IL: Human Kinetics). Reprinted, by permission, from Center for Science in the Public Interest. Retrieved April 10, 2007, from www.cspinet.org/new/pdf/liquid_candy_final_w_new_supplement.pdf.

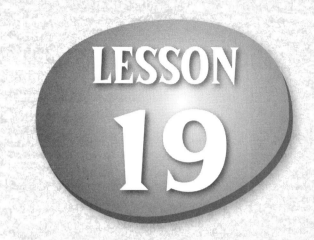

Snack Decisions

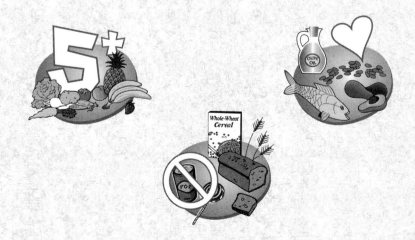

BACKGROUND

There are no 'bad' foods that should never be eaten. But most Americans eat too many foods that are high in saturated and trans fat, salt, and added sugar, and most Americans do not eat enough fruits, vegetables, and whole grains. Snack foods tend to have a lot of saturated and trans fat, salt, and added sugars and few vitamins or minerals. The purpose of this lesson is to help students make better snack choices by teaching them to recognize sources of unhealthy fat—namely, sources of saturated fat (which is solid at room temperature) and trans fat (partially hydrogenated vegetable oils and shortening). Remember that most saturated fat comes from animal sources (including beef, chicken, pork, and dairy products). The few exceptions are coconut oil and palm oil, which are also rich in saturated fat. Since many commercial baked or fried foods are prepared with partially hydrogenated vegetable oils, they also are sources of trans fat. Reading food labels and ingredient lists is an effective way to compare the fat and nutrient content of various snack foods.

The column on the Nutrition Facts label headed % Daily Value (% DV) can quickly tell you if a food is high or low in the nutrients listed. If the % DV for a nutrient is 5 or less, the food is considered low in that nutrient. If the % DV is 20 or more, the food is high in that nutrient.

Whether or not a food fits into your diet depends on what other foods you eat. For most people, the daily goal is to choose foods that add up to 100% of the DV for total dietary fiber, vitamins, and minerals (especially vitamins A and C, calcium, and iron). For saturated fat and sodium, the goal is to choose foods that add up to less than 100% of the DV. (To calculate the % DV for saturated fat, see lesson 17.) The % DV is based on a diet of 2,000 calories per day.

There is no % DV for trans fat because it is unclear if there is any safe level of intake. But food labels list the number of grams of trans fat per serving. It is best to avoid foods that contain trans fat. Keep in mind that products made with partially hydrogenated oils can still claim "0 grams trans fat" if the product contains less than 0.5 grams of trans fat per serving. These small amounts of trans fat can add up over the day. So make sure to watch out for the words *partially hydrogenated vegetable oil;* or *partially hydogenated soybean, cottonseed,* or other oils; or *shortening* in the ingredients list. Choose an alternative product that does not contain partially hydrogenated oil, especially if it is a product you consume regularly.

Added sugar comes in many forms—sugar (or sucrose), high fructose corn syrup, dextrose, and honey are all examples of added sugar (see worksheet 2 in lesson 7, page 116, for a list of the various names for sugar). The ingredients list on the food package can be used to identify added sugars; since ingredients are listed in descending order of quantity (by weight), we can get an idea of the quantity of added sugars from their relative position on the ingredients list. A good rule of thumb is to avoid snacks and other foods that list sugar (in some form) as one of the first three ingredients.

ESTIMATED TEACHING TIME AND RELATED SUBJECT AREA

Estimated teaching time: 1 hour, 10 minutes

Related subject area: language arts

OBJECTIVES

1. Students will examine a list of food selections to identify those with high nutritional value.

2. Students will be able to apply the Collect-Consider-Compare-Decide model when choosing snack foods.

3. Students will write a formal letter in support of healthy snacks.

MATERIALS

1. Decision-making steps written on a large poster board:
   Collect information.
   Consider nutrients.
   Compare to other choices.
   Decide what to choose.

2. Transparency 1, Reading Food Labels

3. Worksheet 1, Healthy Snacks Vending Machine Company

4. Worksheet 2, Take a Stand!

5. Worksheet 3, Investigating TV Ads (for extension activity)

6. Handout 1, Common Snacks Nutrient Chart

7. Handout 2, Snack Food Comparison Labels (for extension activity)

8. Sample snack food labels (have a variety available plus ask students to bring some from home)

PROCEDURE

PART I

1. Tell the students that sometimes during work or school hours, people take a break. This break may be called a *snack break, rest break,* or *time-out.*

2. Have the students say what they think happens during a break from work or play. List the students' suggestions on the board.

3. Have the students tell why a pause or break is a healthy practice. Emphasize that the body's needs—such as rest and food—may be addressed during breaks.

4. Have students name some snacks they might enjoy during a work or play break. Write down the students' choices on the board.

PART II

1. Explain to the students that they will be in charge of choosing snacks for the snack machines of the Healthy Snacks Vending Machine Company. Tell the students, "The workers need snacks that will strengthen their bones and muscles and give them lots of vitamins A, B, and C. Since the workers do a

lot of lifting and have to work for long hours, they want snacks that will also give them energy."

2. Display the decision-making steps (on poster board).

3. Show transparency 1, Reading Food Labels. Discuss % DV with students and tell them that it is a good tool for choosing healthy snacks.

The % DV that appears on food labels lets people find out whether a food is high or low in a nutrient. Regarding saturated fat, if the % DV is 5 or less for an individual food, then the food is considered low in saturated fat. The more foods chosen that have a % DV of 5 or less for saturated fat, the easier it is to eat a heart-healthy diet. The overall daily goal (for all the foods eaten in 1 day) is to select foods that add up to less than 100% of the DV for saturated fat.

The % DV also lets people find out whether a food is high or low in other nutrients, like vitamins A and C, calcium, and iron. If the % DV for any of these nutrients is 5 or less, the food is considered low in that nutrient. If the % DV is 20 or higher, the food is considered high in that nutrient. The overall daily goal (for all the foods eaten in 1 day) is to select foods that together reach 100% of the DV for these beneficial nutrients.

4. Distribute handout 1, Common Snacks Nutrient Chart. Select one of the snacks from the list and lead the students in applying the following step-by-step process to determine if the snack is a healthy choice:

Collect information: Study the label or read the nutrient chart (handout 1).

Consider nutrients: Think about the nutrient content. Healthful snacks need to be (1) low in saturated fat and free of trans fat, (2) good sources of vitamins and minerals, (3) moderate to low in added sugar, and (4) moderate to low in salt (foods with a % DV of 5 or less are considered low in sodium).

Compare other choices: What other choices do I have? Is there a better selection?

Decide what to choose: What is best for the body? Is this selection low in saturated and trans fat? Does it have added sugars? Does it contain whole grains? Is it a fruit or vegetable or a low-fat or nonfat dairy product?

5. Distribute worksheet 1, Healthy Snacks Vending Machine Company, and refer students to handout 1, Common Snacks Nutrient Chart, or to sample labels of snack foods (or to both). Have the students work in pairs or small groups to examine selections from the list of snacks. Ask the students to apply the decision-making process to come up with several healthy snacks for the vending machine, along with some snacks that should stay out. Students should be able to explain why they decided certain snacks were healthy and others were not.

6. After the pairs or groups have decided which snacks will be in their vending machines, have them share some of their findings with the rest of the class, referring to the steps of the decision-making model to explain their choices.

For example, students might say, "One of the snacks we analyzed was an orange. We consider this a good choice because we want something that is loaded with nutrients. We found that an orange has a lot vitamin C, about 100% of the DV. An orange can help workers meet the Principles of Healthy Living goal to eat 5 or more servings of fruits and vegetables each day, and it is a natural source of sugar that provides a quick but healthy boost of energy."

Students might also say, "We examined M&M candies as a snack. M&M's have a lot of added sugar, so they do provide energy, but the energy probably won't last long. Also, they have no vitamins or minerals, so they won't give our bodies any healthy nutrients. We decided that M&Ms wouldn't be a healthy choice."

SUMMARY

Ask students to write a formal letter using one of the following scenarios (distribute worksheet 2 so that the students may select their scenario—or you may assign scenarios if you like):

1. The school committee is considering a vending machine policy that prohibits unhealthy snacks and soft drinks. Some members of the committee, however, think that students should be able to make their own decisions, and they know that snack sales bring in a lot of money. You know that it is sometimes difficult to find healthy choices in the vending machine and you want to be able to eat well when at school. Write a letter to the school committee explaining why you support a healthy vending machine policy, and include some examples of healthy snacks that you would eat if they were available.

2. You went to the local football game for the first time and were surprised that chips, candy bars, soft drinks, and fruit punch were the only things available from the school-sponsored snack bar. Write a letter to the manager of the snack bar explaining why children and teenagers need snacks that provide vitamins and minerals without added sugars, saturated fat, and trans fat. Recommend some healthy snacks that the manager can sell.

3. You are part of a community group that needs to raise money. Some people want to sell candy bars, but you just learned that candy bars are a source of saturated and trans fat, a lot of sugar, and no beneficial nutrients. Write a letter to the fundraising leader to explain why selling candy is not a good idea for the children or the adults in the community. Come up with 1 or 2 other fundraising ideas that do not promote unhealthy foods.

EXTENSION ACTIVITIES

1. Distribute worksheet 3, Investigating TV Ads, and have students record the number of snacks advertised on television during a 30-minute program.

    a. Discuss the types of unhealthy snacks advertised. Were any healthy snacks advertised? For additional ideas on discussing advertisements with students, refer to lesson 18, Teacher Resource Page 1, Evaluating Media Advertising, page 279.

    b. Group the students and have them create an advertisement for one of the healthy snack choices they selected while completing worksheet 1. The advertisement may be a poster (for a magazine or billboard) or a skit, rap, or song (for radio or television).

    c. Write a letter to the cafeteria manager (this may be done as a class) requesting permission to display the healthy snack posters in the cafeteria. For groups who created a television ad, provide a time for them to put on their skits for the class. Groups that created a radio ad may also write a letter to the principal requesting permission to deliver their radio message on the school's public announcement system.

2. Have students create a nutrition crossword puzzle that reinforces the important aspects of choosing healthful snacks. The puzzle may also contain nutrition and physical activity information learned in previous lessons.

3. Distribute handout 2, Snack Food Comparison Labels, or present two actual food labels (one food should be high in saturated and trans fat and one low in saturated and trans fat). Have the students write a paragraph explaining why one is a better choice than the other for a person trying to eat a diet low in saturated and trans fat.

Reading Food Labels

Nutrition Facts

Serving Size (1 cup) (228g) ——————————— | Serving size |

Servings Per Container (2) ——————————— | Servings per container |

Amount Per Serving

Calories 250   Calories from Fat 120

| | % Daily Value* |

Total Fat 13g — 20%

Saturated fat per serving — Saturated Fat (3g) — (15%)

Trans fat per serving: Choose foods that have 0g of *trans* fat — *Trans* Fat (3g)

Cholesterol 31mg — 10%

Sodium 470mg — 20%

Total Carbohydrate 31g — 10%

   Dietary Fiber 0g — 0%

   Sugars 5g

Protein 5g

Vitamin A 4%   •   Vitamin C 2%

Calcium 15%   •   Iron 4%

% DV of saturated fat:
Foods with a DV for saturated fat of 5 or less are low in saturated fat. Foods with a % DV for saturated fat of 20 or more are high in saturated fat. The daily goal is to choose foods that together contain less than 100% of the DV for saturated fat.

% DV of vitamins and minerals:
The daily goal is to choose foods that add up to 100% of the DV for vitamins A and C and for iron and calcium. Foods with a % DV of 5 or less are low in these nutrients. Foods with a % DV of 20 or more are high in these nutrients.

*Percent Daily Values are based on a 2,000 calorie diet. Your daily values may be higher or lower depending on your calorie needs:

	Calories	2,000	2,500
Total Fat	Less than	65g	80g
Sat. Fat	Less than	20g	25g
Cholesterol	Less than	300mg	300mg
Sodium	Less than	2,400mg	2,400mg
Total Carbohydrate		300g	375g
Dietary Fiber		25g	30g

Calories per gram:
Fat 9 • Carbohydrate 4 • Protein 4

From L.W.Y. Cheung, H. Dart, S. Kalin, and S.L. Gortmaker, 2007, *Eat Well & Keep Moving*, 2nd ed. (Champaign, IL: Human Kinetics). http://cfsan.fda.gov/~dms.labtr.html.

Name _____

Healthy Snacks Vending Machine Company

You need to stock snacks in a company for workers who need snacks that will strengthen their bones and muscles and give them lots of vitamins A, B, and C. Since workers need to do a lot of lifting and have to work for long hours, they want snacks that will also give them lasting energy.

Directions

Review the list of snack options and use the Collect-Consider-Compare-Decide method to come up with four healthy snacks to put in the vending machines and two snacks to leave out. Write your final snack choices on the Healthy Vending Machine Company Order Form. Explain why or why not you included each food in the vending machine.

▶**TABLE 19.1 Healthy Vending Machine Company Order Form**

YES! Put these healthy snacks in!

NO! Keep these snacks out!

From L.W.Y. Cheung, H. Dart, S. Kalin, and S.L. Gortmaker, 2007, *Eat Well & Keep Moving,* 2nd ed. (Champaign, IL: Human Kinetics).

Name _____

Take a Stand!

Write a formal letter that addresses one of the following problems and provides the person who will receive the letter with information that supports your case. Choose one of the following scenarios (or address the one your teacher assigned to you):

1. The school committee is considering a vending machine policy that prohibits unhealthy snacks and soft drinks. Some members of the committee, however, think that students should be able to make their own decisions, and they know that snack sales bring in a lot of money. You know that it is sometimes difficult to find healthy choices in the vending machine and you want to be able to eat well when at school. Write a letter to the school committee explaining why you support a healthy vending machine policy, and include some examples of healthy snacks that you would eat if they were available.

2. You went to the local football game for the first time and were surprised that chips, candy bars, soft drinks, and fruit punch were the only things available from the school-sponsored snack bar. Write a letter to the manager of the snack bar explaining why children and teens need snacks that provide vitamins and minerals without added sugars, saturated fat, and trans fat. Recommend some healthy snacks that the manager can sell.

3. You are part of a community group that needs to raise money. Some people want to sell candy bars, but you just learned that candy bars are a source of saturated and trans fat, a lot of sugar, and no beneficial nutrients. Write a letter to the fundraising leader to explain why selling candy is not a good idea for the children or the adults in the community. Come up with 1 or 2 other fundraising ideas that do not promote unhealthy foods.

Following are some tips for getting started:

▶ Include a return address and date on your letter.

▶ Include the name and title of the person you are writing (for example, begin with "Dear Mr. Smith" or "Dear Snack Bar Manager").

▶ State why you are writing the letter; what is the issue?

▶ State what the problem is and provide information for the reader to understand why you feel the way you do.

▶ Offer your recommendation.

▶ Close the letter ("Sincerely," your name) and sign and print your full name.

From L.W.Y. Cheung, H. Dart, S. Kalin, and S.L. Gortmaker, 2007, *Eat Well & Keep Moving,* 2nd ed. (Champaign, IL: Human Kinetics).

Name _____

Investigating TV Ads

The next time you watch television, use table 19.2, TV Ad Tracking Chart, to record the food advertisements that are shown during a 30-minute program. Each time you see a food or drink advertisement, mark the appropriate column (healthy drinks, sugary drinks, healthy snacks and other foods, unhealthy snacks or fast foods). At the end of the show, write the number of ads that you saw in each category and the total number of food ads that you viewed during the 30-minute television show.

Name of show: _____ Day: _____ Time: _____

▶ TABLE 19.2 TV Ad Tracking Chart

Healthy drinks	Sugary drinks
Examples: milk, 100% fruit juice, water	Examples: soft drinks, fruit punches, sports drinks, energy drinks
Healthy snacks and other foods	**Unhealthy snacks or fast foods**
Examples: fruits, vegetables, whole-grain crackers or cereal, yogurt	Examples: chips, candy bars, fruit leathers or roll-ups, fast-food restaurants or meals

Number of advertisements for healthy drinks: _____

Number of advertisements for sugary drinks: _____

Number of advertisements for healthy snacks and other foods: _____

Number of advertisements for unhealthy snacks or fast foods: _____

Total number of food advertisements: _____

From L.W.Y. Cheung, H. Dart, S. Kalin, and S.L. Gortmaker, 2007, *Eat Well & Keep Moving,* 2nd ed. (Champaign, IL: Human Kinetics).

▶ TABLE 19.3 Common Snacks Nutrient Chart

Snack	Total calories	Added sugars (g)	Fat (g)	% DV	Saturated fat (g)	% DV	Trans fat (g)	Vitamin A (IU)	% DV	Vitamin C (mg)	% DV	Calcium (mg)	% DV	Iron (mg)	% DV	Sodium (mg)	% DV
Lay's potato chips (1 oz., or 30g, bag)	150	—	10	15%	3	15%	—	—	—	10	17%	8	1%	0.55	3%	207	9%
Cheetos (1 oz., or 30g, bag)	160	—	10	15%	1.5	8%	***	83	2%	1	2%	17	17%	0.75	4%	368	15%
Chocolate cupcakes (2)	360	34	12	18%	2.5	12%	***	2	0%	—	—	43	4%	1.37	8%	490	20%
Popcorn, unbuttered (1 cup)	54	—	0.7	1%	—	—	—	—	—	0.06	0%	2	0%	.4	2%	Trace	—
Almonds, unsalted (3 tbsp, or 15g)	180	—	16	25%	1	5%	—	Trace	—	Trace	—	10	1%	—	—	138	6%
Mixed nuts (30 nuts)	179	—	15	23%	2	10%	—	—	—	Trace	—	14	1%	0.5	3%	2	0%
Pear (1 medium)	98	—	0.7	1%	—	—	—	33	0%	7	12%	19	2%	0.41	2%	1	0%
Spinach (1 cup)	19	—	—	—	—	—	—	5,354	129%	13	23%	86	8%	1.9	11%	—	—
Oreo cookies (34g)	160	14	7	11%	2	10%	—	30	0%	—	—	24	2%	0.38	2%	114	5%

(continued)

*** These products have zero grams of trans fat per serving but list partially hydrogenated oil in their ingredients.

From L.W.Y. Cheung, H. Dart, S. Kalin, and S.L. Gortmaker, 2007, *Eat Well & Keep Moving*, 2nd ed. (Champaign, IL: Human Kinetics). Nutrition information from brand name foods retrieved from company Web sites, March 18, 2007: Pepperidge Farm Goldfish, www.campbellwellness.com/product-list.asp?brandID=4&brandCatID=821&productID=120276&catID=373; Ritz Bitz Cheese Crackers, www.nabiscoworld.com/Brands/brandlist.aspx?SiteId=1&CatalogType=1&BrandKey=ritzbits&BrandLink=/ritzbits/&BrandId=82&PageNo=1; Cheetos, www.fritolay.com/fl/flstore/cgi-bin/products_cheetos.htm; Coca-Cola, www.thecoca-colacompany.com/us_nutrition.html; Dunkin' Donuts, www.dunkindonuts.com/aboutus/nutrition/; Lay's potato chips, www.fritolay.com/fl/flstore/cgi-bin/products_lays.htm; M&M, http://us.mms.com/us/about/products/; Oreos, www.nabiscoworld.com/Brands/default.aspx; Snyder's 12-grain pretzels, www.snydersofhanover.com/en/products.php?cat=1&id=11; Triscuit, www.nabiscoworld.com/Brands/brandlist.aspx?SiteId=1&CatalogType=1&BrandKey=triscuit&BrandLink=/triscuit/&BrandId=91&PageNo=1; York, www.hersheys.com/products/details/york.asp.

(continued)

► TABLE 19.3   Common Snacks Nutrient Chart   (continued)

Snack	Total calories	Added sugars (g)	Fat (g)	% DV	Saturated fat (g)	% DV	Trans fat (g)	Vitamin A (IU)	% DV	Vitamin C (mg)	% DV	Calcium (mg)	% DV	Iron (mg)	% DV	Sodium (mg)	% DV
Peanut butter sandwich cookies (28g)	130	8	5	8%	1.5	8%	***	—	—	—	—	—	—	0.75	4%	110	5%
Coca-Cola (12 oz., or 375 ml)	145	40.5	—	—	—	—	—	—	—	—	—	—	—	—	—	33	2%
Spring water (12 oz., or 375 ml)	—	—	—	—	—	—	—	—	—	—	—	—	—	—	—	1	0%
Fig bar cookies (2)	130	9.6	2.5	4%	~0.5	3%	***	—	—	~0.06	0%	14	1%	—	—	138	6%
York Peppermint Pattie (1)	160	25	3	5%	1.5	8%	—	—	—	—	—	—	—	—	—	—	—
M&M candies (1.7 oz., or 51g)	240	31	10	15%	6	30%	0	—	—	—	—	—	—	—	—	—	—
Chocolate chip cookies (34g)	160	11	8	12%	2.5	13%	***	—	—	—	—	—	—	0.7	4%	110	5%
Sunflower seeds (1 oz., or 30g)	161	1	14	22%	1	7%	0	—	—	14	23%	34	3%	1.99	11%	220	10%
Orange (1 medium)	59	0	0.4	0%	—	—	0	278	6%	59	98%	48	5%	0.11	1%	—	—
Orange juice, frozen (8 oz., or 250 ml)	112	0	0.1	0%	—	—	0	194	4%	97	162%	22	2%	0.24	1%	2	0%

(continued)

*** These products have zero grams of trans fat per serving but list partially hydrogenated oil in their ingredients.

From L.W.Y. Cheung, H. Dart, S. Kalin, and S.L. Gortmaker, 2007, *Eat Well & Keep Moving*, 2nd ed. (Champaign, IL: Human Kinetics). Nutrition information from brand name foods retrieved from company Web sites, March 18, 2007: Pepperidge Farm Goldfish, www.campbellwellness.com/product-list.asp?brandID=4&brandCatID=821&productID=120276&catID=373; Ritz Bitz Cheese Crackers, www.nabiscoworld.com/Brands/brandlist.aspx?SiteId=1&CatalogType=1&BrandKey=ritzbits&BrandLink=/ritzbits/&BrandId=82&PageNo=1; Cheetos, www.fritolay.com/fl/flstore/cgi-bin/products_cheetos.htm; Coca-Cola, www.thecoca-colacompany.com/us_nutrition.html; Dunkin' Donuts, www.dunkindonuts.com/aboutus/nutrition/; Lay's potato chips, www.fritolay.com/fl/flstore/cgi-bin/products_lays.htm; M&M, http://us.mms.com/us/about/products/; Oreos, www.nabiscoworld.com/Brands/default.aspx; Snyder's 12-grain pretzels, www.snydersofhanover.com/en/products.php?cat=1&id=11; Triscuit, www.nabiscoworld.com/Brands/brandlist.aspx?SiteId=1&CatalogType=1&BrandKey=triscuit&BrandLink=/triscuit/&BrandId=91&PageNo=1; York, www.hersheys.com/products/details/york.asp.

(continued)

▶ TABLE 19.3   Common Snacks Nutrient Chart (continued)

Snack	Total calories	Added sugars (g)	Fat (g)		Saturated fat (g)		Trans fat (g)	Vitamin A (IU)		Vitamin C (mg)		Calcium (mg)		Iron (mg)		Sodium (mg)	
				% DV		% DV			% DV		% DV		% DV		% DV		% DV
Carrots (1 large)	42	0	0.2	0%	—	—	0	11,000	220%	8	13%	37	4%	0.7	4%	37	2%
Beef hot dog (1)	140	0	13	20%	6	30%	1	—	—	11	18%	75	8%	1.5	8%	868	36%
Celery sticks (1 stalk)	8	0	0.01	0%	—	—	0	120	2%	5	8%	20	2%	0.2	1%	63	3%
Snyder's multi-grain pretzels (1 oz., or 30g)	120	2	2	3%	—	—	0	—	—	—	—	—	1%	—	4%	170	28%
Dunkin' Donuts doughnut (with sugar icing) (1)	180	6	8	12%	1.5	8%	4	3	0%	—	—	—	—	0.7	4%	250	10%
Whole-grain Triscuit snack crackers (28g)	120	0	4.5	7%	0.5	4%	0	—	—	—	—	—	—	1.7	10%	180	7%
Banana (1 medium)	105	0	0.6	1%	—	—	0	92	2%	10	17%	7	1%	0.35	2%	1	0%
Apple (1 medium)	81	0	0.5	0%	—	—	0	74	1%	8	13%	10	1%	0.25	1%	1	0%
1% milk (1 cup)	110	0	2.5	4%	1.5	8%	0	500	10%	6	10%	300	30%	0.12	0%	125	5%
Grapes (1 cup)	58	0	0.3	0%	—	—	0	92	2%	4	7%	13	1%	0.27	2%	2	0%
Hamburger	260	7	9	14%	3.5	17%	0.5	82	5%	2	13%	51	22%	15	87%	530	11%

*** These products have zero grams of trans fat per serving but list partially hydrogenated oil in their ingredients.

Snack Food Comparison Labels

Pepperidge Farm Whole-Grain Goldfish Crackers

Nutrition Facts

Serving Size 55 pieces (30 g/1.1 oz)

Amount Per Serving

Calories 140   Calories from Fat 45

	% DV*
Total Fat 5g	**8%**
Saturated Fat 1g	**5%**
Trans Fat 0g	
Polysaturated Fat 1.5g	
Monounsaturated Fat 2.5g	
Cholesterol <5mg	**1%**
Sodium 250mg	**10%**
Total Carbohydrate 19g	**6%**
Dietary Fiber 2g	**7%**
Sugars <1g	
Protein 4g	

Calcium 4%   •   Iron 4%

*Percent Daily Values are based on a 2,000 calorie diet. Your daily values may be higher or lower depending on your calorie needs.

Ritz Bits Cracker Sandwiches Cheese

Nutrition Facts

Serving Size 42g
Servings per Container about 1

Amount Per Serving

Calories 220   Calories from Fat 110

	% DV*
Total Fat 13g	**20%**
Saturated Fat 4.5g	**23%**
Trans Fat 0g	
Cholesterol 5mg	**1%**
Sodium 480mg	**20%**
Total Carbohydrate 24g	**8%**
Dietary Fiber 1g	**2%**
Sugars 6g	
Protein 3g	

Calcium 8%   •   Iron 6%

*Percent Daily Values are based on a 2,000 calorie diet. Your daily values may be higher or lower depending on your calorie needs.

Ingredients: whole-grain wheat flour, unbleached enriched wheat flour (flour, niacin, reduced iron, thiamin mononitrate [vitamin B$_1$], riboflavin [vitamin B$_2$], folic acid), cheddar cheese ([pasteurized milk, cheese cultures, salt, enzymes], water, salt), vegetable oils (canola, sunflower, and/or soybean), contains 2% or less of: salt, yeast, autolyzed yeast, spice, leavening (baking soda, monocalcium phosphate, ammonium bicarbonate), annatto (color), onion powder, butter (milk), enzymes, sodium phosphate

Ingredients: enriched flour (wheat flour, niacin, reduced iron, thiamine mononitrate [vitamin B$_1$], riboflavin [vitamin B$_2$], folic acid), soybean and or palm oil, whey, sugar, partially hydrogenated cottonseed oil, high fructose corn syrup, milkfat and/or sunflower oil, salt, cheddar cheese (made from cultured milk, salt, and enzymes), leavening (baking soda, calcium phosphate), buttermilk, contains less than 0.5% of the following: disodium phosphate, natural flavor, soy lecithin (emulsifier), maltodextrin, artificial color (includes yellow 6), modified cornstarch

From L.W.Y. Cheung, H. Dart, S. Kalin, and S.L. Gortmaker, 2007, *Eat Well & Keep Moving,* 2nd ed. (Champaign, IL: Human Kinetics). Nutrition information retrieved from package and/or company Web sites on July 6, 2007: Campbell's, www.campbellwellness.com/product-list.asp?brandID=4&brandCatID=821&productID=120276&catID=373.; Nabisco, www.nabiscoworld.com/./Brands/ProductInformation. aspx?BrandKey=ritzbits&Site=1&Products=4400000958.

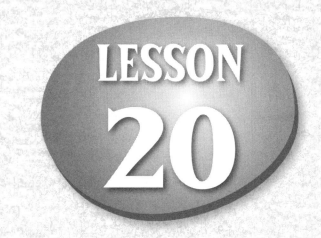

Snacking and Inactivity

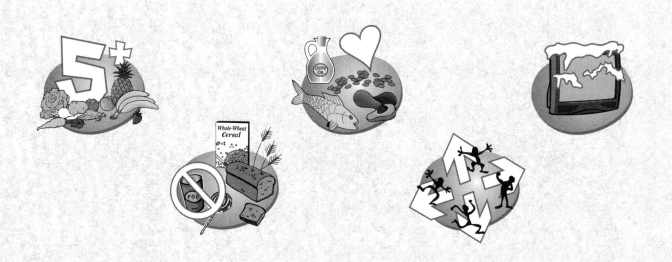

BACKGROUND

Students need energy to think, learn, and grow. Snacks are a very important part of a growing child's diet. The usual snacks students choose, however, are not optimal for good health. Students most frequently snack on chips, soft drinks, and other foods high in sugar, salt, and saturated or trans fat. But they should choose snacks that are low in saturated and trans fat and high in the nutrients the body needs for good health (like fruits, vegetables, whole grains, low-fat dairy products, and 100% juices; limit juice to no more than 8 ounces per day).

At the same time, students must be encouraged to be physically active—to keep moving. Children should get at least 60 minutes of physical activity every day; these 60 minutes should include moderate- and vigorous-intensity activities and can be accumulated throughout the day in sessions of 15 minutes or longer. Yet more and more students spend their days in inactive ways. In an average year, students spend more time watching TV than they spend attending school.

Students should not only snack on nutritious foods but also choose to be physically active every day. This lesson stresses making healthy snack choices and being physically active every day. In the first part of the lesson, the teacher and class discuss the students' actual snacking and physical activity habits. In the second part of the lesson, students play the Snack-n-Act game, in which they pick out healthful snacks and activities from a pile of healthful and unhealthful choices. Before the game, students are guided through a warm-up exercise. After the game, students are guided through a cool-down session.

ESTIMATED TEACHING TIME AND RELATED SUBJECT AREAS

Estimated teaching time: 1 hour

Related subject areas: physical education, language arts

OBJECTIVES

1. The students will be able to choose a variety of healthy snacks.
2. The students will identify snacks that are less nutritious.
3. The students will identify active and inactive after-school pastimes.
4. The students will perform an endurance workout while pacing themselves during the fitness activity.
5. The students will demonstrate a pace that works for them so that they can move for a long time without stopping.

MATERIALS

1. Nutritious (low in saturated and trans fat, high in fiber, or a whole grain) and less nutritious (high in saturated and trans fat, high in sugar, or a refined grain) snack choices cards (provided)
2. Active and inactive after-school pastime cards (provided)

3. Ten boxes (places for students to put cards)—five with smiling faces, five with frowning faces

4. Diagrams of stretches (see appendix A, pages 565-567)

PROCEDURE

1. Discuss the following with students: Do they snack after school? Why do they snack after school? What snacks do they eat?

2. Review the five food groups and name snacks that come from the different food groups (see page 8 for an overview of the best choice foods in each food group).

3. Discuss the following with students: What do they do after school? Do they have active lifestyles or inactive lifestyles?

4. If students are snacking for energy, what are they doing with the energy? Are they sitting around or are they using the extra energy?

5. Lead the students in warm-up and stretching exercises.

    a. Warm-up—The first part of the safe workout, in which slow movements get the body ready for stretching and the fitness activity.
    What to Emphasize
    - Car analogy: Your body is like a cold car—warm it up and then move it!
    - If you do not warm up, you are more likely to get injured.
    - You should always warm up before exercising, even when you are at home.
    - Always do the movements very slowly to warm up.
    - For example, when beginning a bike ride, warm up by riding slowly at first.
    - Likewise, when throwing a ball, throw slowly at first.

    b. Stretch—The part of the safe workout in which you do exercises that improve flexibility fitness and get the body ready for the fitness activity (see diagrams in appendix A, pages 565-569).
    What to Emphasize
    - Stretching improves flexibility fitness.
    - Activities such as riding a bike or doing push-ups do not improve flexibility.
    - Even if you aren't going to start a fitness activity, stretch at home while watching TV or when doing nothing in particular.
    - Hold stretches for 10 or more seconds.
    - Use slow movements; don't bounce.

6. Explain the Snack-n-Act game to students. This game stresses the importance of healthy snacking and physical activity. We are also playing the game so that we can learn the importance of nonstop movement. Endurance fitness activities are crucial for a healthy body. Remind students that they should get at least 1 hour of physical activity every day.

7. Have the students form five groups and have them stand in lines. Place a variety of the nutritious snack cards, less nutritious snack cards, active after-school pastime cards, and inactive after-school pastime cards on the opposite side of the room.

8. In front of each group line, place a box with a smiling face and one with a frowning face. Tell the students about the food and activity cards located on the opposite side of the room.

9. Tell the students that to play the game, each group member (one by one) will jog across the room, pick a food or activity card, jog back to the line, and place the card in the appropriate box. Each group has a box with a smiling face on it and a box with a frowning face—the frowning box is for the unhealthy snack and inactive after-school pastime choices, while the smiling box is for the healthy snack and active after-school pastime choices.

10. Begin the game. Tell the students to jog in place while waiting for their turn. Remember to stress that students should pace themselves.

11. Keep the game going until each group has received 4 or 5 turns, or until each student has had a turn (depending on how much time you have).

12. When the game is over, lead the students in a cool-down.

    a. Cool-down—The part of the safe workout in which your body slows down and recovers from the fitness activity.
       What to Emphasize
       - Move slowly. Walking is an excellent cool-down activity.
       - Remember to cool down after exercising at home.

    b. Cool-down stretch—The last part of the safe workout, in which you do exercises that improve flexibility fitness (see appendix A, pages 565-569).
       What to Emphasize
       - Stretching after an activity is especially important; it improves flexibility fitness and helps you recover faster.
       - Activities such as riding a bike or doing push-ups do not improve flexibility.
       - Hold stretches for 10 or more seconds.
       - Use slow movements; don't bounce.

13. After the cool-down, review the contents of the boxes. Discuss any wrong choices.

Nutritious Snack Choices

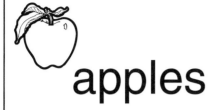 apples

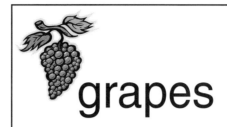 grapes

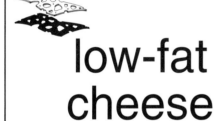 100% fruit juice

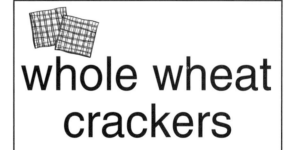 frozen fruit bars

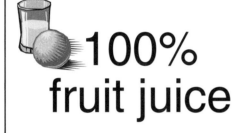 low-fat cheese

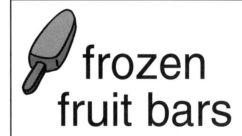 whole wheat crackers

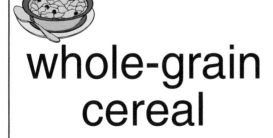 whole-grain cereal

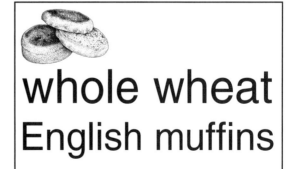 whole wheat English muffins

From L.W.Y. Cheung, H. Dart, S. Kalin, and S.L. Gortmaker, 2007, *Eat Well & Keep Moving*, 2nd ed. (Champaign, IL: Human Kinetics).

(continued)

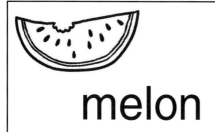 melon

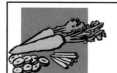 carrots

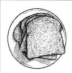 whole wheat toast

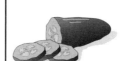 cucumber slices

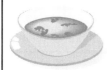 vegetable soup

 low-fat yogurt

 multigrain bagel

 orange

From L.W.Y. Cheung, H. Dart, S. Kalin, and S.L. Gortmaker, 2007, *Eat Well & Keep Moving*, 2nd ed. (Champaign, IL: Human Kinetics).

(continued)

whole-wheat pretzels

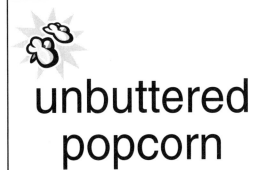

unbuttered popcorn

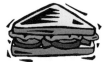

banana

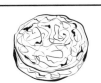

brown rice cakes

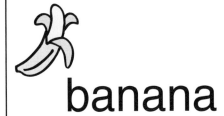

turkey sandwich
on
whole wheat bread

From L.W.Y. Cheung, H. Dart, S. Kalin, and S.L. Gortmaker, 2007, *Eat Well & Keep Moving*, 2nd ed. (Champaign, IL: Human Kinetics).

Less Nutritious Snack Choices

 soft drink

 potato chips

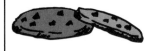 cookies

 cake

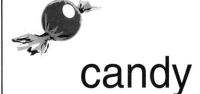 candy

 cheese puffs

 brownies

 cupcakes

From L.W.Y. Cheung, H. Dart, S. Kalin, and S.L. Gortmaker, 2007, *Eat Well & Keep Moving*, 2nd ed. (Champaign, IL: Human Kinetics).

(continued)

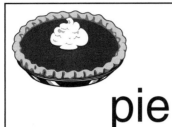 pie

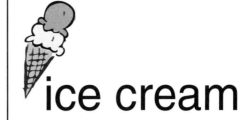 ice cream

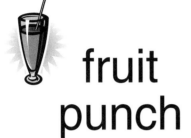 fruit punch

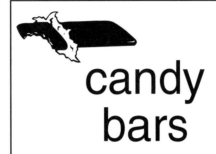 candy bars

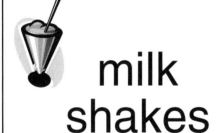 milk shakes

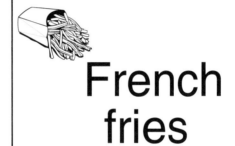 French fries

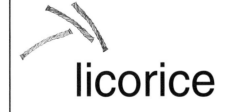 licorice

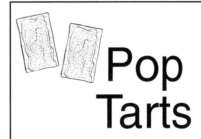 Pop Tarts

Active After-School Pastimes

bike riding	jumping rope
walking	running
skating	swimming
playing basketball	dancing
playing hockey	doing yoga

From L.W.Y. Cheung, H. Dart, S. Kalin, and S.L. Gortmaker, 2007, *Eat Well & Keep Moving*, 2nd ed. (Champaign, IL: Human Kinetics).

(continued)

doing chores	playing catch
tossing a Frisbee	playing baseball
playing kickball	playing soccer
playing tag	playing hopscotch

From L.W.Y. Cheung, H. Dart, S. Kalin, and S.L. Gortmaker, 2007, *Eat Well & Keep Moving*, 2nd ed. (Champaign, IL: Human Kinetics).

Inactive After-School Pastimes

watching TV	sitting on the couch
playing video games	watching music videos
watching movies	sitting around doing nothing
napping	getting a ride everywhere
playing computer games	surfing the Web

From L.W.Y. Cheung, H. Dart, S. Kalin, and S.L. Gortmaker, 2007, *Eat Well & Keep Moving*, 2nd ed. (Champaign, IL: Human Kinetics).

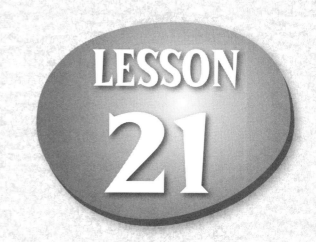

Freeze My TV

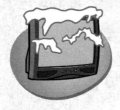

BACKGROUND

In the United States, children watch about 4 hours of TV every day. And this doesn't even count other screen time, like surfing the Web, instant messaging, and playing video games. When added up, TV and other screen time have basically become a full-time job!

And our children are suffering because of it. On average, American youths spend more time watching television each year than they spend in school. This tendency toward an inactive or sedentary lifestyle is a contributing factor to more and more children being overweight. The more television a child watches, the more likely he will be overweight. The increase in television viewing has also been associated with elevated cholesterol levels and poor cardiorespiratory fitness in youths and less time spent reading and doing homework.

To combat inactivity, young people should be encouraged to consider healthy alternatives to television viewing and other screen activities, particularly choices that involve more physical activity. Children should limit television and other screen time to no more than 2 hours per day; less is better.

ESTIMATED TEACHING TIME AND RELATED SUBJECT AREAS

Estimated teaching time: 1 hour, 15 minutes

Related subject areas: math, language arts, art, social studies

OBJECTIVES

1. Students will analyze their leisure time to identify hours spent watching television as well as participating in other screen activities like surfing the Web, instant messaging, and playing video games.

2. Students will create a list of alternative activities to consider instead of watching television.

MATERIALS

1. Transparency 1, Couch Potato
2. Transparency 2, Instead of Watching TV, I Could
3. TV guide or TV section of the newspaper
4. Worksheet 1, Time to Get Active
5. Worksheet 2, Television Blackout Tracking
6. Colored stick-on dots (optional)
7. Worksheet 3, Tell Your Friend About TV Blackout Time
8. Worksheet 4, What Did You Do Instead of Watching TV?

PROCEDURE

PART I: MOTIVATION

1. Display transparency 1, Couch Potato, and ask students to discuss the message.

2. Have students suggest as many words or phrases as possible to describe a couch potato. You may want to use a Web or other graphic organizer to record their suggestions.

3. Have students comment on their television habits by identifying shows that they frequently watch.

4. Ask students if they think they can be called a *couch potato*. Have them explain why or why not.

PART II: CONCEPT DEVELOPMENT

1. Display a television guide and have students brainstorm a list of their favorite weekday and weeknight television programs.

   As the list is compiled, help students add to it by recalling programs that may have been left out.

2. Record the student responses on a blackboard chart with columns for each of the 7 days of the week. Be certain to list shows under the appropriate day of the week.

3. Have students review the list of programs and write down their 3 to 5 favorites for each day. Have them rate the shows, placing a number 1 next to their favorite show and a number 5 next to their fifth favorite show, and so on.

4. After days 1 and 2 have been completed, have students circle the numbers indicating the two shows (one per day) they would have the least difficulty giving up. (These will probably be the shows they ranked as their fourth or fifth favorites.)

   This activity may be lengthy. You may initiate it in class but then have the students finish it independently when they have completed other assigned work. Be certain that students have identified their 3 to 5 favorites for at least day 1 and day 2.

5. Briefly discuss with students why watching less TV and participating more in active alternatives might benefit their health. Encourage them to include the ideas that they are inactive and may tend to snack more than usual while watching television. Watching TV also provides less time to socialize with friends or family.

PART III: APPLICATION

1. Display transparency 2, Instead of Watching TV, I Could. Ask the students to brainstorm a list of alternative activities that they could do if they were not watching television. Encourage them to include all sorts of alternatives, such as hobbies, games, music, sports, reading, exercising, and so on. Let them know that other screen activities (watching DVDs, instant messaging, playing video games, and so on) do not count as TV alternatives and, in fact, should be limited (see the bonus activity described in part IV). Video games that require users to engage in moderate to vigorous physical activity, such as Dance, Dance Revolution (DDR), do count as an alternative to television. DDR is also a heart-healthy activity.

2. Write the student suggestions on the transparency. Have the students indicate whether each alternative involves physical activity (such as dancing, running, or playing basketball) or no physical activity (such as reading or playing a board game).

3. After the students have evaluated and described each activity, discuss the activities in terms of whether they are heart healthy (exercise the heart).

4. Distribute worksheet 1, Time to Get Active. Have the students estimate the number of waking hours in their day that could be classified as active and how many could be classified as inactive. (Have a student discuss the meaning of "inactive.") Have students make bar graphs to compare their inactive waking hours to their active hours. Ask the students to estimate the amount of time they have spent watching television and participating in other screen activities in their lifetimes, and have them explain how they came up with their answers. These graphs or charts and lifetime estimates can be used to emphasize the need to increase physical activity.

PART IV: TELEVISION BLACKOUT TRACKING

1. Refer the students to their previous list of their favorite 3 to 5 shows for each day and have them write the names of the shows on worksheet 2, Television Blackout Tracking. Instruct the students to circle the name of at least one show that they agree to give up each day.

2. Have the students review the list they made for transparency 2, Instead of Watching TV, I Could, and select those activities that they would like to try instead of watching television during one of their blackout times. Each student will write the alternative activities in the Alternatives spaces that follow the shows to be missed (on worksheet 2).

3. Ask the students to give up at least one 30-minute TV program each day. This is their TV blackout time. Explain that the following day each student will share with the rest of the class what she did as an alternative to watching TV. As a bonus activity, students can also give up 30 minutes of other screen activities like surfing the Web, instant messaging, and playing video games.

4. If you like, students may place a red sticker over the blackout selection on the tracking sheet if they successfully give up at least one 30-minute show per night. Give the students one sticker for every 30 minutes of TV they give up. You can give an additional sticker for each day a student gives up another screen activity.

Students who are not successful should be encouraged to try again the next day.

PART V: FOLLOW-UP

1. Discuss the Freeze My TV promotion with the students (see lesson 27).

2. Have the students create a poster that illustrates their involvement in an alternative activity during a TV blackout time and that encourages others to try similar activities instead of watching TV.

3. Distribute worksheet 3, Tell Your Friend About TV Blackout Time. Have the students write a letter to a friend discussing their self-selected alternatives

to watching television and how changing their television habits could affect their lives.

4. Have the students interview older relatives or neighbors about what they did as children to entertain themselves instead of watching television. As a class, have the students generate five questions to ask their older relatives or neighbors. Students can record the interview questions and the interviewees' answers on worksheet 4, What Did You Do Instead of Watching TV?

When students have gathered this information, have them work in small groups or as a class to organize the information into relevant categories and compile a Catalog of Activities. For example, the activities could be organized by time period in which the person grew up (1940s, 1950s, 1960s, 1970s, etc.) or location (city, state, or even country); by type of entertainment (hobbies, games, sports, reading, and so on); by whether the entertainment is active or inactive; or by whether the entertainment is something that students today would or would not enjoy.

For an extension to this activity, have students do additional research in the library/media center or on the Web about children's television-free pastimes throughout history.

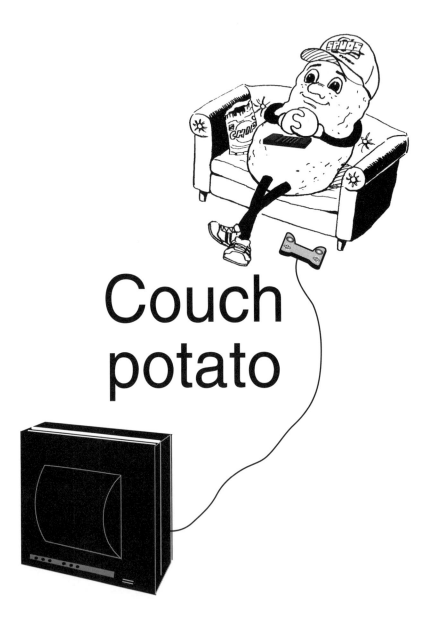

Couch potato

From L.W.Y. Cheung, H. Dart, S. Kalin, and S.L. Gortmaker, 2007, *Eat Well & Keep Moving,* 2nd ed. (Champaign, IL: Human Kinetics).

Instead of Watching TV, I Could

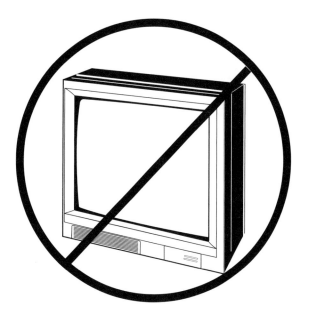

_____   _____
_____   _____
_____   _____
_____   _____
_____   _____
_____   _____
_____   _____
_____   _____
_____   _____
_____   _____

From L.W.Y. Cheung, H. Dart, S. Kalin, and S.L. Gortmaker, 2007, _Eat Well & Keep Moving_, 2nd ed. (Champaign, IL: Human Kinetics).

Name _____

Time to Get Active

1. Estimate the number of hours you spend sleeping each day, and the number of hours you spend awake.

2. Estimate how many of your waking hours could be classified as active.

3. Estimate how many of your waking hours could be classified as inactive.

4. Using the blank graph provided, create a bar graph to compare your active waking hours to your inactive waking hours. Use different colored pencils to represent active time and inactive time.

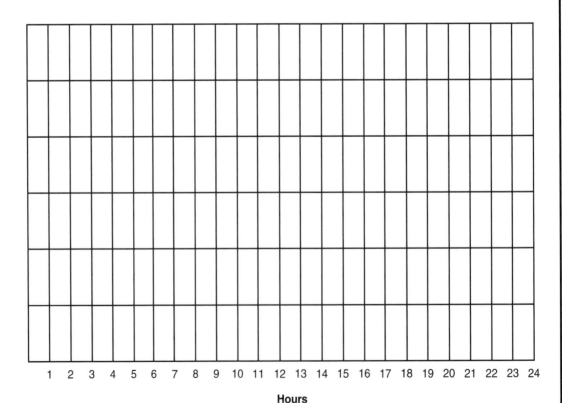

Hours

From L.W.Y. Cheung, H. Dart, S. Kalin, and S.L. Gortmaker, 2007, *Eat Well & Keep Moving,* 2nd ed. (Champaign, IL: Human Kinetics).

(continued)

5. Estimate how much time you have spent watching television and participating in other screen activities in your lifetime. Explain how you came up with your estimate.

6. Do you think you need to increase your active time and decrease your screen time?

(Circle one)   Yes   No

Write a statement explaining your answer.

_____

_____

_____

_____

_____

_____

_____

_____

_____

_____

Name _____

Television Blackout Tracking

Directions

For each day, write in the television shows you usually watch. For each day, circle one show to give up.

▶**TABLE 21.1 Television Blackout Tracking Chart**

Monday	Tuesday	Wednesday	Thursday	Friday	Saturday	Sunday
Alternatives						
Bonus: Mark the box for the day you also gave up 30 min. of other screen activities (like surfing the Web, instant messaging, watching DVDs, and playing video games).						

Tell Your Friend About TV Blackout Time

Directions

Write an informal letter to a friend that discusses your experiences during TV blackout time.

Following are some tips for getting started:

▶ Include a return address and date on your letter.

▶ Include the first name of the friend you are writing ("Dear Lee" or "Dear Maria").

▶ State why you are writing the letter.

▶ Write about your personal experience giving up television. Was it difficult for you to give up watching television? What did you do instead of watching TV? Did you miss watching TV? Give details to support your description of your TV blackout experience.

▶ Write about how changing TV habits could affect your life.

▶ Close the letter ("Sincerely," or "Best regards," or "Your friend") and sign your name.

From L.W.Y. Cheung, H. Dart, S. Kalin, and S.L. Gortmaker, 2007, *Eat Well & Keep Moving,* 2nd ed. (Champaign, IL: Human Kinetics).

Name _____

What Did You Do Instead of Watching TV?

Directions

Interview an older relative or neighbor about what they did to entertain themselves without television when they were young. Write down the questions you are going to ask, and then write down the person's response to each question. Be sure to ask the person's name and current age, and ask where the person grew up.

Name of person interviewed: _____

Age of person interviewed: _____

Where did this person grow up? (City, State, and Country) _____

_____

Question 1: _____

Response to Question 1:

_____

_____

_____

_____

_____

Question 2 : _____

Response to Question 2:

_____

_____

_____

_____

_____

(continued)

Question 3: _____

Response to Question 3:

_____

_____

_____

_____

_____

Question 4: _____

Response to Question 4:

_____

_____

_____

_____

_____

Question 5:_____

Response to Question 5:

_____

_____

_____

_____

_____

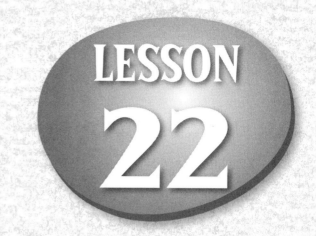

Menu Monitoring

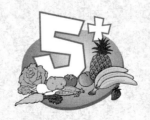

BACKGROUND

Whole-grain products, vegetables, and fruits are key parts of a varied and healthful diet. They provide vitamins, minerals, fiber, and other substances that are vital for good health. They are also generally low in saturated and trans fat, depending on how they are prepared and what is added to them at the table. Most Americans eat fewer than the recommended number of servings of whole-grain products, vegetables, and fruits, even though the consumption of these foods is associated with a substantially lower risk for many chronic diseases, including heart disease, high blood pressure, and possibly some cancers.

Fruits and vegetables are naturally low in unhealthy fat and provide many essential nutrients and other food components important for health. These foods are excellent sources of vitamin C, vitamin B_6, carotenoids (including those that form vitamin A), and folate. The antioxidants found in plant foods (e.g., vitamin C, carotenoids, vitamin E, and certain minerals) are of great interest to scientists and the public because of their potentially beneficial role in reducing the risk for some cancers and other chronic diseases. Scientists are also trying to determine if other substances in plant foods (phytochemicals) protect against high blood pressure, heart disease, and possibly some cancers.

THE GET 3 AT SCHOOL AND 5⁺ A DAY promotion, which encourages students to eat more fruits and vegetables, can be used as an extension of this lesson. See lesson 28 in part III, Promotions for the Classroom, for details.

WHAT ARE THE MAIN BENEFITS OF FRUITS AND VEGETABLES?

▶ They are major sources of vitamins and minerals.
▶ They are important sources of fiber.
▶ They are low in saturated and trans fat.
▶ Research has shown that they reduce the risk of heart disease, stroke, and possibly certain forms of cancer.

The availability of fresh fruits and vegetables varies by season and by region of the country, but frozen and canned fruits and vegetables ensure a plentiful supply of these healthful foods throughout the year.

The Principles of Healthy Living promote the consumption of at least 5 servings of fruits and vegetables every day; more is always better. In this lesson, encourage students to choose vegetables other than potatoes to meet this goal. Potatoes contain vitamins and minerals, but they are digested quickly and are similar to refined grains in their effects on blood sugar. They should only be eaten, at most, a few times a week, and in small portions. (For more information on potatoes and refined carbohydrates, see the background section of Lesson 2, Carb Smart, pp. 26-27)

ESTIMATED TEACHING TIME AND RELATED SUBJECT AREAS

Estimated teaching time: 50 minutes

Related subject areas: math, science, language arts, music

OBJECTIVES

1. Students will design a day's menu of fruits and vegetables, making sure that their menu choices include at least 5 servings of fruits and vegetables.
2. Students will identify the nutritional values of certain fruits and vegetables.

MATERIALS

1. Handout 1, What They Do for Me
2. Worksheet 1, Plan a Menu
3. Worksheet 2, Create a Frozen Food
4. Transparency 1, Principles of Healthy Living
5. Transparency 2, Vegetables and Fruits
6. Solutions to worksheet 1
7. Green and orange crayons or markers
8. Tape recorder or digital recorder (optional, to record students' songs and raps about the fruits and vegetables)

PROCEDURE

PART I

1. Have the students form pairs. Distribute worksheet 1, Plan a Menu, and explain to the students that each pair will plan a healthful, full day's menu of fruits and vegetables.
2. Display transparency 1, Principles of Healthy Living, to the class. Review the recommendation to eat daily at least 5 servings of fruits and vegetables in a rainbow of colors; remind the students that more is always better. Explain that they will evaluate their menu to determine if they are reaching their goal.
3. Ask students why potatoes are not the best choice for reaching this goal. (Answer: Potatoes are not the best choice because, like white bread and white rice, potatoes are digested quickly and give us a quick boost of energy that does not last. Most other fruits and vegetables provide a longer energy boost because the sugar and starches in the food take longer to be digested and enter the blood stream. Potatoes should only be eaten, at most, a few times a week, and in small portions.)
4. Display transparency 2, Vegetables and Fruits, to the class. Encourage the students to think of creative ways to include several fruit and vegetable servings in their menus. Encourage students to pick whole fruit rather than juice, since whole fruit contains more fiber and is easy to grab on the go. Note that students should limit 100% fruit juice consumption to no more than 8 ounces per day, since juice is high in natural sugars.
5. Explain to the students that some dishes are mixed dishes—dishes that contain fruits or vegetables along with other foods. Mixed dishes may include stir-fries, vegetable pizza, and chicken salad. The fruits and vegetables in

mixed dishes can add up to a serving (or more). For example, the vegetables on two slices of vegetable pizza are likely to equal 1 serving of cooked vegetables (1/2 cup).

6. Give the pairs 10 to 15 minutes to design their menus and record their selections on worksheet 1, Plan a Menu. If desired, students can plan an entire week's menu on a separate sheet.

7. After 10 to 15 minutes have passed, distribute handout 1, What They Do for Me, which lists the benefits of some of the vitamins and minerals found in fruits and vegetables (iron, calcium, vitamins A and C). Go over the chart with the class and discuss why we need these vitamins and minerals.

PART III

Although healthy foods from other food groups will have been chosen for the menu, they should not receive any points. The objective of the exercise is to highlight and reward selections of fruits and vegetables.

1. Have the students score their menu selections by using the How Do You Rate? evaluation scale on the Plan a Menu worksheet. Have the students color in the Vita-Miner Meter, using green crayons or markers to represent the number of vegetable points and orange crayons or markers to represent the number of fruit points.

2. Have the students review and discuss their rating and decide whether they need to increase the number of fruits and vegetables in their menu. Have the students set a goal for increasing (or maintaining if they already eat at least 5 servings a day) the number of fruits and vegetables they eat daily.

PART IV

1. Distribute and review worksheet 2, Create a Frozen Food.

2. Have the students write their own songs or raps about fruits and vegetables. Ask the music teacher to suggest well-known songs that children can write new lyrics to, or to help come up with new melodies. If possible, record the songs or raps so they can be played in the cafeteria during the Get 3 At School and 5+ A Day promotion (see lesson 28).

What They Do for Me

▶TABLE 22.1 Vitamins and Minerals

Nutrient	Healthy sources	Role
VITAMINS		
Vitamin A	Dark-green, yellow, and orange vegetables and fruits such as kale, spinach, broccoli, romaine lettuce, carrots, cantaloupe, apricots	Helps with night vision, bone growth, and tissue maintenance
Vitamin C	Oranges, grapefruit, tangerines, cantaloupe, mangoes, papaya, strawberries, broccoli, tomatoes, bell peppers	Keeps skin and tissue healthy
Vitamin E	Almonds, sunflower seeds, sunflower oil, safflower oil, peanut butter, corn oil, soybean oil, canola oil, spinach, broccoli, dandelion greens, tomato sauce	Helps protect cells from damage (antioxidant)
MINERALS		
Calcium	Low-fat or skim milk, low-fat cheese, low-fat or fat-free yogurt, low-fat or fat-free cottage cheese, kale, broccoli, greens, tofu (bean curd), fortified 100% juice, fortified nondairy milks	Helps keep bones and teeth strong
Potassium	Sweet potatoes, tomatoes, winter squash, peaches, cantaloupe, bananas, greens, spinach, dried beans (white beans, lentils, kidney beans), low-fat or nonfat yogurt	Helps the body maintain fluid balance, electrolyte balance, and acid–base balance
Iron	Lean red meat, whole wheat bread, spinach, liver, lima beans	Allows blood to carry oxygen to all parts of the body

From L.W.Y. Cheung, H. Dart, S. Kalin, and S.L. Gortmaker, 2007, *Eat Well & Keep Moving,* 2nd ed. (Champaign, IL: Human Kinetics).

Name _____

Plan a Menu

Directions

Design a fruit and vegetable menu that allows you to get 5 or more servings of fruits and vegetables each day. Be sure to write down fruits and vegetables you could eat for breakfast, lunch, and dinner.

▶ TABLE 22.2 Spotlight on Fruits and Vegetables

	Breakfast	**Lunch**	**Dinner**
Day 1			

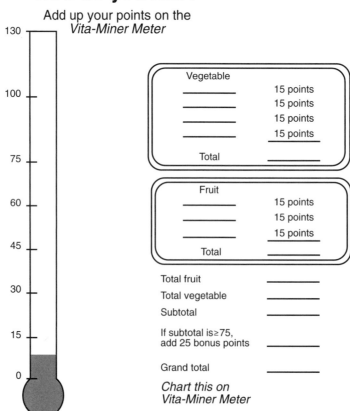

How do you rate?

Add up your points on the
Vita-Miner Meter

130
100
75
60
45
30
15
0

Vegetable
_____ 15 points
_____ 15 points
_____ 15 points
_____ 15 points
Total _____

Fruit
_____ 15 points
_____ 15 points
_____ 15 points
Total _____

Total fruit _____
Total vegetable _____
Subtotal _____
If subtotal is ≥75, add 25 bonus points _____
Grand total _____

Chart this on Vita-Miner Meter

Create a Frozen Food

You are the cook in charge of creating a new frozen food. Your assignment is to make the new food product with ingredients that will help your body build strong bones, help you have healthy skin, and help your body get the oxygen it needs. (Use handout 1, What They Do for Me, for guidance.)

1. Give your food product a name.
2. Write a short description of your new food product.
3. Write down the different types of ingredients you used (fruits, vegetables, and grains) and what each of these foods does for your body (for example, builds strong bones and healthy skin).
4. On the back of this page, design a container for your product.
5. Also on the back of this page, create a food label that includes the ingredients and nutrients in your food product.

New Product Name

_____

Description

_____
_____
_____
_____
_____
_____
_____
_____
_____
_____
_____
_____
_____
_____
_____
_____

From L.W.Y. Cheung, H. Dart, S. Kalin, and S.L. Gortmaker, 2007, *Eat Well & Keep Moving*, 2nd ed. (Champaign, IL: Human Kinetics).

Principles of Healthy Living

Go for 5 Fruits and Veggies—More Is Better!

Eat 5 or more servings of fruits and vegetables each day! Eat a variety of colors—try red, orange, yellow, green, blue, and purple.

Get Whole Grains and Sack the Sugar!

Choose healthy whole grains for flavor, fiber, and vitamins. Limit sweets. Candy, soft drinks, and other sugary drinks have almost nothing in them that is good for you—no vitamins or minerals or other healthy things. They contain just sugar.

Keep the Fat Healthy!

We need fat in our diets, but not all types of fat are good for us. Our bodies like the healthy fat that tends to come from plants and is liquid at room temperature. Examples are olive oil, canola oil, vegetable oil, and peanut oil. Our bodies do not like unhealthy fat, which is solid at room temperature. Examples include saturated fat (usually found in animal products such as meat and whole milk) and trans fat (found in fast-food fries and store-bought cookies). Of the unhealthy fats, trans fat is the worst and should rarely, if ever, be eaten.

Start Smart With Breakfast!

Eating breakfast helps you focus on schoolwork and gives you energy to play. Breakfast is a great meal for adding whole grains, fruit, and low-fat or nonfat milk to your day!

Keep Moving!

Being active is a very important part of healthy living. Do what you like most, and keep your body moving for at least an hour per day!

Freeze the Screen!

Watching TV, playing video games, or playing on the computer keeps your body still. Keep screen time as low as it can go, and never let it add up to more than 2 hours per day.

From L.W.Y. Cheung, H. Dart, S. Kalin, and S.L. Gortmaker, 2007, *Eat Well & Keep Moving*, 2nd ed. (Champaign, IL: Human Kinetics).

Vegetables and Fruits

Vegetables	Fruits
Artichokes	Apples
Asparagus	Apricots
Beans (string and lima)	Avocados
Beets	Bananas
Broccoli	Blueberries
Brussels sprouts	Cantaloupes
Cabbage	Cherries
Cauliflower	Figs
Carrots	Grapes
Celery	Grapefruits
Cucumbers	Kiwi fruits
Eggplant	Lemons
Greens	Mangoes
Kale	Nectarines
Leeks	Oranges
Lettuce	Pears
Onions	Pineapples
Okra	Peaches
Peas	Raspberries
Potatoes	Strawberries
Radishes	Tangerines
Rhubarb	Watermelons
Seed sprouts	
Spinach	
Sweet corn	
Squash	
Sweet potatoes	
Tomatoes	
Turnips	
Yams	
Zucchini	

From L.W.Y. Cheung, H. Dart, S. Kalin, and S.L. Gortmaker, 2007, *Eat Well & Keep Moving*, 2nd ed. (Champaign, IL: Human Kinetics).

Plan a Menu

▶ **TABLE 22.3 Spotlight on Fruits and Vegetables Example**

	Breakfast	**Lunch**	**Dinner**
Day 1	Orange	Celery Carrots Banana	Spinach Sweet potato Cherries

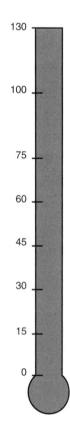

Vegetables:

Spinach	15 points
Sweet potatoes	15 points
Celery	15 points
Carrot	15 points
Total	60 points

Fruit:

Orange	15 points
Cherries	15 points
Banana	15 points
Total	45 points

Total vegetable	60 points
Total fruit	45 points
Subtotal	105 points
If subtotal is 75, add 25 bonus points	25 points
Grand total	130 points

Chart this on Vita-Miner Meter

From L.W.Y. Cheung, H. Dart, S. Kalin, and S.L. Gortmaker, 2007, *Eat Well & Keep Moving,* 2nd ed. (Champaign, IL: Human Kinetics).

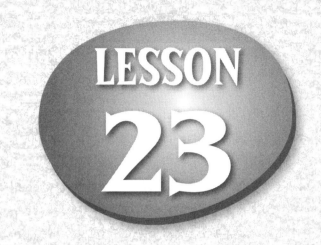

Veggiemania

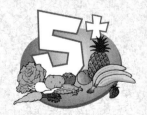

BACKGROUND

The four most popular vegetables in the United States are potatoes, tomatoes, iceberg lettuce, and onions. These vegetables, unfortunately, often end up as French fries, onion rings, or potato chips and as ketchup, lettuce, and onions on fast-food hamburgers.

While there is no such thing as a bad vegetable, some vegetables are more nutrient dense than others, meaning they contain more nutrients such as vitamins and minerals. The question, then, is which vegetables are more nutrient dense than others. All vegetables are good, but in this lesson, students will learn about which vegetables are the densest in nutrients.

Components that can be used to rate the nutrient density of vegetables include vitamins like vitamin C and folate; minerals like potassium, calcium, and iron; carotenoids (which act as antioxidants); and fiber.

- ▶ The top vegetables (based on nutrient density) are broccoli, cabbage, carrots, chard, collard greens, winter squash, sweet potatoes, kale, spinach, and tomatoes.
- ▶ Good vegetables (all the rest) are asparagus, avocado, cauliflower, celery, corn on the cob, romaine lettuce, parsley, squash, green beans, beets, corn (fresh or frozen), eggplant, mushrooms, onions, radishes, and turnips.

The basic message is that all vegetables are good to eat, but some are better than others in terms of the nutrients and benefits they provide the body. Of the four most popular vegetables in the United States (potatoes, tomatoes, iceberg lettuce, and onions), only tomatoes could be categorized as a top vegetable. Students (as well as everyone else) should be encouraged to eat more vegetables from the top category.

ESTIMATED TEACHING TIME AND RELATED SUBJECT AREAS

Estimated teaching time: 1 hour

Related subject areas: math, science

OBJECTIVES

1. The students will understand that all vegetables are good but that some are more nutrient dense (and therefore more nutritious) than others.
2. Students will be able to distinguish those vegetables that are very nutrient dense.
3. Students will demonstrate the parts of a safe workout while learning about nutrient density.

MATERIALS

1. Five containers (such as bags or boxes)
2. Worksheet 1, Let's Get to the Points
3. Veggiemania cards (cards displaying names of vegetables)

   (Two copies of each card should be made so that there are 50-60 cards that can be spread out, faceup, at the opposite end of the room.)

PROCEDURE

PART I

1. Ask the students to raise their hands if they have ever eaten any of the following vegetables: broccoli, cabbage, carrots, chard, collard greens, winter squash, sweet potatoes, kale, spinach, or tomatoes.
2. Explain to the students that if they have eaten any of those vegetables, then they have eaten some of the best, the healthiest, and the most nutrient-dense vegetables available.
3. Explain to the students that a nutrient-dense vegetable contains a lot of the vitamins and minerals our bodies need to grow, to be healthy, and to work right.
4. Discuss additional benefits of eating vegetables that are nutrient dense. Such vegetables contain a lot of nutrients, especially vitamins A and C and fiber, which can help protect the body against heart disease and other diseases.

PART II

As in previous lessons, this lesson should follow the format of the safe workout.

1. Lead the students through a warm-up and stretch.

   Warm-up—The first part of the safe workout, in which slow movements get the body ready for stretching and the fitness activity.

   Stretch—The part of the safe workout in which you do exercises that improve flexibility fitness and get the body ready for a fitness activity (see appendix A, pages 565-569).

2. Explain to the students that they are going to participate in a fitness activity focusing on nutrient-dense vegetables.

   Fitness activity—The part of the safe workout in which strength and endurance fitness exercises are performed.

3. Have the students form five groups.
4. Each group will be moving nonstop in a line, one student behind another—thus on one side of the classroom there should be five lines moving nonstop (pacing). Remind the students that eating right is only half the story—they must also be active!
5. Place a container next to each line into which the students will put their Veggiemania cards. (This and the next step can be done beforehand.)

6. On the opposite side of the classroom, spread out the Veggiemania cards on the floor, with the vegetable names facing up (see figure 23.1).

7. Explain to the students that when you say "Go," the first person in each line should jog or walk to the other side of the room, choose a Veggiemania card naming the most nutrient-dense vegetable she can find (without taking too much time), return (jogging or walking) to the line, put the card into the container, and then go to the end of the line, where she should continue pacing (marching or jogging in place). The next student in line should take a turn as soon as the card is put in the bag.

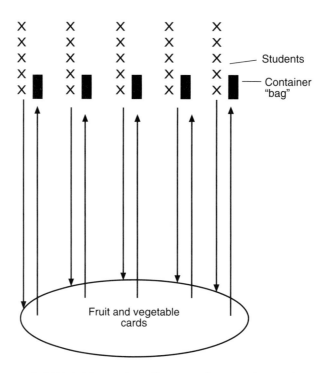

▶ FIGURE 23.1 Line diagram for Veggiemania.

8. Conclude the game once all the cards have been picked up or when time is up (the length of time is up to you).

9. Lead the students in a cool-down and a cool-down stretch.

   Cool-down—The part of the safe workout in which your body slows down and recovers from the fitness activity.

   Cool-down stretch—The last part of the safe workout, in which you do exercises that improve flexibility fitness.

10. Have each group sit around their container and remove the Veggiemania cards.

11. Distribute worksheet 1, Let's Get to the Points, to each group. Explain the vegetable point system to students and have each group add up the points on their cards and share their answers with the other groups.

12. Have each group share their 100-point (Top Vegetables) cards and write these on the board. Encourage students to eat more of these nutrient-dense vegetables.

Name _____

Let's Get to the Points

Date _____

Group members _____

_____

Directions

Using the following point system, determine the points for each of your vegetable cards. Then add up the total points for all the cards.

▶TABLE 23.1 Veggiemania Card Points

100-point cards	Top vegetables (very nutrient dense)
	Broccoli, cabbage, carrots, chard, collard greens, winter squash, sweet potatoes, kale, spinach, tomatoes
50-point cards	**Good vegetables (all the rest)**
	Asparagus, avocado, celery, cauliflower, corn (fresh or frozen), romaine lettuce, parsley, squash, beets, cucumbers, eggplant, mushrooms, onions, radishes, turnips

▶TABLE 23.2 Veggiemania Scorecard

Vegetable	Points	Vegetable	Points

Total points for all vegetables: _____

From L.W.Y. Cheung, H. Dart, S. Kalin, and S.L. Gortmaker, 2007, *Eat Well & Keep Moving,* 2nd ed. (Champaign, IL: Human Kinetics).

Veggiemania Cards

Top Vegetables

spinach	kale
collard greens	tomatoes
carrots	winter squash
broccoli	cabbage
Swiss chard	sweet potatoes

From L.W.Y. Cheung, H. Dart, S. Kalin, and S.L. Gortmaker, 2007, *Eat Well & Keep Moving*, 2nd ed. (Champaign, IL: Human Kinetics).

(continued)

Good Vegetables

asparagus	avocado
cauliflower	celery
corn (fresh or frozen)	parsley
zucchini	romaine lettuce
cucumbers	beets

From L.W.Y. Cheung, H. Dart, S. Kalin, and S.L. Gortmaker, 2007, *Eat Well & Keep Moving*, 2nd ed. (Champaign, IL: Human Kinetics).

(continued)

mushrooms	eggplant
radishes	onions
	turnips

From L.W.Y. Cheung, H. Dart, S. Kalin, and S.L. Gortmaker, 2007, *Eat Well & Keep Moving*, 2nd ed. (Champaign, IL: Human Kinetics).

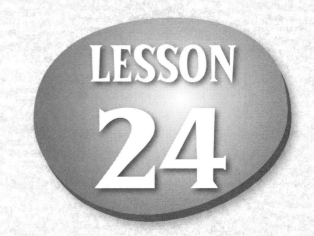

Breakfast Bonanza*

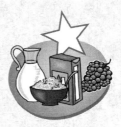

*Lesson adapted from Texas Education Agency Nutrition Education Curriculum Guide Grade 5-8, and a lesson plan developed by Ms. Michele Dorsey.

BACKGROUND*

Breakfast is the most important meal of the day. Eating breakfast gives the body the energy it needs to start the day and perform the morning's tasks, from thinking to doing the dishes to working out. Generally, adults who eat breakfast regularly learned this lifelong good habit when they were children.

National studies show that children who eat breakfast are better prepared for the school day. They perform better in school, are tardy less often, and miss fewer days of school. Students who eat breakfast have also demonstrated better concentration, faster reaction times, higher energy levels, and better test scores.

To help make breakfast a lifelong habit, students (and adults) should be encouraged to start their day by eating breakfast. Any good, nutritious food can be eaten for breakfast. If people don't like typical breakfast foods, such as whole-grain cereal or toast, they can eat leftovers from dinner, like pizza or a sandwich. The most important thing is to eat a nutritious meal in the morning.

Ideally, breakfast should contain a healthy balance of nutrients including carbohydrate (from foods like whole-grain cereal, toast, fruit, and 100% fruit juice; limit juice to no more than 8 ounces per day) and some protein (preferably from nuts, which also provide healthy fat, or from low-fat dairy products like 1% or nonfat milk or low-fat or nonfat yogurt). This means that foods from each of the food groups can be part of a nutritious breakfast!

The carbohydrate in a nutritious breakfast gives the body energy, and the protein helps stave off a midmorning drop in blood sugar that can make children lethargic before lunchtime. In a healthy person, blood sugar levels indicate how much fuel (in the form of glucose) is immediately available to the body. When blood sugar levels drop, children (and adults) may feel hungry, drowsy, and less energetic as well as have trouble concentrating. Breakfast can help keep blood sugar at the right level throughout the morning until lunchtime.

Foods such as doughnuts, soft drinks, candy bars, and desserts contain a lot of added sugar and are not the best choices for breakfast because they can cause blood sugar levels to drop faster than foods containing both healthy carbohydrate and protein. (For more on healthy carbohydrate, see lesson 2, Carb Smart.)

*Background information partially from Maryland Food Committee.

ESTIMATED TEACHING TIME AND RELATED SUBJECT AREAS

Estimated teaching time: 1 hour
Related subject areas: math, science

OBJECTIVES

1. Students will describe why they should eat a healthy breakfast.
2. Students will be able to name nutritious breakfast foods.
3. Students will demonstrate their ability to calculate the measurements of an orange and to calculate the average of their findings.

MATERIALS

1. Blank sheets of drawing paper
2. Pencils, crayons, or colored markers
3. Rulers
4. Twine or string
5. Scale (1 or more)
6. Calculators
7. Oranges (2 oranges for each group of 4 students)
8. Worksheet 1, Measure Up!
9. Passages, Oranges for Each Day's Journey, and Have You Ever Heard of Pineapple Oranges?

PROCEDURE

PART I: IMPORTANCE OF BREAKFAST

1. Ask the students why they think it is important to eat a nutritious breakfast. Write their responses on the board. Following are some examples of what studies have shown about breakfast:
   - People who skip breakfast do not perform as well in tasks of concentration as those who eat breakfast.
   - People who skip breakfast have shorter attention spans.
   - People who skip breakfast may feel drowsy by midmorning.
   - People who skip breakfast score lower on tests than those who eat breakfast.
   - People who skip breakfast are less energetic.

2. Explain to the students that the body needs fuel in order to perform well. For example, you could have the fastest car in the world, but if it doesn't have any gas (fuel), it won't go anywhere.

3. Explain to students that the word *breakfast* means *breaking the fast*. A fast is going for a long time without eating. After dinner and sleeping overnight, the body has gone 10 to 12 hours without food. By eating breakfast, you are breaking the overnight fast and giving your body the fuel (food) it needs to play, think, and have fun. If appropriate, remind students that breakfast is available to them before school in the cafeteria.

4. Ask students to name foods they enjoy eating for breakfast. Tell them that any nutritious foods may be eaten for breakfast—they don't have to eat only breakfast foods. For example, leftover vegetable pizza, a turkey sandwich on whole wheat bread, brown rice and beans, and casseroles are all foods they can eat for breakfast.

5. Give each student a blank piece of paper. Instruct the students to write the letters of their name vertically. Have students write, next to each letter in their name, the name of a food beginning with that letter. Suggest that they write down foods that they enjoy eating for breakfast, and encourage them to think of healthy foods.

Following is an example of a name with healthy foods:

Dates
Apples
Raisins
Yogurt
Loganberries

6. Pick a few students to share their answers. Ask some students who have an *O* in their name to share their answers. Did any of them come up with *orange* for the *O*? An orange or a small glass of 100% orange juice is a good part of a nutritious breakfast. Remind students to limit consumption of 100% fruit juice to no more than 8 ounces per day.

7. Have students read aloud (in unison) the two short passages, Oranges for Each Day's Journey and Have You Ever Heard of Pineapple Oranges? (on pages 346-347). Discuss the following questions relating to the passages:
   - Why do you think the author wrote the passage?
   - What is the main idea of the passage?
   - Name the places in the world where oranges grow.
   - What is meant by the term *Valencia?*
   - How did the blood orange get its name?
   - Why is it important to have vitamin C in your body?
   - How does vitamin C protect you?

PART II: EXAMINING AN ORANGE

For part II, the class must be able to use oranges. If oranges (or similar fruit) are unavailable, part II can be postponed until they are available.

1. Tell the students that now that they know why oranges are good for them nutritionally, they are going to learn even more about oranges by examining them scientifically.

2. Demonstrate to the students how the circumference is the distance around the orange.

3. Show the students that by placing a piece of string around the orange and then using a ruler to measure the length of the string, they will get an approximation of the circumference of the orange.

ADDITIONAL INFORMATION

Explain the math formulas that can be used to determine the circumference of a circle:

$$\text{Circumference} = \text{diameter} \times \pi.$$
$$\text{Circumference} = 2\pi r,$$
where $\pi = 3.1416$; r = radius.

To help the students approximate the weight of the orange, it may be helpful to mention how much some similarly sized items (such as an apple or a tennis ball) weigh.

4. Distribute worksheet 1, Measure Up!, and divide students into groups of four. Give 2 oranges to each group. Have the students work cooperatively to complete the questions, chart, and graph. Their goal is to gather data and present their findings in an organized chart and graph.

5. If students have been keeping journals, have students write in their journals what they learned about breakfast and oranges.

LESSON EXTENSIONS

SCIENCE

Use the orange (or another fruit with seeds) to examine how fruit reproduce. The following Web site offers a resource for teachers:

▶ www.urbanext.uiuc.edu/gpe/index.html

▶ The University of Illinois curriculum called *The Great Plant Escape* contains several lessons on plant structure; case 4 discusses the propagation of flowers and includes some references to fruit. The curriculum is available in English and Spanish.

SOCIAL STUDIES

Go to the library and research the travels of the orange, from its origins in Asia and the West Indies to its current production around the world (particularly in Brazil and Florida). Create maps and tie the orange into discussions of European explorations and the settlement of the New World.

Name _____

Measure Up!

Date _____

Group members _____

_____

Step 1

Answer these questions:

▶ How much do you think an average orange weighs? _____

▶ How many sections do you think are in an average orange? _____

▶ How many seeds do you think are in an average orange? _____

▶ What do you think is the circumference of an average orange? _____

Step 2

Write the answers from step 1 in the column labeled *Your estimates* in table 24.1.

▶TABLE 24.1 Orange Attributes

	Your estimates	Your measurements	Average of estimates made by group members
Weight (ounces)			
Sections (number)			
Seeds (number)			
Circumference (inches)			

From L.W.Y. Cheung, H. Dart, S. Kalin, and S.L. Gortmaker, 2007, *Eat Well & Keep Moving,* 2nd ed. (Champaign, IL: Human Kinetics).

(continued)

Step 3

Examine an actual orange to determine its weight (use the scale), circumference (use the ruler and string), and number of seeds and sections. Write these findings in the column labeled *Your measurements* on table 24.1. Now average the findings of your group (use calculators). Put these answers in the column labeled *Average of estimates made by group members* on table 24.1.

Step 4

Using the blank graphs provided, make bar graphs to display your estimates and actual measurements of the orange.

Attributes of an orange

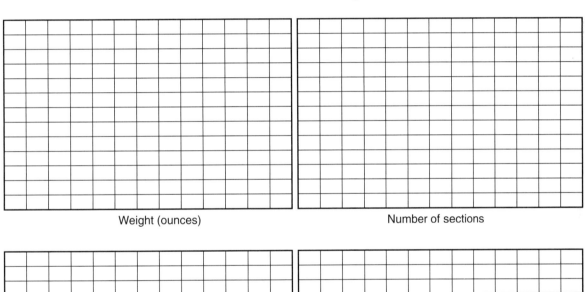

Weight (ounces)   Number of sections

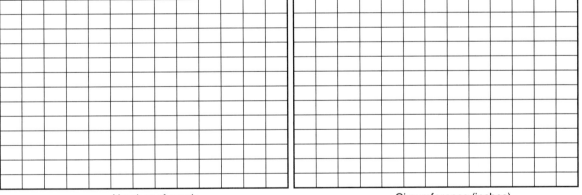

Number of seeds   Circumference (inches)

☐ Estimated   ■ Actual measurement

From L.W.Y. Cheung, H. Dart, S. Kalin, and S.L. Gortmaker, 2007, *Eat Well & Keep Moving*, 2nd ed. (Champaign, IL: Human Kinetics).

Passages

Oranges for Each Day's Journey

Originally, oranges grew in Asia and the East Indies—do you know where these areas are on the map? Oranges were brought to Europe and then to the New World (North America) by explorers. Orange trees were first planted in the San Gabriel Mission in San Gabriel, California, in 1804. In 1841, William Wolfskill planted a commercial orange grove in Los Angeles. By 1849, this entrepreneur sold oranges to gold rushers to prevent scurvy, a disease marked by overall weakness, spots on the skin, and, in the worst cases, bleeding gums.

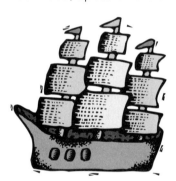

The vitamin C in oranges and other citrus fruits (like lemons, limes, and grapefruit) helped keep the gold rushers and the early explorers, like Columbus, Magellan, and Marco Polo, healthy during their long journeys. Just like the explorers, you can keep healthy and strong on your daily journeys (to school, to home, and to the store) by eating oranges and other citrus fruit. It's as easy as pouring a small glass of 100% orange juice or eating the orange wedges served in the cafeteria. You'll have energy for playing, and the vitamin C will help you grow strong, heal cuts and bruises, and fight off infections.

From L.W.Y. Cheung, S.L. Gortmaker, H. Dart, and S. Kalin, 2007, *Eat Well & Keep Moving,* 2nd ed. (Champaign, IL: Human Kinetics).

From L.W.Y. Cheung, H. Dart, S. Kalin, and S.L. Gortmaker, 2007, *Eat Well & Keep Moving,* 2nd ed. (Champaign, IL: Human Kinetics).

(continued)

Have You Ever Heard of Pineapple Oranges?
(How About Valencia, Temple, Navel, or Blood Oranges?)

The oranges you usually see in the cafeteria are called *pineapple oranges.* Pineapple oranges are popular because they have few seeds and have the familiar bright orange skin.

All types of oranges are sweet and juicy, but each type has a different name and looks a little bit different from the others. Some are light orange on the inside, some are bright orange on the inside, and some are even bright red on the inside (these oranges are called *blood oranges).*

Some oranges have thin skin, like Valencia oranges, which also have few seeds and so are great for juicing, and some have thick, easily peeled skin, like navel oranges. Oranges also come in different sizes, ranging from the smaller temple to the larger navel.

Because oranges are so delicious, they make a great snack and a sweet dessert! You can eat them peeled or cut into wedges, or you can drink them as a small glass of 100% orange juice. Eating oranges in any of these ways lets you enjoy them and gives you a boost of vitamin C that helps you grow, play, and learn.

From L.W.Y. Cheung, S.L. Gortmaker, H. Dart, and S. Kalin, 2007, *Eat Well & Keep Moving,* 2nd ed. (Champaign, IL: Human Kinetics).

From L.W.Y. Cheung, H. Dart, S. Kalin, and S.L. Gortmaker, 2007, *Eat Well & Keep Moving,* 2nd ed. (Champaign, IL: Human Kinetics).

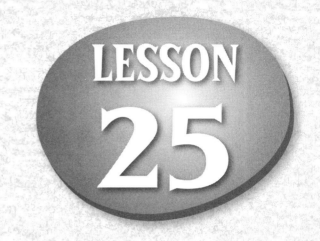

Foods From Around the World: Italy, China, Mexico, and Ethiopia

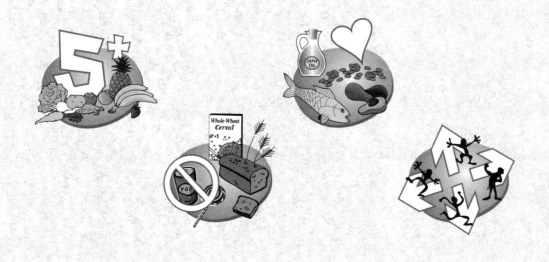

BACKGROUND

Although all people of the world eat food because it provides them with nutrients and energy, they get their nutrients from many different types of foods prepared in many different ways. In Italy, Mexico, China, and Ethiopia, the types of foods and patterns of eating differ greatly from those in the United States. Yet the traditional diets of each country provide the people with the nutrients they need to grow and stay healthy.

In Italy, the midday meal is the largest meal of the day. It consists of several courses, including an appetizer course called *antipasto.* Evening meals are traditionally light. Pizza was first served in Naples, a city in southern Italy, as bread topped with tomatoes and mozzarella cheese. It is eaten as a light evening meal or as a snack. The Italians have given us not only pizza but also pastas and delicious cheeses.

Traditional foods in Mexico include corn tortillas, tomatoes, beans, rice, chocolate, and cheese. Canned milk and powdered milk are common. Traditionally, Mexicans eat breakfast, a main midday meal, and a light evening meal or snack. Tortillas are generally served at every meal as bread.

In China, especially in the southern regions, people usually eat rice with every meal. Many cooks prepare it each morning and keep it on the stove ready to eat all through the day. Along with rice, meals often include seafood, chicken, soybean products, noodles, and vegetables.

People in Ethiopia typically eat one main meal in the evening. Lentils, other beans, teff (a kind of grain), bread, potatoes, fruit, and vegetables are a big part of their diets.

Experimenting with dishes from other countries can bring excitement to a meal as well as provide a whole new range of foods that fit into a healthful diet.

ESTIMATED TEACHING TIME AND RELATED SUBJECT AREAS

Estimated teaching time: 1 hour

Related subject areas: social studies, geography

OBJECTIVES

1. Students will understand that different foods are eaten in different countries around the world.
2. Students will be able to identify foods from Mexico, China, Italy, and Ethiopia.
3. Students will discuss what food groups the different foods for each country belong in.
4. Students will perform a safe workout while learning about multiethnic foods.

MATERIALS

1. Cards listing foods from each country (duplicate the cards to create four sets)

2. Maps of Mexico, China, Italy, and Ethiopia (see figures 25.1-25.4)
3. Four bags to hold the food cards

PROCEDURE

As in previous lessons, this lesson should follow the format of the safe workout.

1. Lead the students through a warm-up and stretch.

   Warm-up—The first part of the safe workout, in which slow movements get the body ready for stretching and the fitness activity.

   Stretch—The part of the safe workout in which you do exercises that improve flexibility fitness and get the body ready for a fitness activity.

2. Explain to the students that they are going to participate in a fitness activity focusing on foods from Italy, Mexico, China, and Ethiopia. Remind students that they should get at least 1 hour of physical activity every day.

   Fitness activity—The part of the safe workout in which strength and endurance fitness exercises are performed.

3. Have the class form four groups.

4. The students will be moving nonstop with their group in a line in the center of the room.

5. On the floor in each corner of the room, place one of the four maps. (This can be done beforehand.) Tell the students which map has been placed in which corner or hang a sign above each map.

6. Place a bag of food cards in front of each group. (For a summary of the food cards and the food groups to which they belong, see table 25.1, Food Groups.)

7. Tell the students that on your signal, the first person in each line should take a food card out of his bag, walk or jog carefully to the map of the country from which that food comes, and place the card on it.

8. All students should continue to move in place nonstop until all the food cards have been distributed about the room. Remind the students to continue to move throughout the entire fitness activity.

9. After all the food cards have been placed on the maps, assign a country to each of the four groups.

10. Have each group go to their map and lead them in a cool-down and cool-down stretch.

    Cool-down—The part of the safe workout in which your body slows down and recovers from the fitness activity.

    Cool-down stretch—The last part of the safe workout, in which you do exercises that improve flexibility fitness.

11. Have each group review the foods placed on its map to make sure that all the foods belong there. If the students in a group have questions about the placement of a food, they can ask you individually or discuss them with the entire class during step 12.

12. Move to each map in the room and discuss the foods of each country and the food groups to which they belong (see table 25.1). Discuss the Principles of Healthy Living—specifically those related to fruits, vegetables, whole grains, and healthy fat—and discuss which foods from each country best fit those principles. Also discuss combination foods (foods containing more than one food group).

13. Using the food cards, discuss how the eating habits and choices of people in these other countries are different from or similar to the eating habits and food choices of people in the United States.

▶TABLE 25.1 Food Groups

Italian food cards	
Farro (whole grain)	Grains
Calamari (squid)	Meat, fish, and beans
Bigoli (whole wheat pasta with anchovy sauce)	Meat, fish, and beans; grains
Polenta (cornmeal)	Grains
Focaccia (flat bread)	Grains
Risotto (rice)	Grains
Fruits	Fruits
Vegetables	Vegetables
Olive oil	Healthy fat
Pasta primavera (pasta with vegetables)	Grains, vegetables
Chinese food cards	
Bean sprouts	Vegetables
Fresh fruit	Fruits
Chicken (roasted, baked, steamed)	Meat, fish, and beans
Mi fan (rice noodles)	Grains
Vegetable lo mein (noodles)	Grains, vegetables
Sautéed vegetables in peanut oil	Vegetables, healthy fat
Chow fan (noodles)	Grains
Tofu (bean curd)	Meat, fish, and beans
Congee (rice pudding)	Grains
Chinese cabbage	Vegetables
Fish	Meat, fish, and beans
Brown rice	Grains
Mexican food cards	
Beans	Meat, fish, and beans
Corn	Vegetables
Beans and rice	Meat, fish, and beans; grains
Pork	Meat, fish, and beans
Amaranth	Grains
Rice	Grains
Salsa	Fruits, vegetables
Tortillas (beans, meat, and cheese)	Meat, fish, and beans; grains; milk
Cheese	Milk
Tostadas	Grains
Chicken enchiladas	Meat, fish, and beans; grains

(continued)

Ethiopian food cards	
Beans	Meat, fish, and beans
Injera (whole-grain bread)	Grains
Fruits	Fruits
Lentils	Meat, fish, and beans
Gomen (collard greens)	Vegetables
Misir wat (lentil stew)	Meat, fish, and beans
Potatoes	Vegetables
Shero wat (pea stew)	Vegetables
Teff (whole grain)	Grains
Vegetables	Vegetables

Food Cards

farro (whole grain)	**pasta primavera** (pasta with vegetables)
focaccia (flat bread)	**polenta** (cornmeal)
fruits	**risotto** (rice)
olive oil	**vegetables**
bigoli (whole wheat pasta)	**calamari** (squid)

From L.W.Y. Cheung, H. Dart, S. Kalin, and S.L. Gortmaker, 2007, *Eat Well & Keep Moving,* 2nd ed. (Champaign, IL: Human Kinetics).

(continued)

bean sprouts	fresh fruit
chicken (roasted, baked, steamed)	mi fan (rice noodles)
vegetable lo mein (noodles)	sautéed vegetables (in peanut oil)
chow fan (noodles)	tofu (bean curd)
congee (rice pudding)	Chinese cabbage

From L.W.Y. Cheung, H. Dart, S. Kalin, and S.L. Gortmaker, 2007, *Eat Well & Keep Moving,* 2nd ed. (Champaign, IL: Human Kinetics).

(continued)

fish	brown rice
beans	corn
beans and rice	pork
amaranth	rice
salsa	tortillas (beans, meat, and cheese)

From L.W.Y. Cheung, H. Dart, S. Kalin, and S.L. Gortmaker, 2007, *Eat Well & Keep Moving*, 2nd ed. (Champaign, IL: Human Kinetics).

(continued)

cheese

tostadas

chicken enchiladas

injera
(whole-grain bread)

beans

potatoes

From L.W.Y. Cheung, H. Dart, S. Kalin, and S.L. Gortmaker, 2007, *Eat Well & Keep Moving,* 2nd ed. (Champaign, IL: Human Kinetics).

(continued)

fruits	**shero wat** (pea stew)
lentils	**teff** (whole grain)
gomen (collard greens)	**vegetables**
misir wat (lentil stew)	

(continued)

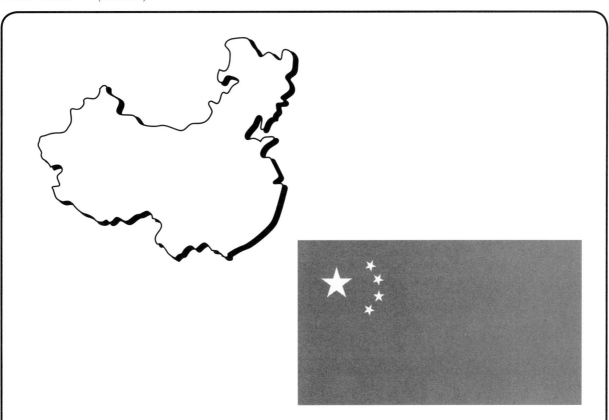

▶ FIGURE 25.1   Map of China and its flag.

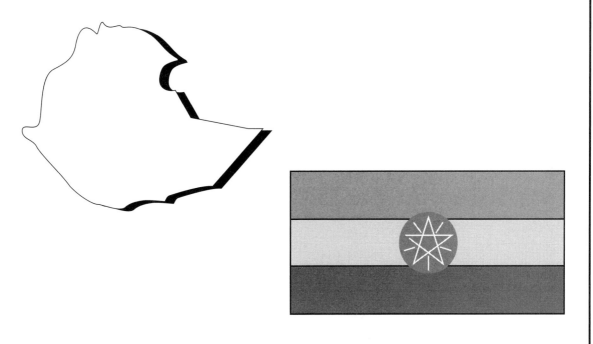

▶ FIGURE 25.2   Map of Ethiopia and its flag.

From L.W.Y. Cheung, H. Dart, S. Kalin, and S.L. Gortmaker, 2007, *Eat Well & Keep Moving,* 2nd ed. (Champaign, IL: Human Kinetics).

(continued)

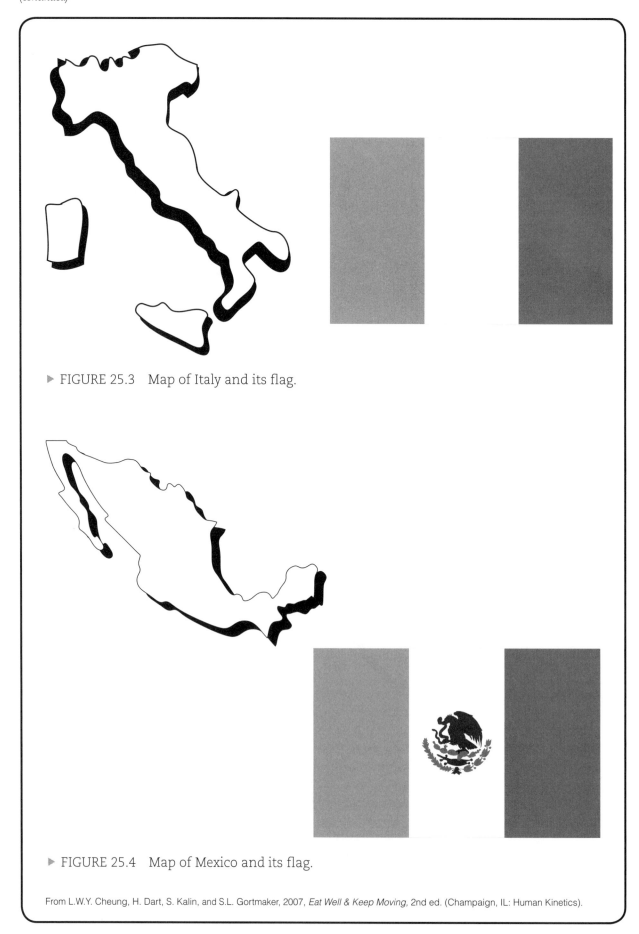

▶ FIGURE 25.3 Map of Italy and its flag.

▶ FIGURE 25.4 Map of Mexico and its flag.

From L.W.Y. Cheung, H. Dart, S. Kalin, and S.L. Gortmaker, 2007, *Eat Well & Keep Moving,* 2nd ed. (Champaign, IL: Human Kinetics).

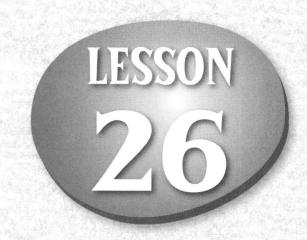

Fitness Walking

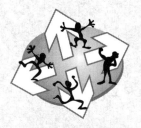

This lesson is a duplicate of lesson 13 in the fourth-grade lesson set. While the walking program aspect is the same for both grades, the fourth- and fifth-grade lessons can be kept distinct by choosing a different social studies theme around which to plan the walking program; there is also an additional science extension suggested for the nature walk for fifth grade.

BACKGROUND

Walking is one of the healthiest, safest, and easiest ways to begin a fitness program, and it can be a big step toward improving your health. Fitness or aerobic walking uses all the major muscle groups in the upper and lower body in a gentle, dynamic, rhythmic action, which is what an ideal exercise should do. Children should get at least 60 minutes of physical activity every day, and walking is a great way for them to reach that goal.

Walking is also free! There are no machines or membership fees, no fancy packaging or expensive clothes. Walking requires only that you pace yourself and do your personal best. What's important is feeling good about yourself and setting your own goals.

Walking can be done with friends or family. It can also be done as an adventure with a school class. An active lifestyle can make you feel better, give you more energy, and enhance your health. We want you and your class to get hooked on walking. It's fun, and it's good for you!

OVERVIEW

This lesson introduces students to the benefits and fun of walking for fitness. The lesson also serves as a kickoff for an ongoing class walking club that can be integrated into geography activities throughout the year.

ESTIMATED TEACHING TIME AND RELATED SUBJECT AREAS

Estimated teaching time: 1 hour

Related subject areas: science, social studies, math, physical education

OBJECTIVES

1. Students will learn the importance of regular exercise and will establish an ongoing class walking club.
2. Students will be exposed to the benefits of walking with family, friends, and classmates.
3. Students will learn walking techniques and learn about the health benefits of raising their heart rate through regular aerobic activity.
4. Students will learn about a particular geographic region of the world.

MATERIALS

1. Comfortable shoes (students and teacher)
2. Worksheet 1, Teacher Classroom Walking Log
3. Worksheet 2, Student Classroom Walking Log (duplicate for students)

4. Worksheet 3, Student Home Walking Log (duplicate for students)
5. Worksheet 4, Dichotomous Key Worksheet (optional extension, duplicate for students)
6. Maps
7. Map pins or thumbtacks
8. Tape recorder, binoculars, bird identification book or field guide (optional, for use during optional nature walk extension)
9. Pedometers* (optional)

PLANNING A WALKING CLUB

In addition to introducing students to how important and fun walking can be, this lesson focuses on organizing a class walking club.

When planning a walking club, first consider where and when your students can walk. The walks can take place before, during, or after school and can be done in the hallways, gym, playground, or neighborhood—whenever and wherever such a program works best for your school.

An effective way to introduce a walking club into your school is to integrate it with your curriculum. One option is to integrate the club with your social studies curriculum. For example, you can combine walking with lessons on the state in which you live, on the entire United States, or on other countries around the world. If there is an area of the world your students would like to learn about, use the walking club to talk about that area. As a class or individually, design the itinerary of a fitness walk across the region you have chosen, and then pretend you are walking across that region. Students could walk across America together, walk across a specific region of the United States, or walk around the world. Students could even walk across a region during a specific time period in history: For example, students could walk across North America prior to colonization, duplicating the migration patterns of the first Native Americans; they could walk across at a later time period exploring the different Native American tribes, as well as the natural resources and shelters of each tribe; or they could walk through the American colonies, studying people, religion, governments, and their interactions with Native Americans. Students could create posters to illustrate these time periods or write journal entries or fictionalized accounts of what they see along their walk. The design is completely open.

Give your program a name, such as Walk Across America or Walk Across the World, or let the students choose a name.

Obtain maps of the area you chose to study, and tie in the students' walking progress with movement on the map. Each time the class walks for a certain length of time, equate that time with a particular distance on the map (for example, 5 minutes walked could equal 50 miles, or 80 kilometers). Each student can have a map to follow, or all of the students can plot their travels on one map. The amount of time the class walks and the distance traveled will depend on the part of the world or country on which you chose to focus. For example, if you decided on a large area of the world, such as Africa, then 5 minutes might equal 200 miles (322 kilometers) traveled. If you chose the state of Maryland, however, 5 minutes might equal 50 miles (80 kilometers).

*Low-cost pedometers are available from many sources on the Web. Consult with your school's physical education director to get recommendations for accurate, easy-to-use, low-cost models. In some communities, local health departments, health centers, or health insurers may provide pedometers for free.

Keep track of your class walks on the logs provided. There is a log for each class as well as for each student. The class log can be made larger and displayed in the classroom for all to see. A map of the region or country that they are traveling across should be displayed along with the class log. Displaying the map and log will motivate the class and keep everyone more involved.

If it is possible to supply students with pedometers, consider tracking their number of steps instead of tracking walking time. Pedometers can also be a fun way to motivate students to increase their activity. Have students keep track of the number of steps they take each day for a week, and then have them determine their average number of steps per day. Set a goal for students to increase their average number of steps per day by 10%.

Possible extensions for combining geography with the walking program include having students learn the state's or country's capital, natural resources, climate, unique features, major monuments, and historical sites. Similar to the social studies extensions, students could create posters to illustrate these geographic features or write journal entries or fictionalized accounts of what they "see" along their walk.

Another way to integrate walking with the curriculum is to link an outdoors nature walk with science lessons (see Extension Activity: Taking a Nature Walk, page 367, which gives suggestions and worksheets for taking a bird observation walk). Students can collect samples, describe a habitat, or look for evidence of human effects on the environment. Have students follow up in the classroom with posters or journal entries describing what they saw.

Encourage students to take on the walking program as an after-school, family-and-friend adventure. Have the students keep a log of the dates and times of their after-school walks (see worksheet 3, Student Home Walking Log). They can plot their travels on the maps with pins or thumbtacks. Get the whole school involved in walking—principals, office staff, custodians, and other teachers and students can join the program. The more the students see others participating, the more they will want to become involved.

PROCEDURE

1. FITNESS WALKING

Explain to the students that fitness walking is walking at a pace (speed) that makes the heart, lungs, and blood vessels work harder than usual. This type of aerobic workout makes the heart muscle pump harder because the body's other muscles—the leg and arm muscles—are working harder and need more blood to keep them going.

Blood delivers energy and oxygen to working muscles. When muscles work hard, such as when you're fitness walking, they need more energy and oxygen. During exercise, the heart works harder to pump blood to these muscles. When the heart works harder, it gets stronger.

Explain to the students that they can check their pulse rate before they begin exercising and again during their fitness workout in order to see firsthand how the heart muscle works harder. (See details on how to do this in the section on Finding a Pulse on page 366.)

Also explain to the students the importance of completing an hour of physical activity on all or most days of the week. It is okay to do this activity a little bit at a time, so a 15-minute or longer walk can help them reach their hour-a-day goal.

2. BENEFITS OF FITNESS WALKING

Ask the students to list the benefits of fitness walking. These can include the following:

a. Walking is an excellent and safe way to improve aerobic fitness. Aerobic exercises like walking strengthen the heart, lungs, and blood vessels. Walking lets you do this with less wear and tear on the body compared to many other types of conditioning.

b. Walking, like other aerobic exercises, can give you more energy and reduce fatigue.

c. Walking can help relieve stress.

d. Walking can improve mood and mental function.

e. Walking can help slow down the progression of osteoporosis (bone loss), which can occur as the body ages.

f. Walking can be performed with friends and family.

3. HOW TO FITNESS WALK

a. Make sure students wear sneakers or comfortable shoes.

b. Review with students the following (and consult figure 26.1):

1. Arm swing: Try to keep the arms swinging faster than they swing when walking normally. The faster the arms swing, the faster the legs will move. Bend the arms 90 degrees at the elbow. Concentrate on moving the arms faster and swinging them from the shoulder. Remember, when you shorten your arms (bending them 90 degrees at the elbow), you can swing them faster and your legs will move faster. Keep your shoulders relaxed. Beginners tend to tense up around the shoulders. Relax!

2. Hands: Form a loose fist. Do not clench your fist and put tension in the arm muscles.

3. Foot placement and toe-off: The power of the step comes from the toe-off. With each step, land the foot on the heel, then roll forward to the toe and push off.

Tell the students that following these instructions for fitness walking should help them enjoy their walking more. They should do what feels comfortable for them. Do it right, but make it *fun!*

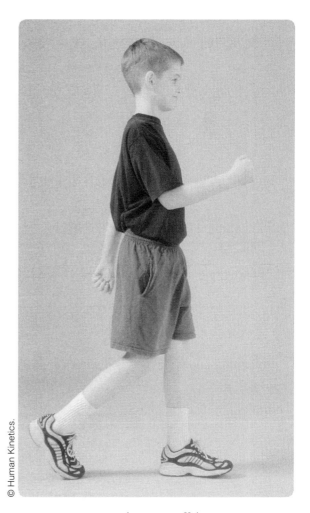

© Human Kinetics.

▶ FIGURE 26.1 Fitness walking.

4. FINDING A PULSE

On the first day of fitness walking (or however often you would like), remind the students that their pulse rate will increase when they exercise and teach them how to find their pulse (refer to figure 26.2). Explain to the students, "During an aerobic workout, you want your heart, lungs, and blood vessels to work harder than they are used to working. Your pulse can help you know what is going on inside your body. On the side of your neck, just below the jawbone, is a major blood vessel bringing blood to the brain. Put your index and middle fingers together and place them gently on that blood vessel on the side of your neck to feel the pulse. During exercise, the pulse is usually very easy to find." To demonstrate how the pulse rate changes from the warm-up to the fitness activity to the cool-down, have the students try to feel their pulse before, during, and after aerobic walking.

Tell the students, "The heart is a muscle that has a huge job to do. It must always be working every second, minute, hour, day, week, month, and year of your lives. Once you understand that this heart muscle of yours has such a huge job, hopefully you will want to take care of it so it can do its job.

"Walking is one way to keep the heart muscle healthy. Likewise, eating right and being active are both a big part of helping the heart stay healthy. If, during the fitness activity, the heart is working harder than it's used to working, then with time the heart will get stronger and stay healthy. The more you include exercise and eating right in your daily lives, the better the body can work and feel!"

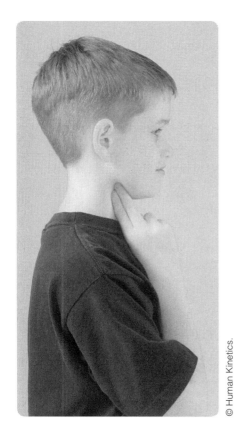

▶ FIGURE 26.2   Finding a pulse.

© Human Kinetics.

5. THE SAFE WORKOUT

Following the steps of the safe workout will help students prevent injuries. The five steps are the following:

Step 1: Warm-up. Start each fitness walk with a slow walk to get the body ready for harder work. Emphasize to the students the importance of warming up and stretching before doing any type of physical activity. During the warm-up, talk about the adventure for the day and review the important facts about the warm-up. (Refer to lesson 3, The Safe Workout: An Introduction.)

Step 2: Stretch. After the warm-up, stretch out and work on flexibility fitness. Review the importance of stretching and the key parts of safe stretching.

Step 3: Fitness activity. Introduce the walking activity you have chosen for your class, such as walking the first leg of a trip across the United States. Have the class set a goal for that particular day. For example, the class goal for the first day may be to walk for 10 minutes without stopping. If students are using pedometers, the goal may be for each student to walk 1,000 steps. Equate the number of minutes walked or number of steps walked to a particular distance on the map. As students get used to the program, the class can set goals to walk longer and more frequently, or (if using pedometers) to increase their average number of steps per day by 10%. Remember, the more days that students walk, the greater the opportunity they have to learn and become fit.

Take the students on their fitness walk. During the walk, lead the students in a discussion about the geographic region they are pretending to walk through on their program. Other topics to discuss include nutrition and physical activity issues.

Step 4: Cool-down. After their fitness walk, have the students walk slowly to let their bodies recover. Review the benefits of the cool-down.

Step 5: Cool-down stretch. After the cool-down, have the students stretch again to prevent soreness, to improve flexibility, and to decrease their chances of injury. While they are stretching, review the benefits of the cool-down stretch and the proper way to cool down.

The Stay Healthy Corner can be an area of the classroom decorated with pictures or student drawings that represent the Principles of Healthy Living (e.g., healthy foods, children engaged in physical activity, and so on). Or it can be simply a time for discussion and reflection on the health messages of the lesson. After the first walk, gather the class together and review the benefits of walking, stressing the enjoyment the students will get from it. Introduce and fill out together the classroom walking logs—worksheet 1, Teacher Classroom Walking Log, and worksheet 2, Student Classroom Walking Log.

Introduce and distribute worksheet 3, Student Home Walking Log, to the students. Review with them the four parts of the log sheet—(1) Date, (2) Time, (3) Miles, and (4) Where—and how to complete the log.

You and your students can decide how to use worksheet 3. For example, the students can keep track of their after-school walking program completely on their own and track their progress on separate maps. Or the students can integrate their after-school walking experience with their in-school tracking system.

However you approach it, the ultimate goal is to motivate students to exercise at home with family or friends so that they can achieve the goal of being physically active for at least 1 hour every day.

EXTENSION ACTIVITY: TAKING A NATURE WALK

Taking a nature walk is a fun way to introduce additional walking time into the schoolday, to explore your local surroundings, and to enhance a science, math, or social studies unit. You can walk to a local green space near your school, such as a park, an urban wild, an open field, or a wooded area. You can also take a walk in the neighborhood surrounding your school. Keep track of nature walks on the class walking log. In general, nature walks cover about half the distance of fitness walks for the same amount of time because of the frequent stops to observe and discuss.

LEARNING ABOUT BIRDS

Birds are a fascinating group of animals to study. They have many observable behaviors, their migration patterns are interesting to study and track, and often their physical characteristics provide clues to their natural habitats. You might want to review some of the main characteristics of birds with the class at the start of the walk. Birds have feathers of different colors and sizes and beaks of different sizes and shapes, and they lay eggs, build nests, use their wings to fly, and often follow migration patterns.

Take along a few pairs of binoculars on your walk. Depending on the habitat you walk in, you can look for birds nesting in the trees, nesting in tall grass, flying in the sky, flitting in or around bodies of water such as ponds and lakes, and perching on telephone wires and fences.

The changing seasons offer different kinds of explorations and lessons on bird behavior, identification, and observation:

- ▶ In spring through early summer, when birds are claiming breeding territories and attracting mates, they sing the most. Each species has a recognizable song, with different pitches and tempos. Bring along a tape recorder, binoculars, and a bird identification book (a field guide) and ask your class to match a birdsong to the bird singing it and to match a bird's physical characteristics to the name of its species. Back in the classroom, play your recordings of the birdsong and translate these sounds into writing. Compare the written examples and imitate these sounds using the written versions.

- ▶ In the fall, some of the birds in any location migrate north or south, while others are year-round residents or merely passing through as transients. The class can observe the migration of birds by looking for large flocks overhead when the temperature turns colder. How birds know when to begin their journey is a fascinating topic to study. As a class you can explore the aspects of nature that trigger migration and how birds absorb this information. You can also research how birds find their way to their new destinations. The science of bird navigation involves studying the roles of the earth's magnetic field, star constellations, geographic land and water features, and much more.

- ▶ The winter is the best time to search for bird nests abandoned in the spring and summer after the young have learned to fly. They are often revealed when broadleaf (deciduous) trees and shrubs lose their leaves and grasses die off. The nest's size, shape, and materials usually are unique to the bird species. With a field guide, nests are a good way to identify birds that have migrated for the season and those that are wintering over.

You may use the following science extensions of the nature walk to enhance classroom study during any season:

1. Create a field journal

   Field journal entries are a valuable way to capture birding expedition activities, observations, and questions. Observations are usually recorded during the walk. Ask the students to record any distinguishing characteristics such as beak length, size, and shape; bird colors; and bird size (small, medium, or large), and then have the students draw the bird as they see or remember it. Hypotheses, new questions, goals of the expedition, and conclusions are written after the trip.

2. Create a key to identify birds by their physical traits

Scientists use keys to help them identify and classify similarities and differences in the natural world around them. A key leads its user through a series of questions on the characteristics of the subject under observation until the name of the object, plant, or animal is reached. It is easy to create a dichotomous key for a group of living or nonliving subjects that you want to organize by physical traits. The key can be a good method for helping students make observations and understand how physical traits contribute to the classification of plants and animals.

Introduce and distribute worksheet 4, Dichotomous Key Worksheet, to familiarize students with the concept of a key. Then follow these basic rules when making a key and you are on your way:

1. Start by observing the birds to be used in the key.
2. List the most general traits that can be used to divide the birds into categories.
3. Each step in a key involves making a single choice between two characteristics. These characteristics are grouped 1a and 1b, 2a and 2b, and so forth.
4. Each step distributes one or more objects (plants, animals, and so on) into two smaller units.
5. Each unit either identifies an object (plant, animal, and so on) or gives directions as to where to go next in the key.

EXAMPLE OF A SIMPLE KEY

1. Does the bird have a beak?
   a. Yes. Go to question 2.
   b. No. It is not a bird.
2. Does the bird have webbing between its toes?
   a. Yes. It is a duck.
   b. No. Go to question 3.
3. Does the bird have a noticeably downward curved beak?
   a. Yes. Go to question 4.
   b. No. Go to question 5.
4. . . .

Name _____

Teacher Classroom Walking Log

▶ **TABLE 26.1** Teacher Classroom Walking Log

Date	Time or Steps*	Miles	Where

*Log number of steps if your class is using pedometers.

Date: Date of the fitness walk

Time or Steps: Number of minutes walked or number of steps walked

Miles: Number of miles walked (depends on how many minutes or steps your class decided equals 1 mile)

Where: Town, city, state, or country traveled through today

From L.W.Y. Cheung, H. Dart, S. Kalin, and S.L. Gortmaker, 2007, *Eat Well & Keep Moving,* 2nd ed. (Champaign, IL: Human Kinetics).

Name _____

Student Classroom Walking Log

▶ **TABLE 26.2 Student Classroom Walking Log**

Date	Time or Steps*	Miles	Where

*Log number of steps if your class is using pedometers.

Date: Date of the fitness walk

Time or Steps: Number of minutes walked or number of steps walked

Miles: Number of miles walked (depends on how many minutes or steps your class decided equals 1 mile)

Where: Town, city, state, or country traveled through today

From L.W.Y. Cheung, H. Dart, S. Kalin, and S.L. Gortmaker, 2007, *Eat Well & Keep Moving,* 2nd ed. (Champaign, IL: Human Kinetics).

Name _____

Student Home Walking Log

▶ **TABLE 26.3 Student Home Walking Log**

Date	Time or Steps*	Miles	Where

*Log number of steps if your class is using pedometers.

Date: Date of the fitness walk

Time or Steps: Number of minutes walked or number of steps walked

Miles: Number of miles walked (depends on how many minutes or steps your class decided equals 1 mile)

Where: Town, city, state, or country traveled through today

From L.W.Y. Cheung, H. Dart, S. Kalin, and S.L. Gortmaker, 2007, *Eat Well & Keep Moving*, 2nd ed. (Champaign, IL: Human Kinetics).

Dichotomous Key Worksheet

Bird Identification Study

Pick one bird you have observed and write out the sequence of questions and answers you followed to arrive at the name of the bird. You may not need five questions to get to the end of the key. Once you have identified the bird, stop, even if you only have one question!

Question 1: _____

Answer: _____

(a) Yes _____

(b) No _____

Question 2: _____

Answer: _____

(a) Yes _____

(b) No _____

Question 3: _____

Answer: _____

(a) Yes _____

(b) No _____

Question 4: _____

Answer: _____

(a) Yes _____

(b) No _____

Question 5: _____

Answer: _____

(a) Yes _____

(b) No _____

Name of animal: _____

From L.W.Y. Cheung, H. Dart, S. Kalin, and S.L. Gortmaker, 2007, *Eat Well & Keep Moving*, 2nd ed. (Champaign, IL: Human Kinetics).

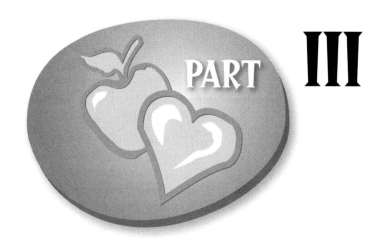

PART III

Promotions for the Classroom

Part III includes four promotions that reinforce the messages of the fourth- and fifth-grade classroom lessons and provide students with an engaging opportunity to put their nutrition and physical activity knowledge into practice. Freeze My TV focuses on limiting television and other screen time. Get 3 At School and 5+ A Day encourages students to get enough fruits and vegetables. Class Walking Clubs offer a fun way to work regular activity into the school day, and Tour de Health uses a game to review the Principles of Healthy Living.

Like most parts of *Eat Well & Keep Moving,* the promotions can be successfully used on their own but are most powerful when combined with the classroom lessons and other *Eat Well & Keep Moving* activities.

- Freeze My TV is an activity in which students track and try to limit their television viewing and other screen time for an entire week. In addition to keeping track of the time they spend watching television and participating in other screen activities (like the surfing the Web and playing video games), students also complete graphing activities, answer questions based on their graphs, and make daily entries in the Freeze My TV Journal.

- Get 3 At School and 5+ A Day allows students to put their knowledge of healthful eating into practice by consuming at least 3 servings of fruits and vegetables while at school. Each student tracks her at-school fruit and vegetable consumption on a large class graph. In addition to getting 3 servings of fruits and vegetables while at school, students are encouraged to get a total of 5 or more servings for the entire day.

- Class Walking Clubs encourages classes to chart walking routes around their school and to go on walks with their teacher at least once a week. To add interest to the club, classes are encouraged to pretend they are walking across a part of the world. Each time they walk, they can accrue a certain number of miles and mark their progress on a map.

• Tour de Health turns the six healthy living messages from *Eat Well & Keep Moving* into a fun and edifying game. Played in groups or as an entire class, Tour de Health can serve as a daily review for the classroom and physical education lessons as well as a refresher of the *Eat Well & Keep Moving* messages throughout the school year. The game consists of question cards relating to the six healthy living messages covered throughout the *Eat Well & Keep Moving* lessons; students also get a Tour de Health scorecard (which emphasizes the healthy living messages) and an Answer Cube. When students answer the questions on nutrition and physical activity correctly, they receive points. The first student or group to reach 20 points (or the student or group with the highest point total) wins the game.

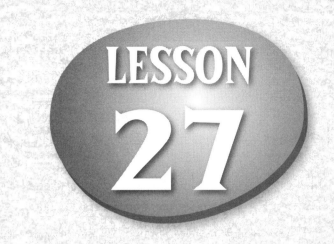

Freeze My TV

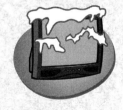

BACKGROUND

Freeze My TV, an extension activity to lessons 9 and 21 of *Eat Well & Keep Moving,* challenges students to track and limit the amount of time they spend watching television and participating in other screen activities in a designated week.

For each day of a 7-day week, students will log the number of hours they spend viewing television, watching DVDs, surfing the Web for fun, instant messaging, and playing video games.* By tracking their own viewing habits, students can then see how they compare to other youths their age as well as to the Principles of Healthy Living, which suggest limiting television and other screen time to no more than 2 hours each day. In addition to logging their screen time, the students will engage in other activities such as graphing, creating charts, and journaling.

*Dance video games that require users to engage in moderate to vigorous physical activity, such as Dance, Dance Revolution (DDR), do not count as screen time.

OBJECTIVES

1. Fourth- and fifth-grade students will spend a week tracking their time spent viewing television and participating in other screen activities and will apply this information to making graphs and journaling.

2. Students will limit their total screen time (TV, Web, video games, and so on) to no more than 2 hours per day.

3. Students will generate alternatives, especially physically active alternatives, to screen activities. Examples of alternatives are dancing, playing games, moving around, helping with chores, solving puzzles, reading, talking with friends, singing, and writing songs or poems.

MATERIALS

1. Freeze My TV packet (Screen Time Chart; worksheet 1, Graph-It Worksheet; worksheet 2, Graph-It Questions; and Freeze My TV Journal)

2. Pieces of poster board or large paper (for creating large chart of class TV viewing)

3. Contest Participant Checklist (created from teacher example 2)

4. Teacher example 1, Completed Graph-It Worksheets

5. Teacher example 2, Contest Participant Checklist

6. Small prizes (optional)

PROCEDURE

1. Freeze My TV may be run in conjunction with the fourth-grade lesson 9 and the fifth-grade lesson 21 of *Eat Well & Keep Moving.* You also may run the activity independently of the lessons if doing so works better with the class schedule. Another option is to run the promotion multiple times throughout the school year in order to rate changes in students' TV viewing and other screen activities.

2. Distribute the Freeze My TV packet to students (provide one packet for each student) and review the materials in the packet.

3. Have the students take the Screen Time Chart home and keep track of the number of hours they spend watching television and doing other screen activities each day of a 7-day week.

4. Tell the students that their goal for the week is to limit the amount of time they spend watching television and doing other screen activities (e.g., surfing the Web, instant messaging, and playing video games) to 2 hours or less each day and that the class will keep a chart so that they can see how they are all doing with the goal. For students who already spend less than 2 hours per day watching television or doing other screen activities, suggest that they set a goal to reduce their daily television and screen time by 30 minutes.

5. Each day, have students report how much time they spent watching television and doing other screen activities the day before, and record their numbers onto a large class chart. Encourage students who had more than 2 hours of total television and screen time to spend less time watching television or doing screen activities the next day.

6. After each day of trying to limit their television and screen time, have students write an entry in the Freeze My TV Journal. Suggested topics for each day's entry appear in the journal.

7. Remind students that even if they are absent from school, they still need to keep track of their screen time and make entries in their journals.

8. At the end of the 7 days, have the students complete the graphing activities and questions on worksheets 1 and 2.

9. Review the worksheets with the students (see teacher example 1, Completed Graph-It Worksheets).

10. Complete the Contest Participant Checklist (see teacher example 2, Contest Participant Checklist).

> **Tip**
>
> One easy way for students to cut down on screen time is to take the TV out of the room where they sleep (if applicable); be sure that they get help from parents or guardians when moving it out of the room. If they do not want to physically take the TV out of the room, they can just unplug it.

PRIZES

If you have access to small giveaways, you may enter all students who complete the entire Screen Time Chart, the Graph-It worksheets, and the Freeze My TV Journal into a drawing to win small prizes.

SCREEN TIME CHART

Read to students the following instructions on how to use the chart:

1. Your goal for Freeze My TV is to cut back on the amount of time you spend in a full week watching TV and doing other screen activities like surfing the

Web, instant messaging, and playing video games. It is best to get no more than 2 hours of screen time a day, and getting less is even better. See how you can do compared to your classmates.

2. Have your chart with you every time you watch television or do other screen activities (including watching TV or playing video games at a friend's or relative's house).

3. Each time you watch television, watch a DVD, surf the Web, or play a video game, write down how much time you spent doing so. To be sure of the time, mark down the time you started and the time you stopped (see table 27.1).

4. At the end of each day, add up the number of screen hours for that day. At the end of the week, add up the number of hours for the week.

5. Bring this chart with you to school each day.

▶TABLE 27.1 Sample Screen Time Chart

Day of the week/ time of day	Time started watching TV, watching DVDs, playing video games, surfing the Web	Time stopped watching TV, watching DVDs, playing video games, surfing the Web	Total hours
Monday			
Morning	7:00 a.m.	7:30 a.m.	0.5 hour
Afternoon	3:00 p.m.	3:30 p.m.	0.5 hour
Evening	8:00 p.m.	9:00 p.m.	1 hour
		TOTAL TIME FOR THE DAY	2.0 hours

Screen Time Chart

▶ **TABLE 27.2 Screen Time Chart**

Day of the week	Time started watching TV, watching DVDs, playing video games, surfing the Web	Time stopped watching TV, watching DVDs, playing video games, surfing the Web	Total hours
_____ Morning Afternoon Evening	_____ _____ _____	_____ _____ _____	_____ _____ _____
	TOTAL TIME FOR THE DAY _____		
_____ Morning Afternoon Evening	_____ _____ _____	_____ _____ _____	_____ _____ _____
	TOTAL TIME FOR THE DAY _____		
_____ Morning Afternoon Evening	_____ _____ _____	_____ _____ _____	_____ _____ _____
	TOTAL TIME FOR THE DAY _____		
_____ Morning Afternoon Evening	_____ _____ _____	_____ _____ _____	_____ _____ _____
	TOTAL TIME FOR THE DAY _____		
_____ Morning Afternoon Evening	_____ _____ _____	_____ _____ _____	_____ _____ _____
	TOTAL TIME FOR THE DAY _____		
_____ Morning Afternoon Evening	_____ _____ _____	_____ _____ _____	_____ _____ _____
	TOTAL TIME FOR THE DAY _____		
_____ Morning Afternoon Evening	_____ _____ _____	_____ _____ _____	_____ _____ _____
	TOTAL TIME FOR THE DAY _____		

From L.W.Y. Cheung, H. Dart, S. Kalin, and S.L. Gortmaker, 2007, *Eat Well & Keep Moving,* 2nd ed. (Champaign, IL: Human Kinetics).

1

Name _____

 # Graph-It Worksheet

1. Using the information from your Screen Time Chart, graph the number of hours you spent in screen activities each day.

2. Using the information from your Screen Time Chart, create a graph that compares the number of hours you spent in screen activities each day during the Freeze My TV week with the daily 2-hour (or less) goal.

(continued)

3. Create a graph comparing the total number of hours you spent in screen activities for the entire week with the maximum number of hours you should watch in 1 week based on the recommendation of no more than 2 hours per day.

4. Create a graph comparing the total number of hours you spent in screen activities for the entire week with the total number of hours you spent in school for the entire week.

Name _____

Graph-It Questions

1. Were you able to reach the Freeze My TV goal of no more than 2 hours of screen time on any of the days? Were you able to reach the goal for the entire week? How much over or under the goal were you?

2. What activities did you do instead of watching television, surfing the Web, instant messaging, or playing video games? Which of these activities did you enjoy most? Which were active (kept you moving around)?

3. Do you think you got a lot of screen time compared to the amount of time you spent at school? What do you think about this?

4. **Extra credit:** About how much total time have you spent in screen activities throughout your lifetime? How did you figure this out? Explain your answer.

From L.W.Y. Cheung, H. Dart, S. Kalin, and S.L. Gortmaker, 2007, *Eat Well & Keep Moving*, 2nd ed. (Champaign, IL: Human Kinetics).

Instructions for Assembling the Freeze My TV Journal

When finished, the Freeze My TV Journal will look like a booklet. To create this booklet, complete the following steps:

1. Line up the dots that appear in the corner of every sheet so that they are all in the same corner. Some sheets will be inverted.

2. Place this packet into the photocopier and make double-sided copies of the packet.

3. Fold the packet on the dotted line.

The instructions for assembling the journal are not necessary if you print the journal straight from the full book text on the CD-ROM. The pages there are chronologically ordered. However, use these instructions if you are photocopying the journal from this book.

From L.W.Y. Cheung, H. Dart, S. Kalin, and S.L. Gortmaker, 2007, *Eat Well & Keep Moving,* 2nd ed. (Champaign, IL: Human Kinetics).

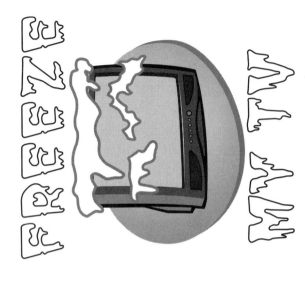

Journal

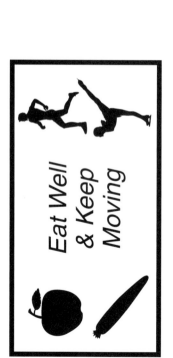

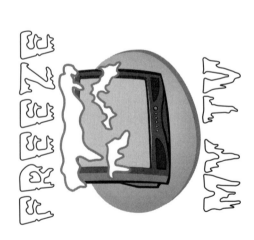

Name _____

Instructions

For each day of Freeze My TV, write a paragraph in this journal. Be sure to read the instructions for each day before you start writing.

Screen Time Alternatives

Acting	Hockey
Babysitting	Hopscotch
Baseball	Inviting friends over
Basketball	Jogging
Bike riding	Jumping rope
Board games	Kickball
Bowling	Lacrosse
Camping	Laundry
Capture the flag	Legos
Checkers	Listening to music
Chess	Painting
Cleaning the house	Planting flowers
Computer work	Playing an instrument
Cooking	Playing Dance, Dance
Dancing	Revolution
Doing each other's hair	Pull-ups
Drawing	Reading
Fishing	Roller skating
Four square	Singing
Frisbee	Sit-ups
Grocery shopping	Skipping
Going to the gym	Stretching
Gymnastics	Tag
Hacky Sack	Swimming
Hide-and-seek	Studying
Hiking	Visiting a museum

From L.W.Y. Cheung, H. Dart, S. Kalin, and S.L. Gortmaker, 2007, *Eat Well & Keep Moving,* 2nd ed. (Champaign, IL: Human Kinetics).

From L.W.Y. Cheung, H. Dart, S. Kalin, and S.L. Gortmaker, 2007, *Eat Well & Keep Moving,* 2nd ed. (Champaign, IL: Human Kinetics).

Day 1

Date _____

Write a paragraph describing how you feel about trying to decrease the amount of time you spend in screen activities for an entire week.

_____

_____

_____

_____

_____

_____

_____

_____

_____

_____

_____

_____

_____

_____

FREEZE MY TV

Day 7

Date _____

A friend of yours wants to try to cut back on screen time. Write a paragraph to your friend with some tips that helped you cut back on your screen time.

_____

_____

_____

_____

_____

_____

_____

_____

_____

_____

_____

_____

_____

Day 2

Date _____

Write a paragraph describing what day 1 of Freeze My TV was like. Did you like getting less screen time? Did you not like it?

_____

_____

_____

_____

_____

_____

_____

_____

_____

_____

_____

_____

_____

Day 6

Date _____

Have you missed all the screen time you usually spend in a typical week? Why or why not?

_____
_____
_____
_____
_____
_____
_____
_____
_____
_____
_____
_____
_____

From L.W.Y. Cheung, H. Dart, S. Kalin, and S.L. Gortmaker, 2007, *Eat Well & Keep Moving*, 2nd ed. (Champaign, IL: Human Kinetics).

Day 3

Date _____

Write a paragraph about what you did during day 1 and day 2 when you weren't watching television or doing other screen activities. How do you think you will spend this time for the rest of the week?

_____
_____
_____
_____
_____
_____
_____
_____
_____
_____
_____
_____
_____
_____

From L.W.Y. Cheung, H. Dart, S. Kalin, and S.L. Gortmaker, 2007, *Eat Well & Keep Moving,*

Day 4

Date _____

Do you like to eat food while you watch television? If yes, what kinds of foods do you eat? Name some healthy snacks you could eat (or already eat) while watching television.

_____

_____

_____

_____

_____

_____

_____

_____

_____

_____

_____

_____

Day 5

Date _____

Write a paragraph describing what you think people did for entertainment before television and computers were invented. How do you think people spent their time back then?

_____

_____

_____

_____

_____

_____

_____

_____

_____

_____

_____

_____

Name _____

Completed Graph-It Worksheets

1. Using the information from your Screen Time Chart, graph the number of hours you spent in screen activities each day.

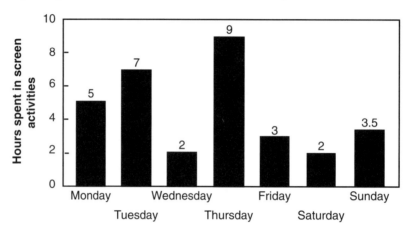

Days of the week

2. Using the information from your Screen Time Chart, create a graph that compares the number of hours you spent in screen activities each day during the Freeze My TV week with the daily 2-hour (or less) goal.

Example 1

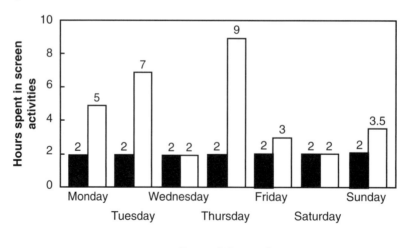

Days of the week

■ 2 hour per day recommendation □ Screen time

(continued)

Example 2

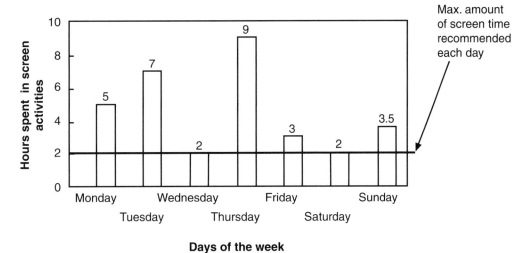

Max. amount of screen time recommended each day

Days of the week

3. Create a graph comparing the total number of hours you spent in screen activities for the entire week with the maximum number of hours you should watch in 1 week based on the recommendation of 2 hours per day.

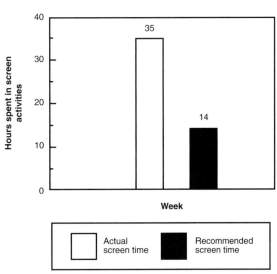

Total recommended and actual hours spent in screen activities for a week

| Actual screen time | Recommended screen time |

(continued)

4. Create a graph comparing the total number of hours you spent in screen activities for the entire week with the total number of hours you spent in school for the entire week.

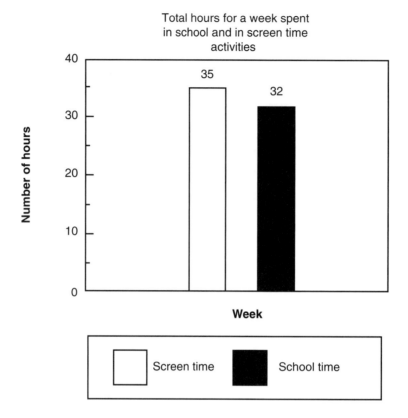

Total hours for a week spent in school and in screen time activities

From L.W.Y. Cheung, H. Dart, S. Kalin, and S.L. Gortmaker, 2007, *Eat Well & Keep Moving*, 2nd ed. (Champaign, IL: Human Kinetics).

Contest Participant Checklist

Teacher _____

School _____ Grade_____

Contest start date _____ Contest end date _____

▶**TABLE 27.3 Teacher Example of Contest Participant Checklist**

Student name	Screen Time Chart	Graph-It worksheets 1 and 2	Freeze My TV Journal
1.	Completed ❑	Completed ❑	Completed ❑
2.	Completed ❑	Completed ❑	Completed ❑
3.	Completed ❑	Completed ❑	Completed ❑
4.	Completed ❑	Completed ❑	Completed ❑
5.	Completed ❑	Completed ❑	Completed ❑
6.	Completed ❑	Completed ❑	Completed ❑
7.	Completed ❑	Completed ❑	Completed ❑
8.	Completed ❑	Completed ❑	Completed ❑
9.	Completed ❑	Completed ❑	Completed ❑
10.	Completed ❑	Completed ❑	Completed ❑
11.	Completed ❑	Completed ❑	Completed ❑
12.	Completed ❑	Completed ❑	Completed ❑
13.	Completed ❑	Completed ❑	Completed ❑
14.	Completed ❑	Completed ❑	Completed ❑
15.	Completed ❑	Completed ❑	Completed ❑
16.	Completed ❑	Completed ❑	Completed ❑
17.	Completed ❑	Completed ❑	Completed ❑
18.	Completed ❑	Completed ❑	Completed ❑
19.	Completed ❑	Completed ❑	Completed ❑
20.	Completed ❑	Completed ❑	Completed ❑

(continued)

From L.W.Y. Cheung, H. Dart, S. Kalin, and S.L. Gortmaker, 2007, *Eat Well & Keep Moving,* 2nd ed. (Champaign, IL: Human Kinetics).

(continued)

▶ **TABLE 27.3** *(continued)*

Student name	Screen Time Chart	Graph-It worksheets 1 and 2	Freeze My TV Journal
21.	Completed ❏	Completed ❏	Completed ❏
22.	Completed ❏	Completed ❏	Completed ❏
23.	Completed ❏	Completed ❏	Completed ❏
24.	Completed ❏	Completed ❏	Completed ❏
25.	Completed ❏	Completed ❏	Completed ❏
26.	Completed ❏	Completed ❏	Completed ❏
27.	Completed ❏	Completed ❏	Completed ❏
28.	Completed ❏	Completed ❏	Completed ❏
29.	Completed ❏	Completed ❏	Completed ❏
30.	Completed ❏	Completed ❏	Completed ❏
31.	Completed ❏	Completed ❏	Completed ❏
32.	Completed ❏	Completed ❏	Completed ❏
33.	Completed ❏	Completed ❏	Completed ❏
34.	Completed ❏	Completed ❏	Completed ❏
35.	Completed ❏	Completed ❏	Completed ❏
36.	Completed ❏	Completed ❏	Completed ❏
37.	Completed ❏	Completed ❏	Completed ❏
38.	Completed ❏	Completed ❏	Completed ❏

From L.W.Y. Cheung, H. Dart, S. Kalin, and S.L. Gortmaker, 2007, *Eat Well & Keep Moving,* 2nd ed. (Champaign, IL: Human Kinetics).

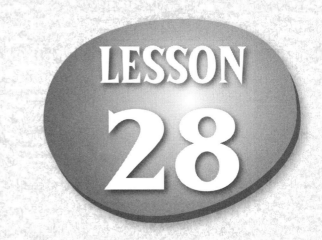

Get 3 At School and 5⁺ A Day

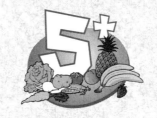

BACKGROUND

Get 3 At School and 5⁺ A Day is an activity that encourages students to eat at least 5 servings of fruits and vegetables each day, with a particular focus on getting at least 3 servings of fruits and vegetables during school breakfast and lunch; getting more is always better. The activity reinforces, in an educational and engaging manner, many of the nutrition messages students have received throughout the year as part of *Eat Well & Keep Moving*.

ACTIVITY LENGTH

The activity runs for an entire school week, beginning on a Monday and ending on a Friday.

GOAL

To help students think about and put into practice the Principles of Healthy Living recommendation that they have been exposed to in the classroom and cafeteria, namely, to eat at least 5 servings of fruits and vegetables every day.

MATERIALS

1. Large Class Tracking Graph example
2. Worksheet 1, My Go for 5⁺ Tracking Chart
3. Fruit and vegetable recipes for each student. Recipes are available online at the following Web sites:
   - Fruits and Veggies—More Matters (Produce for Better Health Foundation): fruitsandveggiesmorematters.org/?page_id=102
   - FruitsandVeggiesMatter.gov (CDC): apps.nccd.cdc.gov/dnparecipe/recipesearch.aspx
   - American Institute for Cancer Research: www.aicr.org/site/PageServer?pagename=dc_rc_veggies
4. Group Tracking Chart
5. Eat Well cards (black and white copies are included in appendix B, pages 572-591)
6. Optional: Recordings of students' songs about fruits and vegetables (if created in lesson 22, menu monitoring; see page 324)

PROCEDURE

PREPARATION DAY

1. On Monday, announce to the students that they will be taking part in a fruits and vegetables activity over the next 4 days (Tuesday-Friday). The students' goal is to eat at least 3 servings of fruits and vegetables every

day at school (including school lunch and breakfast). They will keep track of the servings they eat on a class chart, and they will try to eat at least 2 additional servings of fruits and vegetables outside of school so that they eat at least 5 servings for the entire day.

2. Review the To Nourish Your Body as Well as Your Soul . . . At Least 5 A Day Should Be Your Goal! Eat Well card. Remind the students of the benefits of eating fruits and vegetables (especially dark-green and orange vegetables). Highlight that fruit provides energy for playing and growing and can help heal cuts and bruises. Likewise, let the students know that vegetables can help them fight infections and see better at night.

3. Create a Large Class Tracking Graph (see example on page 401).

4. During lunch (on Day 1 and throughout the week), you may want to ask the cafeteria manager to play students' songs about fruits and vegetables (created in lesson 22) over the cafeteria's public address system; alternatively, you may want to play the songs in the classroom while students write down the number of servings of fruits and vegetables they have had each day (optional).

DAY 1

1. Before lunch, divide the students into small groups and distribute the Group Tracking Charts (for an example, see page 403). Explain that the students in each group will help each other keep track of the fruits and vegetables they eat at lunch. (This activity may also be done individually.)

2. Also before lunch, discuss the What a Treat to Eat a Sweet Peach! Eat Well card.

3. After lunch, have the groups write down on their Group Tracking Chart the number of servings of fruits and vegetables each individual in the group ate. Remind the students that they may also count any fruits or vegetables they ate for breakfast (at school or home). Remind the students that potatoes are not the best choice for reaching their 3 At School or 5⁺ A Day goal. (Potatoes have vitamins and minerals, but they are digested quickly, like white bread or white rice. They should only be eaten, at most, a few times a week, and in small portions. For more information on potatoes and refined carbohydrate, see the background section of Lesson 2, Carb Smart.) Also explain that a small glass of 100% juice can count toward one of the students' servings of fruits and vegetables during the day, but that whole fruit is an even better choice, since it contains more fiber and is easy to grab on the go (see related Eat Well card, Punch Out Fruit Punch—Pick Whole Fruit). Explain that students should limit 100% juice consumption to no more than 8 ounces per day, since juice is high in natural sugars.

4. Mark the students' progress on the Large Class Tracking Graph (see example on page 401). You are encouraged to track your consumption along with that of your students.

5. Explain to the students that they should not stop eating fruits and vegetables once they reach the 3 At School goal. They should strive to get at least 5 servings of fruits and vegetables each day. More is always better.

The Eat Well cards listed for each day are only recommendations. There may be more appropriate Eat Well cards for your Get 3 At School and 5⁺ A Day week— such as those that correspond to the week's lunch menu. You can get a copy of the menu from the cafeteria manager and determine which of the Eat Well cards (in appendix B) would work well with the lunch for each day.

One "serving" can be defined as any time a student consumes the entire amount of a fruit or vegetable served in the cafeteria. If a student consumes only part of the fruit or vegetable served, it can count as a half serving. If a student just tastes a fruit or vegetable, it can count as a quarter serving. A small glass of 100% juice counts as a serving, but note that students should limit juice consumption to no more than 8 ounces (375 milliliters) per day.

6. Distribute worksheet 1, My Go for 5⁺ Tracking Chart, to each student and tell the students that this chart can help them make sure they get at least 5 servings for each day. Explain how to use the chart and encourage them to use their charts at home.

DAY 2

1. Before lunch, discuss the Pick Peppers Eat Well card.

2. After lunch, have the student groups write down on their Group Tracking Chart the number of servings of fruits and vegetables each individual in the group ate. Remind the students that they may also count any fruits or vegetables they ate for breakfast (at school or home).

3. Mark the students' progress on the Large Class Tracking Graph.

4. Remind the students that they should not stop eating fruits and vegetables once they reach the 3 At School goal. They should strive to eat at least 5 servings of fruits and vegetables each day; more is always better.

DAY 3

1. Before lunch, discuss the Punch Out Fruit Punch—Pick Whole Fruit Eat Well card. You can introduce this card by asking the students who had 100% orange juice or a whole orange for breakfast.

2. After lunch, have the student groups write down on their Group Tracking Chart the number of servings of fruits and vegetables each individual in the group ate. Remind the students that they may also count any fruits or vegetables they ate for breakfast (at school or home).

3. Mark the students' progress on the Large Class Tracking Graph.

4. Remind the students that they should not stop eating fruits and vegetables once they reach the 3 At School goal. They should strive to eat at least 5 servings of fruits and vegetables each day; more is always better.

THE FINAL DAY—DAY 4

1. Before lunch discuss the A Message From Bobby Broccoli Eat Well card.

2. After lunch, have the student groups write down on their Group Tracking Chart the number of servings of fruits and vegetables each individual ate. Remind the students that they may also count any fruits or vegetables they ate for breakfast (at school or home).

3. After lunch, complete the Large Class Tracking Graph and review the final results with the students.

4. Remind the students that eating their fruits and vegetables at lunch and getting at least 5 servings each day is vital for their health and will give them the energy they need to think, run, and play.

Distribute recipes to each participant as a prize for participation. Explain that the students may want to try these recipes at home with the help of their parents or other family members.

EAT WELL CARDS

To complement the Get 3 At School and 5⁺ A Day activity, you may discuss Eat Well cards with students right before they go off to lunch on each day of the activity. A black and white copy of each card is provided in appendix B (pages 572-591).

SCHEDULE FOR EAT WELL CARDS

Review the Eat Well cards with your students just before they go to lunch.

► Monday, Preparation Day: To Nourish Your Body as Well as Your Soul . . . At Least 5 A Day Should Be Your Goal!

► Tuesday, Day 1: What a Treat to Eat a Sweet Peach!

► Wednesday, Day 2: Pick Peppers

► Thursday, Day 3: Punch Out Fruit Punch—Pick Whole Fruit

► Friday, Day 4: A Message From Bobby Broccoli

LARGE CLASS TRACKING GRAPH EXAMPLE

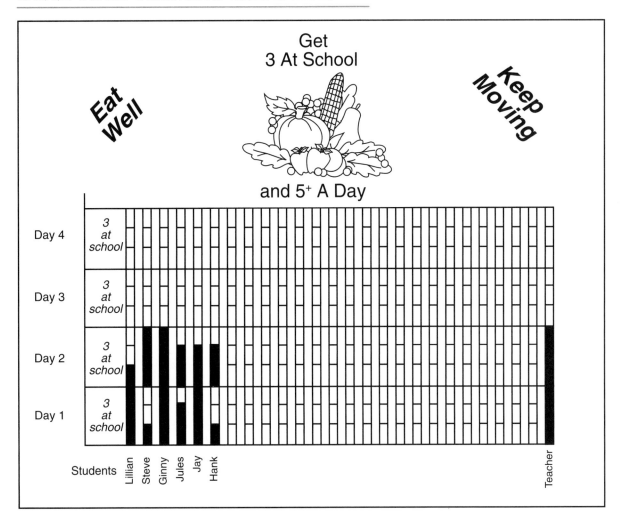

Name _____

My Go for 5⁺ Tracking Chart

Use this chart to track your fruit and vegetable intake during the Get 3 At School and 5⁺ A Day promotion. Write down the names of each fruit and vegetable you eat on each day of the promotion. Remember: The goal is to get at least 3 servings of fruits and vegetables at school, and at least 5 a day. More is always better!

	Day 1	Day 2	Day 3	Day 4
1.				
2.				
3.				
4.				
5.				
6.				
7.				
8.				
9.				
10.				
11.				
12.				
Total				
Check this box if you met the 5⁺ A Day goal				

Group Tracking Chart

School _____ Grade _____

Teacher _____

Group Name _____

Group members	Servings (day 1)	Servings (day 2)	Servings (day 3)	Servings (day 4)	Total servings

From L.W.Y. Cheung, H. Dart, S. Kalin, and S.L. Gortmaker, 2007, *Eat Well & Keep Moving*, 2nd ed. (Champaign, IL: Human Kinetics).

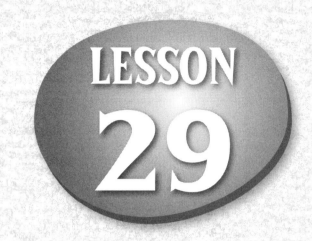

Class Walking Clubs

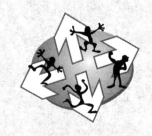

BACKGROUND

This description also appears as part of the Fitness Walking lessons (lesson 13 for fourth grade and lesson 26 for fifth grade) in parts I and II of *Eat Well & Keep Moving.*

This document describes how you can begin an ongoing walking club with your students. Such a walking club will be not only educational but also fun and healthful for your students.

OBJECTIVES

1. Students will participate regularly in a walking activity and establish an ongoing class walking club.

2. Students will learn about the benefits of walking with family, friends, and classmates.

3. Students will learn walking techniques and the health benefits of raising the heart rate through regular aerobic activity.

4. Students will learn about a particular geographic region of the world.

MATERIALS

*Low-cost pedometers are available from many sources on the Web. Consult with your school's physical education director to get recommendations for accurate, easy-to-use, low-cost models. In some communities, local health departments, health centers, or health insurers may provide pedometers for free.

1. Comfortable shoes (students and teacher)
2. Worksheet 1, Teacher Classroom Walking Log
3. Worksheet 2, Student Classroom Walking Log (duplicate for students)
4. Worksheet 3, Student Home Walking Log (duplicate for students)
5. Maps
6. Pedometers* (optional)

WHY WALKING?

Walking is one of the healthiest, safest, and easiest ways to begin a fitness program, and it can be a big step toward improving your health. Fitness or aerobic walking uses all the major muscle groups in the upper and lower body in a gentle, dynamic, rhythmic action, which is what an ideal exercise should do. Children should get at least 60 minutes of physical activity every day, and walking is a great way for them to reach that goal.

Walking is also free! There are no machines or membership fees, no fancy packaging or expensive clothes. Walking requires only that you pace yourself and do your personal best. What's important is feeling good about yourself and setting your own goals.

Walking can be done with friends or family. It can also be done as an adventure with a school class. An active lifestyle can make you feel better, give you more energy, and enhance your health. We want you and your class to get hooked on walking. It's fun, and it's good for you!

PLANNING A WALKING CLUB

When planning a walking club, first consider where and when your students can walk. The walks can take place before, during, or after school and can be done in the hallways, gymnasium, playground, or neighborhood—whenever and wherever such a program works best for your school.

An effective way to introduce a walking club into your school is to integrate it with your curriculum. One option is to integrate the club with your social studies curriculum. For example, you can combine walking with lessons on the state in which you live, on the entire United States, or on other countries around the world. If there is an area of the world your students would like to learn about, use the walking club to talk about that area. As a class or individually, design the itinerary of a fitness walk across the region you have chosen, and then pretend you are walking across that region. Students can walk across America together, walk across a specific region of the United States, or walk around the world. The design is completely open.

Give your program a name, such as Walk Across America or Walk Across the World, or let the students choose a name.

Obtain maps of the area you chose to study, and tie in the students' walking progress with movement on the map. Each time the class walks for a certain length of time, equate that time with a particular distance on the map (for example, 5 minutes walked could equal 50 miles, or 80 kilometers). Each student can have a map to follow, or all of the students can plot their travels on one map. The amount of time the class walks and the distance traveled will depend on the part of the world or country on which you chose to focus. For example, if you decided on a large area of the world, such as Africa, then 5 minutes might equal 200 miles (322 kilometers) traveled. If you chose the state of Maryland, however, 5 minutes might equal 50 miles (80 kilometers).

Keep track of your class walks on the logs provided. There is a log for each class as well as for each student. The class log can be made larger and displayed in the classroom for all to see. A map of the region or country that the students are traveling across should be displayed along with the class log. Displaying the map and log will motivate the class and keep everyone more involved.

If it is possible to supply students with pedometers, consider tracking their number of steps instead of tracking walking time. Pedometers can also be a fun way to motivate students to increase their activity. Have students keep track of the number of steps they take each day for a week, and then have them determine their average number of steps per day. Set a goal for students to increase their average number of steps per day by 10%.

Possible extensions for combining geography with the walking program include having students learn the state's or country's capital, natural resources, climate, unique features, major monuments, and historical sites. Students could create posters to illustrate these features or write journal entries or fictionalized accounts of what they "see" along their walk.

Another way to integrate walking with the curriculum is to link an outdoor nature walk with science lessons (see Extension Activity: Taking a Nature Walk in lessons

13 and 26, pages 193 and 367, which gives suggestions and worksheets for taking a bird observation walk). Students can collect samples, describe a habitat, or look for evidence of human effects on the environment. Have students follow up in the classroom with posters or journal entries describing what they saw.

EXTENSION IDEAS

As an extension of the class walking club, encourage students to take the walking club home as an after-school, family-and-friend adventure. Have the students keep a log of their dates and times of their after-school walks (see Student Home Walking Log on page 414). They can plot their travels on the maps with pins or thumbtacks.

Get the whole school involved in walking—principals, office staff, custodians, and other teachers and students can join the program. The more the students see others participating, the more they will want to become involved.

DAY 1

1. WHAT IS FITNESS WALKING?

Explain to the students that fitness walking is walking at a pace (speed) that makes the heart, lungs, and blood vessels work harder than usual. This type of aerobic workout makes the heart muscle pump harder because the body's other muscles—the leg and arm muscles—are working harder and need more blood to keep them going.

Blood delivers energy and oxygen to working muscles. When muscles work hard, such as when you're fitness walking, they need more energy and oxygen. During exercise, the heart works harder to pump blood to these muscles. When the heart works harder, it gets stronger.

Explain to the students that they can check their pulse rate before they begin exercising and again during their fitness workout in order to see firsthand how the heart muscle works harder. (See details on how to do this in the section on Finding a Pulse on pages 409-410.) Also explain to the students the importance of completing an hour of physical activity on all or most days of the week. It is okay to do that activity a little bit at a time, so a 15-minute or longer walk can help them reach their hour-a-day goal.

2. BENEFITS OF FITNESS WALKING

Ask the students to list the benefits of fitness walking. These can include the following:

a. Walking is an excellent and safe way to improve aerobic fitness. Aerobic exercises, like walking, strengthen the heart, lungs, and blood vessels. Walking lets you do this with less wear and tear on the body compared to many other types of conditioning.

b. Walking and other aerobic exercises can give you more energy and reduce fatigue.

c. Walking can help relieve stress.

d. Walking can improve mood and mental function.

e. Walking can help slow down the progression of osteoporosis (bone loss), which can occur as the body ages.

f. Walking can be performed with friends and family.

3. HOW TO FITNESS WALK

a. Make sure the students wear sneakers or comfortable shoes.

b. Review with students the following (and consult figure 29.1):

1. Arm swing: Try to keep the arms swinging faster than they swing when walking normally. The faster the arms swing, the faster the legs will move. Bend the arms 90 degrees at the elbow. Concentrate on moving the arms faster and swinging them from the shoulder. Remember, when you shorten your arms (bending them 90 degrees at the elbow), you can swing them faster and your legs will move faster. Keep your shoulders relaxed. Beginners tend to tense up around the shoulders. Relax!

2. Hands: Form a loose fist. Do not clench your fist and put tension in the arm muscles.

3. Foot placement and toe-off: The power of the step comes from the toe-off. With each step, land the foot on the heel, and then roll forward to the toe and push off.

Tell the students that following these instructions for fitness walking should help them enjoy their walking more. They should do what feels comfortable for them. Do it right, but make it *fun!*

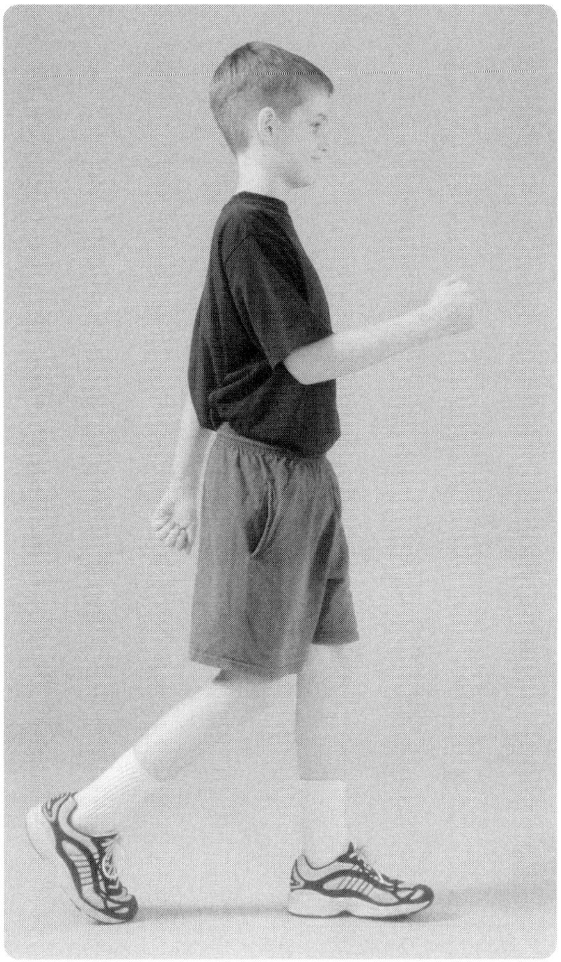

4. THE FITNESS WALK

Step 1: Finding a Pulse

© Human Kinetics.

▶ FIGURE 29.1 Fitness walking.

On the first day of fitness walking (or however often you would like), remind the students that their pulse rate will increase when they exercise and teach them how to find their pulse (refer to figure 29.2). Explain to the students, "During an aerobic workout, you want your heart, lungs, and blood vessels to work harder than they are used to working. Your pulse can help you know what is going on inside your body. On the side of your neck, just below the jawbone, is a major blood vessel bringing blood to the brain. Put your index and middle fingers together and place them gently on that blood vessel on the side of your neck to feel the pulse. During exercise, the pulse is usually very easy to find." To demonstrate how the pulse rate changes from the warm-up to the fitness activity to the cool-down, have the students feel their pulse before, during, and after aerobic walking.

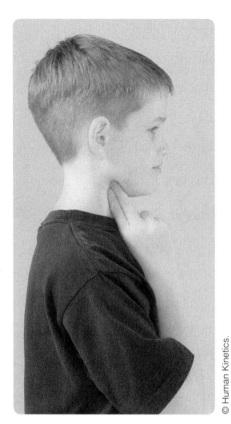

▶ FIGURE 29.2   Finding a pulse.

Tell the students, "The heart is a muscle that has a huge job to do. It must always be working every second, minute, hour, day, week, month, and year of your lives. Once you understand that this heart muscle of yours has such a huge job, hopefully you will want to take care of it so it can do its job.

"Walking is one way to keep the heart muscle healthy. Likewise, eating right and being active are both a big part of helping the heart stay healthy. If during the fitness activity the heart is working harder than it's used to working, then with time the heart will get stronger and stay healthy. The more you include exercise and eating right in your daily lives, the better the body can work and feel!"

Step 2: The Walk

Introduce the walking activity you have chosen for your class, such as walking the first leg of a trip across the United States. Have the class set a goal for that particular day. For example, the class goal for the first day may be to walk for 10 minutes without stopping. If students are using pedometers, the goal may be for each student to walk 1,000 steps. Equate the number of minutes walked or number of steps walked to a particular distance on the map. As students get used to the program, the class can set goals to walk longer and more frequently or (if using pedometers) to increase their average number of steps per day by 10%. Remember, the more days that students walk, the greater the opportunity they have to learn and become fit.

Start each walking session with a few minutes of slow walking to get the body warmed up. After this, the walking can be faster. During the walk, lead the students in a discussion about the geographic region they are pretending to walk through on their program. Other topics to discuss include nutrition and physical activity issues.

After their main walk, have the students walk more slowly to let their bodies cool down.

If time allows, the class can also stretch after the warm-up and cool-down. Follow the stretching examples in lesson 3 of *Eat Well & Keep Moving*.

Step 3: The Stay Healthy Corner

After the first walk, gather the class together and review the benefits of walking, stressing the enjoyment the students will get from it. Introduce and fill out together the classroom walking logs—worksheet 1, Teacher Classroom Walking Log, and worksheet 2, Student Classroom Walking Log.

Introduce and distribute worksheet 3, Student Home Walking Log, to the students. Review with them the four parts of the log sheet—(1) Date, (2) Time or Steps, (3) Miles, and (4) Where—and how to complete the log.

You and your students can decide how to use worksheet 3. For example, the students can keep track of their after-school walking program completely on their own and track their progress on separate maps. Or the students can integrate their after-school walking experience with their in-school tracking system.

However you approach it, the ultimate goal is to motivate students to exercise at home with family or friends.

DAY 2 AND BEYOND

The walking clubs are intended to continue throughout the school year. Whenever possible, they should be done at least 2 to 3 times a week.

When the class has finished "walking" across one region, it can vote for the next region to walk across. To make the activity even more interesting, the class can also "climb" a mountain—such as Mt. McKinley (Denali) or Mt. Everest—or can "walk" between the planets in the solar system, through the center of the earth, or along the circulatory system of the body.

Name _____

Teacher Classroom Walking Log

▶ **TABLE 29.1 Teacher Classroom Walking Log**

Date	Time or Steps*	Miles	Where

*Log number of steps if your class is using pedometers.

Date: Date of the fitness walk

Time or Steps: Number of minutes walked or steps walked

Miles: Number of miles walked (depends on how many minutes or steps your class decided equals 1 mile)

Where: Town, city, state, or country traveled through today

From L.W.Y. Cheung, H. Dart, S. Kalin, and S.L. Gortmaker, 2007, *Eat Well & Keep Moving,* 2nd ed. (Champaign, IL: Human Kinetics).

Name _____

Student Classroom Walking Log

▶**TABLE 29.2 Student Classroom Walking Log**

Date	Time or Steps*	Miles	Where

*Log number of steps if your class is using pedometers.

Date: Date of the fitness walk

Time or Steps: Number of minutes walked or steps walked

Miles: Number of miles walked (depends on how many minutes or steps your class decided equals 1 mile)

Where: Town, city, state, or country traveled through today

From L.W.Y. Cheung, H. Dart, S. Kalin, and S.L. Gortmaker, 2007, *Eat Well & Keep Moving,* 2nd ed. (Champaign, IL: Human Kinetics).

Name _____

Student Home Walking Log

▶ TABLE 29.3 Student Home Walking Log

Date	Time or Steps*	Miles	Where

*Log number of steps if your class is using pedometers.

Date: Date of the fitness walk

Time or Steps: Number of minutes walked or steps walked

Miles: Number of miles walked (depends on how many minutes or steps your class decided equals 1 mile)

Where: Town, city, state, or country traveled through today

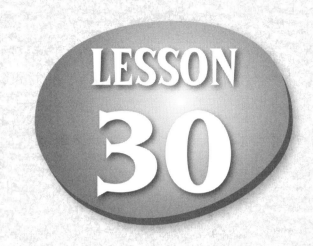

Tour de Health

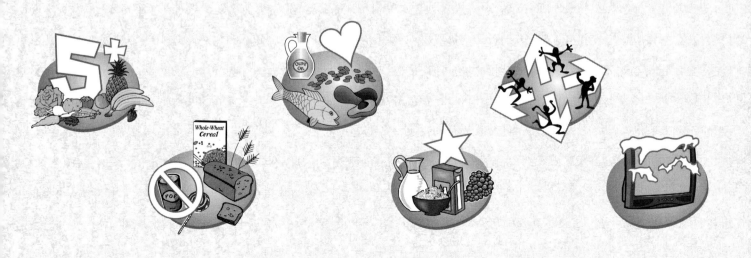

BACKGROUND

A healthy diet and regular physical activity are key to lifelong health. Although the prospect of leading a healthy life is often portrayed as daunting, it is simpler than most people imagine, especially if good habits are started early in life.

Following these six basic guidelines goes a long way toward lowering the risk of disease and improving health:

Principles of Healthy Living

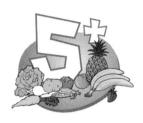

- **Eat 5 or more servings of fruits and vegetables each day.**

Student message: Go for 5⁺ fruits and veggies—more is better!

Fruits and vegetables are packed with vitamins, minerals, antioxidants, and fiber, and they provide healthy carbohydrate that gives us energy. Choose fruits and vegetables in a rainbow of colors (choose especially dark-green and orange vegetables). For more on fruits and vegetables, refer to lessons 10, 11, and 23 and to the school-wide promotion Get 3 At School and 5⁺ A Day (lesson 28).

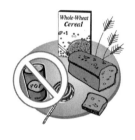

- **Choose whole-grain foods and limit foods and beverages with added sugar.**

Student message: Get whole grains and sack the sugar!

Minimally processed whole grains make better choices than processed or refined grains do. Whole grains contain fiber, vitamins, and minerals, and the refining process strips away many of these beneficial nutrients. Even though some refined grains are fortified with vitamins and minerals, fortification does not replace all the lost nutrients. In addition, refined grains get absorbed very quickly, which causes sugar levels in the blood to spike. In response, the body quickly takes up sugar from the blood to bring sugar levels down to normal; but it can overshoot things a bit, making blood sugar levels a bit low, and this can cause feelings of false hunger even after a big meal. Choose whole grains whenever possible, making sure that at least half of the grain servings you eat each day are made with whole grains. For more on whole grains and healthy carbohydrate, refer to lessons 2 and 12.

In addition to selecting whole-grain foods, limit your intake of sugary beverages such as soft drinks and limit foods with added sugar. Sweetened drinks are said to be filled with empty calories because they provide many calories but few of the nutrients the body needs to stay healthy and grow strong. A growing body of research suggests that consuming sugar-sweetened beverages is associated with excess weight gain in children and adults. For more on sugar-sweetened beverages, refer to lessons 7 and 18.

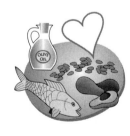

- **Choose healthy fat, limit saturated fat, and avoid trans fat.**

Student message: Keep the fat healthy!

Plant-based foods, including plant oils (such as olive, canola, soybean, corn, sunflower, and peanut oils), nuts, and seeds, are natural sources of healthy fat, as are fish and shellfish. Healthy fat can help lower the risk of heart disease, stroke, and possibly diabetes. Unhealthy fat—namely, saturated fat and trans fat—increases the risk of heart disease, stroke, and possibly diabetes. Much of the fat that comes from animals, including dairy fat, the fat in meat or poultry skin, and lard, is saturated. Saturated fat should make up no more than 10% of your total calorie intake. Trans fat is formed when healthy vegetable oils are partially hydrogenated (a process that makes the oil solid and makes the fat more stable for use in packaged foods). This is the worst type of fat because it raises the risk of heart disease in a number of different ways, and it may raise the risk of diabetes. For more on choosing healthy fat, refer to lessons 5, 6, and 17.

- **Eat a nutritious breakfast every morning.**

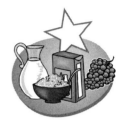

Student message: Start smart with breakfast!

Breakfast is a critical meal since it gives the body the energy it needs to perform at school, work, or home. Studies have shown that breakfast can improve learning, and it helps boost overall nutrition. Many common breakfast foods are rich in whole grains; breakfast is also a great time to get started toward the daily goal of consuming 5 or more servings of fruits and vegetables. For more on eating breakfast, refer to lessons 12 and 24.

- **Be physically active every day for at least an hour per day.**

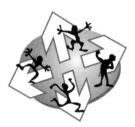

Student message: Keep moving!

Regular physical activity not only improves our physical health (it helps prevent several chronic diseases) but also benefits our emotional well-being. Children should get at least 60 minutes of physical activity every day. This should include moderate- and vigorous-intensity activities, and it can be accumulated throughout the day in sessions of 15 minutes or longer. For more on physical activity, refer to lessons 3, 8, 13, 16, and 26 as well as to the physical education lessons and microunits in parts III through VII.

- **Limit television and other screen time to no more than 2 hours per day.**

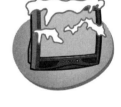

Student message: Freeze the screen!

The more television you watch, the less time you have to engage in physical activity or other healthy pursuits; the same goes for surfing the Web, instant messaging (or text messaging), and playing video games. Watching more television means watching more ads for unhealthy foods, and evidence suggests that this leads to eating extra calories. Such sedentary behavior combined with poor diet can lead to excess weight gain. Children should watch no more than 1 to 2 hours of quality television or videos each day; watching less is better. Children should limit total screen time, including watching television, playing computer games, watching DVDs, and Web surfing, to no more than 2 hours each day. For more on reducing TV viewing and screen time, refer to lessons 9 and 21 and to the school-wide promotion Freeze My TV (lesson 27).

This activity may be used as an assessment for the preceding lessons. The optional extension (part IV), My Tour de Health—How *I* Can Eat Well and Keep Moving, is a great way to bring together all the messages of *Eat Well & Keep Moving* and to involve parents with the program. The My Tour de Health booklet can be completed as a classroom activity; students can bring the completed booklets home to share their health-promoting ideas with their families. Alternatively, students can complete the booklet at home, with family input, as a homework assignment and then bring it to the classroom to share ideas with their peers.

ESTIMATED TEACHING TIME AND RELATED SUBJECT AREA

Estimated teaching time: 1 hour (longer with optional extension)

Related subject area: math

OBJECTIVES

1. Students will review their general knowledge of the Principles of Healthy Living.

2. Students will reinforce their factual knowledge about a healthy lifestyle and appropriate behavior choices.

MATERIALS

1. Handout 1, The Right Style Lifestyle (can be made into a transparency)

2. Game sheet 1, Tour de Health Game Instructions

3. Game sheet 2, Tour de Health Scorecard—one for each person in each group (excluding the question reader) or one for each group, depending on method of play

4. Game sheet 3, Answer Cube

5. Game sheet 4, Building Block for Healthy Living

6. Game sheet 5, Tour de Health Game Cards (to be photocopied)

7. My Tour de Health—How *I* Can Eat Well and Keep Moving booklet (optional extension)

PROCEDURE

PART I

1. Display or distribute handout 1, The Right Style Lifestyle. Review the six healthy lifestyle messages with students and have students recall and fill in the missing words (see the lesson background for more information).

2. Tell the students that they will play a game called *Tour de Health* that quizzes them on the healthy living messages.

PART II

1. Explain the rules for Tour de Health. (See game sheet 1, Tour de Health Game Instructions.)

2. Show the students one of the game cards and read it out loud.

3. Have a student answer using the Answer Cube, and then explain to the class what happens when a correct answer is given.

Keep Moving
How much exercise should you get each week? (3 points)

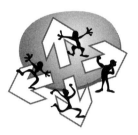

1) About 1 hour
2) About 2 hours
3) About 3 hours
4) About 6 or more hours

Freeze the Screen
What types of food are most often advertised on television? (1 point)

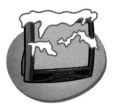

1) Fruits and vegetables
2) Foods made with healthy fat
3) Fast food and junk food
4) Whole grains

PART III

1. Distribute scorecards, the Answer Cube, and game cards to each group leader. You may also keep the game cards up front depending on the version of the game you're playing (see rules).

2. Review the game rules and provide an opportunity for the students to ask questions. Begin the game.

3. At the end of 15 to 20 minutes, if a winner is not declared, you may end the game by announcing, "Last two questions coming up!" The group that ends with the most points is the winner.

4. Review the correct answers to missed game card questions with the students.

PART IV (OPTIONAL EXTENSION)

1. Photocopy and distribute the My Tour de Health—How *I* Can Eat Well and Keep Moving booklet. Discuss ways that students can make changes in their own lives to follow the Principles of Healthy Living.

2. Have the students complete the booklets in class and then take them home to share with their families; alternatively, have the students complete the booklets with family input, as a homework assignment, and then discuss their family's ideas in class once the booklets are completed.

The Right Style Lifestyle

 Go for _____ _____ and _____ —more is better!

 Get _____ _____ and sack the _____!

 Keep the _____ healthy!

 Start smart with _____!

 Keep _____!

 Freeze the _____!

From L.W.Y. Cheung, H. Dart, S. Kalin, and S.L. Gortmaker, 2007, *Eat Well & Keep Moving,* 2nd ed. (Champaign, IL: Human Kinetics).

Tour de Health Game Instructions

Purpose of the Game

In this game, students respond to questions relating to the six healthy living messages covered throughout *Eat Well & Keep Moving.* You may add new questions as new concepts are introduced. The game may also serve as a means of reinforcing previously taught information.

Materials

1. Game cards for each group (to be photocopied from cards provided)
2. Game scorecard
3. Answer Cube (optional)
4. Building Block for Healthy Living (optional)

Setting Up the Game

The general game questions are worth 1 point, 2 points, or 3 points. There is also a select number of bonus questions that are worth 4 points. Photocopy the cards on game sheet 5 and cut them up. There will be approximately 60 general questions and 10 bonus questions in a deck. Shuffle the general deck and place it facedown on the top of a desk or table. The bonus questions should be kept separate from the general questions. You may keep the cards if option 1 of the game is played or give them to the question reader of each group if option 2 is played.

Playing the Game

Here are two ways to play the game:

Option 1: Divide the class into groups of 4, 5, or 6. Assign one person in each group to be the question reader. In this case, the members of each group compete against one another. There will be one winner from each group.

Option 2: Divide the class into groups of 4, 5, or 6. Read the questions to the class and have the members of each group work cooperatively to come up with an answer. In this case, the groups compete against each other.

The reader draws one card at a time, in order from the top, and reads the category of the question (e.g., Whole Grains, Keep Moving). The reader then asks the question of the group or groups. All the questions are either multiple choice, or true

From L.W.Y. Cheung, H. Dart, S. Kalin, and S.L. Gortmaker, 2007, *Eat Well & Keep Moving,* 2nd ed. (Champaign, IL: Human Kinetics).

(continued)

or false. All the players in the group (or all the groups) will then use their Answer Cubes to answer the question. For example, if they think the answer is true, the side of the cube that says "true" should be up, or if they think answer number 1 is correct, the side of the cube that says "1" should be up. (If wanted, players can use their hands to shield their answers until everyone has placed their cube.)

Instead of using Answer Cubes, students can use hand signals to answer questions (thumbs-up for true, thumbs-down for false, and 1, 2, 3, or 4 fingers to indicate answer 1, 2, 3, or 4).

Students who answer correctly receive 1, 2, 3, or 4 points depending on the value of the question. These points are then entered on the scorecard in the related category column. For example, if 2 points are earned for answering a Keep Moving question, then 2 points are entered in the Keep Moving column.

Bonus Round (Optional)

There can be two bonus rounds in each game. The bonus round can be used to quickly add points to the point total and to further reinforce the healthy lifestyle messages of the lessons.

Bonus rounds use the Building Block for Healthy Living from lessons 1 (fourth grade) and 14 (fifth grade). If the game is played under option 1, a Building Block is needed for each group (and is held by the question reader). If the game is played under option 2, only one Building Block is needed (and is held by the teacher).

In the bonus round, the reader picks a card from the bonus card deck. The reader shows the message on the Building Block that corresponds to the message the question will be about (for example, Start smart with breakfast!). The reader asks the question, and students answer just as before, using the Answer Cube or hand signals.

How to Win

Option 1: Play can be timed (for example, for 15 or 20 minutes), and the group or student with the most points at the end wins.

Option 2: First group or player to get 20 total points wins.

From L.W.Y. Cheung, H. Dart, S. Kalin, and S.L. Gortmaker, 2007, *Eat Well & Keep Moving*, 2nd ed. (Champaign, IL: Human Kinetics).

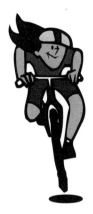

Tour de Health Scorecard

Name (Group Name)_____

When you answer a question correctly, put the number of points for the answer under the appropriate message. At the end of the game, add up the points for each column. Then add all the column totals together to get a grand total.

▶**TABLE 30.1 Tour de Health Scorecard**

POINTS EARNED					
Go for 5⁺ fruits and veggies— more is better!	**Get whole grains and sack the sugar!**	**Keep the fat healthy!**	**Start smart with breakfast!**	**Keep moving!**	**Freeze the screen!**
Total:	Total:	Total:	Total:	Total:	Total:

Grand Total _____

From L.W.Y. Cheung, H. Dart, S. Kalin, and S.L. Gortmaker, 2007, *Eat Well & Keep Moving,* 2nd ed. (Champaign, IL: Human Kinetics).

Answer Cube

Using scissors, cut out the entire cube by cutting along the outside lines. Be sure to cut around the round tabs. Fold the paper so that it forms the cube and tape the round tabs on the inside of the cube to hold it together.

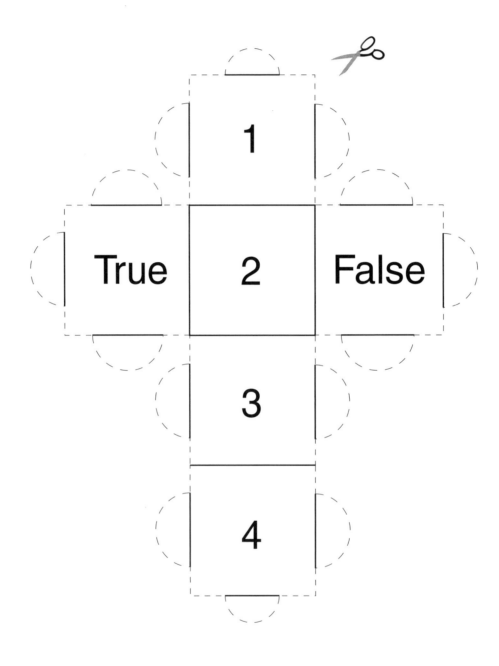

Building Block for Healthy Living

Using scissors, cut out the entire cube on page 426 by cutting along the outside lines. Be sure to cut around the round tabs. Fold the paper so that it forms the cube and tape the round tabs on the inside of the cube to hold it together.

From L.W.Y. Cheung, H. Dart, S. Kalin, and S.L. Gortmaker, 2007, *Eat Well & Keep Moving*, 2nd ed. (Champaign, IL: Human Kinetics).

(continued)

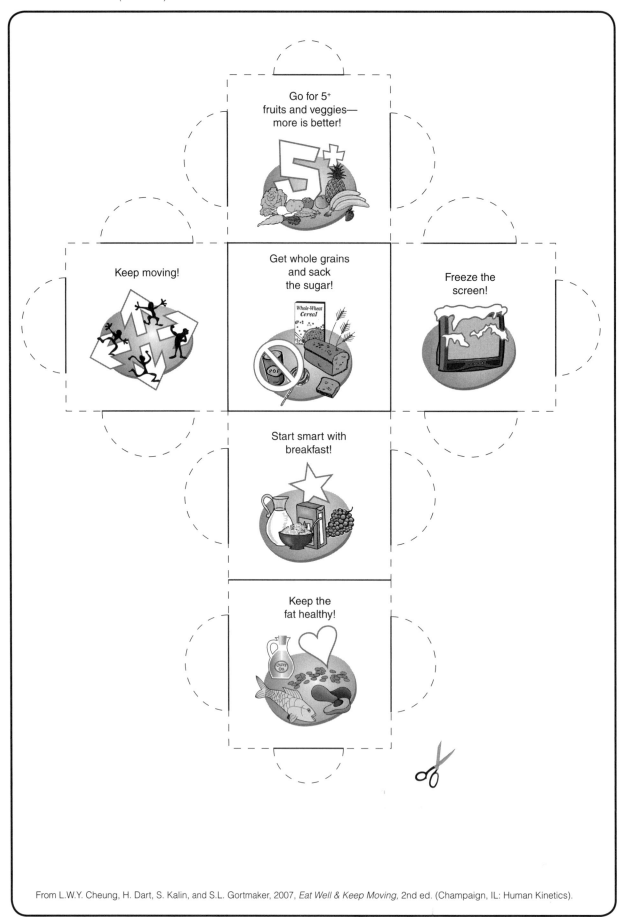

Go for 5+
fruits and veggies—
more is better!

Keep moving!

Get whole grains
and sack
the sugar!

Freeze the
screen!

Start smart with
breakfast!

Keep the
fat healthy!

From L.W.Y. Cheung, H. Dart, S. Kalin, and S.L. Gortmaker, 2007, *Eat Well & Keep Moving,* 2nd ed. (Champaign, IL: Human Kinetics).

Tour de Health Game Cards

Copy and cut out.

Keep Moving
Stretching is part of a safe workout. (1 point)

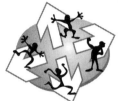

True
False

Freeze the Screen
If I get enough exercise, it doesn't matter how much I watch TV or play video games. (1 point)

True
False

Keep Moving
Exercising with a group of friends is a fun way to stay active. (1 point)

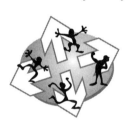

True
False

Freeze the Screen
What do kids spend the most time doing each year? (2 points)

1) Going to school
2) Watching TV and playing video games
3) Playing sports
4) Doing homework

Keep Moving
The first thing you should do before exercising hard is (2 points)

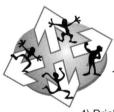

1) Warm up and stretch
2) Eat a huge meal
3) Just sit around
4) Drink a sports drink or energy drink

Freeze the Screen
What's the most time I should spend watching television per day? (1 point)

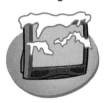

1) 4-5 hours
2) 3-4 hours
3) 2-3 hours
4) 1-2 hours

Keep Moving
How much exercise should you get each week? (3 points)

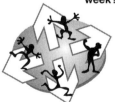

1) About 1 hour
2) About 2 hours
3) About 3 hours
4) About 7 hours (or more)

Freeze the Screen
What types of food are most often advertised on television? (1 point)

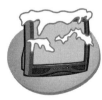

1) Fruits and vegetables
2) Foods made with healthy fat
3) Fast food and junk food
4) Whole grains

From L.W.Y. Cheung, H. Dart, S. Kalin, and S.L. Gortmaker, 2007, *Eat Well & Keep Moving,* 2nd ed. (Champaign, IL: Human Kinetics).

(continued)

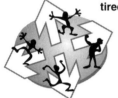

Keep Moving
Which best describes what regular exercise does for you? (1 point)

1) It makes you healthier
2) It helps you feel better about yourself
3) It gives you more energy.
4) It does all of the above.

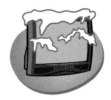

Freeze the Screen
TV time is a great time to stretch and work on my flexibility. (1 point)

True
False

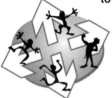

Keep Moving
Exercise helps build strong bones.
(1 point)

True
False

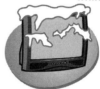

Freeze the Screen
What types of food do most kids eat while watching TV? (1 point)

1) Fruits and vegetables
2) Chips, soft drinks, and other unhealthy snacks
3) Nuts
4) Whole grains

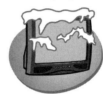

Keep Moving
Exercising regularly will make me feel tired all the time. (1 point)

True
False

Freeze the Screen
Playing video games counts as exercise.
(1 point)

True
False

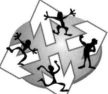

Keep Moving
If I get thirsty while playing or exercising, what is the best thing for me to drink? (2 points)

1) Energy drink
2) Water
3) Soft drink
4) Sports drink

Freeze the Screen
What are some other things you could do instead of playing video games or watching TV? (1 point)

1) Ride bikes with my friends
2) Play in the sprinkler
3) Write a poem
4) All the above

Keep Moving
To be fit, what should you work on?
(2 points)

1) Cardiorespiratory endurance
2) Muscular strength
3) Flexibility
4) All of the above

Freeze the Screen
Most of the food ads on TV try to get me to buy foods that aren't good for me. (1 point)

True
False

From L.W.Y. Cheung, H. Dart, S. Kalin, and S.L. Gortmaker, 2007, *Eat Well & Keep Moving,* 2nd ed. (Champaign, IL: Human Kinetics).

(continued)

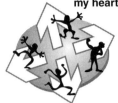

Keep Moving
Lifting weights is the best way to keep my heart healthy. (1 point)

True
False

Freeze the Screen
If you watch 2 hours of TV a day starting when you are very young, how many years will you have spent watching TV by the time you're 65? (3 points)

1) about 1 yr.
2) about 2 yr.
3) about 3 yr.
4) about 5 yr.

Go for 5⁺ Fruits and Veggies–More is Better
One stalk of cooked broccoli has more vitamin C than one tomato has. (2 points)

True
False

Get Whole Grains and Sack the Sugar
Which of these foods does *not* contain whole grain? (2 points)

1) Tabbouleh (bulgur salad)
2) Granola
3) Quinoa pilaf
4) White bread

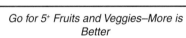

Go for 5⁺ Fruits and Veggies–More is Better
Frozen fruits and vegetables are *not* as good for you as fresh vegetables are. (1 point)

True
False

Get Whole Grains and Sack the Sugar
Which would be the healthiest snack choice? (2 points)

1) Doritos
2) Pretzels made with white flour
3) Sugar cookies
4) Whole wheat crackers

Go for 5⁺ Fruits and Veggies–More is Better
We should try to eat more dark-green and orange vegetables. (1 point)

True
False

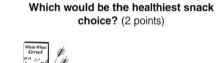

Get Whole Grains and Sack the Sugar
How much sugar is in one regular can of Coke? (2 points)

1) 2 tsp
2) 5 tsp
3) 8 tsp
4) 10 tsp

Go for 5⁺ Fruits and Veggies–More is Better
We should try to eat less dried beans and peas. (1 point)

True
False

Get Whole Grains and Sack the Sugar
Which beverage had no added sugar? (1 point)

1) Coke
2) Sports drink
3) Low-fat chocolate milk
4) Skim milk

From L.W.Y. Cheung, H. Dart, S. Kalin, and S.L. Gortmaker, 2007, *Eat Well & Keep Moving*, 2nd ed. (Champaign, IL: Human Kinetics).

(continued)

Go for 5⁺ Fruits and Veggies–More is Better
What is the maximum amount of 100% fruit juice children should drink in 1 day? (3 points)

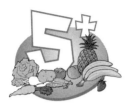

1) 6 oz
2) 8 oz
3) 10 oz
4) 20 oz

Get Whole Grains and Sack the Sugar
Why should we limit how many soft drinks and sugary beverages we drink? (2 points)

1) They are a source of empty calories.
2) They cause blood sugar levels to rise quickly and then fall, leaving us low in energy.
3) They replace more nutritious foods and beverages.
4) They do all of the above.

Go for 5⁺ Fruits and Veggies–More is Better
How much of a watermelon (by weight) is water? (2 points)

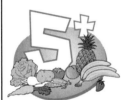

1) 25%
2) 50%
3) 70%
4) 90%

Get Whole Grains and Sack the Sugar
Which of these is a type of sugar that is added to foods and beverages? (2 points)

1) Sucrose
2) High fructose corn syrup
3) Honey
4) All of the above

Go for 5⁺ Fruits and Veggies–More is Better
Which of these fruits are rich in vitamin C? (2 points)

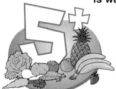

1) Oranges
2) Strawberries
3) Cantaloupe
4) All of the above

Get Whole Grains and Sack the Sugar
How can you tell if a food contains whole grains? (3 points)

1) It's brown
2) It has wheat in the ingredients list.
3) It has a whole grain in the ingredients list.
4) There is no way to tell.

Go for 5⁺ Fruits and Vegetables–More is Better
Which of these vegetables are rich in potassium? (2 points)

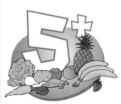

1) Sweet potato
2) Winter squash
3) Spinach
4) All of the above

Get Whole Grains and Sack the Sugar
Why is it important to eat whole grains? (2 points)

1) They are rich in fiber.
2) They are rich in minerals.
3) They are rich in vitamins.
4) They are all of the above.

From L.W.Y. Cheung, H. Dart, S. Kalin, and S.L. Gortmaker, 2007, *Eat Well & Keep Moving,* 2nd ed. (Champaign, IL: Human Kinetics).

(continued)

Go for 5 Fruits and Vegetables–More is Better
Which fruit is an excellent source of fiber? (1 point)

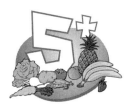

1) Apple
2) Blackberries
3) Grapefruit
4) All of the above

Get Whole Grains and Sack the Sugar
Which of these drinks contains added sugar? (1 point)

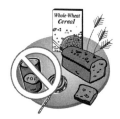

1) 100% orange juice
2) Water
3) Lemonade
4) 1% milk

Go for 5 Fruits and Vegetables–More is Better
Name a large, orange fruit that is popular during an October celebration. (1 point)

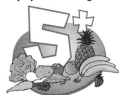

1) Tangerine
2) Peach
3) Pumpkin
4) Apricot

Get Whole Grains and Sack the Sugar
We should eat whole grains once a week. (1 point)

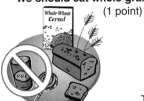

True
False (Every day, at least half of our grains should be whole grains.)

Keep the Fat Healthy
The healthiest person is the one who doesn't eat any fat. (1 point)

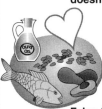

True
False (Healthy fat is an important part of the diet.)

Start Smart With Breakfast
Skipping breakfast so you can sleep late is a good way to start the school day. (1 point)

True
False

Keep the Fat Healthy
Fat that is liquid at room temperature (such as canola oil) is better for your health than is fat that is solid at room temperature (such as stick margarine or butter). (2 points)

True
False

Start Smart With Breakfast
Which breakfast would give you energy to last all the way to lunchtime? (3 points)

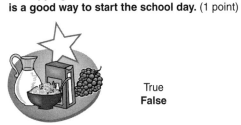

1) A doughnut and a soft drink
2) A bowl of Frosted Flakes with 1% milk
3) White bread toast with jelly
4) Plain (unsweetened) oatmeal with walnuts, apples, and 1% milk.

From L.W.Y. Cheung, H. Dart, S. Kalin, and S.L. Gortmaker, 2007, *Eat Well & Keep Moving*, 2nd ed. (Champaign, IL: Human Kinetics).

(continued)

Keep the Fat Healthy
Which is a healthier food choice? (1 point)

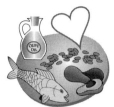

1) Ice cream
2) Milk shake
3) Low-fat frozen yogurt
4) Plain fat-free yogurt with fresh fruit

Start Smart With Breakfast
A turkey sandwich on whole wheat bread with lettuce and tomato is a healthy breakfast. (1 point)

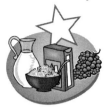

True
False

Keep the Fat Healthy
What is the % Daily Value for saturated fat of a McDonald's Quarter Pounder with cheese? (2 points)

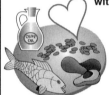

1) 5%
2) 15%
3) 34%
4) 59%

Start Smart With Breakfast
Leftover chicken stir-fry is a healthy breakfast. (1 point)

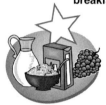

True
False

Keep the Fat Healthy
How many grams of trans fat are in a large order of McDonald's French fries? (2 points)

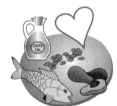

1) 0
2) 2
3) 5
4) 8

Start Smart With Breakfast
A sports drink is a good beverage to have with breakfast. (1 point)

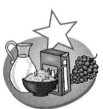

True
False

Keep the Fat Healthy
Which food is a good source of healthy fat? (2 points)

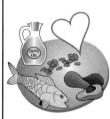

1) Oil and vinegar salad dressing
2) Walnuts
3) Salmon
4) All of the above

Start Smart With Breakfast
Eating a healthy breakfast always takes a long time. (1 point)

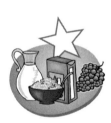

True
False

From L.W.Y. Cheung, H. Dart, S. Kalin, and S.L. Gortmaker, 2007, *Eat Well & Keep Moving,* 2nd ed. (Champaign, IL: Human Kinetics).

(continued)

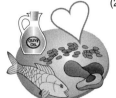

Keep the Fat Healthy
Which snack is a source of healthy fat?
(2 points)

1) Almonds
2) Ice cream
3) Doughnut
4) Pepperoni slices

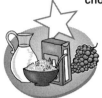

Start Smart With Breakfast
Which of these are healthy breakfast choices? (1 point)

1) Bacon and sausage
2) Sugary breakfast cereal
3) White bread toast with jam
4) None of the above

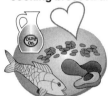

Keep the Fat Healthy
Which of these is a healthy fat choice for cooking broccoli and other vegetables? (1 point)

1) Butter
2) Lard
3) Stick margarine
4) Olive oil

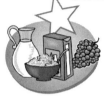

Start Smart With Breakfast
You have to eat breakfast foods at breakfast time. (1 point)

True
False

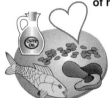

Keep the Fat Healthy
Which of these spreads is a great source of healthy fat? (2 points)

1) Butter
2) Stick margarine
3) Peanut butter
4) Cream cheese

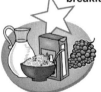

Start Smart With Breakfast
Any healthy food can be a healthy breakfast food. (1 point)

True
False

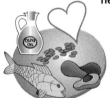

Keep the Fat Healthy
Which salad topping is the best source of healthy fat? (1 point)

1) Olive oil vinaigrette
2) Bacon bits
3) Blue cheese dressing
4) Grated cheddar cheese

Start Smart With Breakfast
Which of these breakfast foods is high in trans fat? (1 point)

1) Fruit salad
2) Oatmeal
3) Doughnut
4) Whole wheat toast

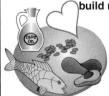

Keep the Fat Healthy
Bonus
Which one of these exercises does not build my cardiorespiratory endurance?

1) Running
2) Dancing
3) Weightlifting
4) Swimming

Keep Moving
Bonus
Walking or running a mile burns about 100 calories. (1 point)

True
False

From L.W.Y. Cheung, H. Dart, S. Kalin, and S.L. Gortmaker, 2007, *Eat Well & Keep Moving,* 2nd ed. (Champaign, IL: Human Kinetics).

(continued)

Freeze the Screen
Bonus
Fast walking burns about 400 Calories an hour. Sitting and watching TV for an hour burns how many calories?

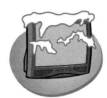

1) 1,000
2) 300
3) 200
4) Less than 100

Freeze the Screen
Bonus
The kids on TV ads for fast food and unhealthy snacks always look fit and healthy and active. Why is this?

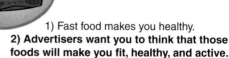

1) Fast food makes you healthy.
2) Advertisers want you to think that those foods will make you fit, healthy, and active.
3) There's no particular reason why advertisers choose these kids for their ads.

Go for 5⁺ Fruits and Veggies–More is Better
Bonus
Name the major vitamin that you get from citrus fruits.

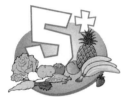

1) Vitamin A
2) Vitamin D
3) Vitamin E
4) Vitamin C

Go for 5⁺ Fruits and Veggies–More is Better
Bonus
Kale, collard greens, and turnip greens have lots of what?

1) Saturated fat
2) Salt
3) Vitamins and minerals
4) Added sugar

Get Whole Grains and Sack the Sugar
Bonus
How can you tell if a beverage contains added sugar?

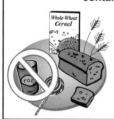

1) Read the Nutrition Facts label.
2) Read the list of ingredients.
3) Taste it.
4) Look at the color of the label.

Get Whole Grains and Sack the Sugar
Bonus
Which of these is a whole grain?

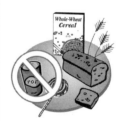

1) Wheat berries
2) Brown rice
3) Barley
4) All of the above

Keep the Fat Healthy
Bonus
Which is the healthiest food choice?

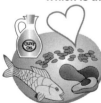

1) Baked chicken with the skin
2) Chicken fried in partially hydrogenated oil
3) Cheeseburger
4) Chicken stir-fried in canola oil

Start Smart With Breakfast
Bonus
Eating breakfast can help you

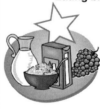

1) Stay more alert until lunch time
2) Do better on tests
3) Have more energy
4) All of the above

From L.W.Y. Cheung, H. Dart, S. Kalin, and S.L. Gortmaker, 2007, *Eat Well & Keep Moving*, 2nd ed. (Champaign, IL: Human Kinetics).

(continued)

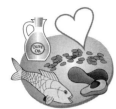

Keep the Fat Healthy
Bonus
Which food has the most trans fat?

1) Almonds
2) Olive oil salad dressing
3) Skim milk
4) French fries

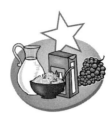

Start Smart With Breakfast
Bonus
**Which of these is a traditional breakfast
food combination in China?**

1) Fish and rice
2) Eggs and whole wheat toast
3) Bran cereal and skim milk
4) Fruit smoothies

Instructions for Assembling My Tour de Health— How *I* Can Eat Well and Keep Moving Booklet

When finished, My Tour de Health—How *I* Can Eat Well and Keep Moving will look like a booklet. To create the booklet, complete the following steps:

1. Line up the dots that appear in the corner of every sheet so that they are all in the same corner. Some sheets will be inverted.

2. Place this packet into the photocopier and make double-sided copies of the packet.

3. Fold the packet on the dotted line.

- -

The instructions for assembling the booklet are not necessary if you are printing the it straight from the full book text on the CD-ROM. The pages there are chronologically ordered. However, use these instructions if you are photocopying the booklet from this book.

From L.W.Y. Cheung, H. Dart, S. Kalin, and S.L. Gortmaker, 2007, *Eat Well & Keep Moving*, 2nd ed. (Champaign, IL: Human Kinetics).

My
Tour de Health—
How *I* Can Eat Well
and Keep Moving

Draw a picture of your favorite healthy food and your favorite activity that gets your body moving.

From L.W.Y. Cheung, H. Dart, S. Kalin, and S.L. Gortmaker, 2007, *Eat Well & Keep Moving*, 2nd ed. (Champaign, IL: Human Kinetics).

From L.W.Y. Cheung, H. Dart, S. Kalin, and S.L. Gortmaker, 2007, *Eat Well & Keep Moving*, 2nd ed. (Champaign, IL: Human Kinetics).

Name _____

Instructions

Review the Principles of Healthy Living. For each message, list three things you can do to be healthier, and then list three things your family can do to be healthier.

Here are three things I can do to cut down on screen time:

1.

2.

3.

Here are three things my family can do to cut down on screen time:

(Examples: Turn off the TV and do fun things together, like play games, take walks, or play sports; take the TVs out of everyone's bedrooms.)

1.

2.

3.

From L.W.Y. Cheung, H. Dart, S. Kalin, and S.L. Gortmaker, 2007, *Eat Well & Keep Moving*, 2nd ed. (Champaign, IL: Human Kinetics)

From L.W.Y. Cheung, H. Dart, S. Kalin, and S.L. Gortmaker, 2007, *Eat Well & Keep Moving*, 2nd ed. (Champaign, IL: Human Kinetics)

Freeze the Screen!

Watching TV, playing video games, or playing on the computer is probably the least active you can be next to sleeping. Do these things too much and you just won't be healthy. Keep screen time as low as it can go, and never let it add up to more than 2 hours per day.

Principles of Healthy Living

 Go for 5⁺ fruits and veggies—more is better!

 Get whole grains and sack the sugar!

 Keep the fat healthy!

 Start smart with breakfast!

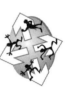 Keep moving!

 Freeze the screen!

From L.W.Y. Cheung, H. Dart, S. Kalin, and S.L. Gortmaker, 2007, *Eat Well & Keep Moving*, 2nd ed. (Champaign, IL: Human Kinetics).

From L.W.Y. Cheung, H. Dart, S. Kalin, and S.L. Gortmaker, 2007, *Eat Well & Keep Moving*, 2nd ed. (Champaign, IL: Human Kinetics).

Go for 5⁺ Fruits and Veggies— More Is Better!

Eat 5 or more servings of fruits and vegetables each day! Eat a variety of colors—try red, orange, yellow, green, blue, and purple.

Here are three fun activities I can do to get my body moving for at least an hour per day:

1.

2.

3.

Here are three fun things my family can do to make sure we are active for at least an hour per day:

(Examples: Go for a walk together after dinner; turn off the TV or computer; do household chores together.)

1.

2.

3.

From L.W.Y. Cheung, H. Dart, S. Kalin, and S.L. Gortmaker, 2007, *Eat Well & Keep Moving*, 2nd ed.

From L.W.Y. Cheung, H. Dart, S. Kalin, and S.L. Gortmaker, 2007, *Eat Well & Keep Moving*, 2nd

Here are three things that I can do to eat 5 or more servings of fruits and vegetables each day:

1.

2.

3.

Here are three things my family can do to eat 5 or more servings of fruits and vegetables each day:

(Examples: Always keep fruit on the counter so it is easy to snack on; add vegetables to sandwiches.)

1.

2.

3.

From L.W.Y. Cheung, H. Dart, S. Kalin, and S.L. Gortmaker, 2007, *Eat Well & Keep Moving*, 2nd ed. (Champaign, IL: Human Kinetics).

Keep Moving!

Being active is a very important part of healthy living. Do what you like most, and keep your body moving for at least an hour per day!

From L.W.Y. Cheung, H. Dart, S. Kalin, and S.L. Gortmaker, 2007, *Eat Well & Keep Moving*, 2nd ed. (Champaign, IL: Human Kinetics).

Get Whole Grains and Sack the Sugar!

Choose healthy whole grains for flavor, fiber, and vitamins. Limit sweets. Candy, soft drinks, and other sugary drinks have almost nothing in them that is good for you. They contain just sugar.

From L.W.Y. Cheung, H. Dart, S. Kalin, and S.L. Gortmaker, 2007, *Eat Well & Keep Moving*, 2nd ed. (Champaign, IL: Human Kinetics)

Here are three things I can do to make sure I eat a healthy breakfast every day:

1.

2.

3.

Here are three things my family can do to make it easy to have a healthy breakfast every day:

(Examples: Buy fruit or juice that is easy to eat on the way to school, such as bananas or apples or a small juice box of 100% juice; have whole-grain breakfast cereals or breads available with healthy spreads such as peanut butter.)

1.

2.

3.

From L.W.Y. Cheung, H. Dart, S. Kalin, and S.L. Gortmaker, 2007, *Eat Well & Keep Moving*, 2nd ed.

Start Smart With Breakfast!

Eating breakfast helps you focus on schoolwork and gives you energy to play. Breakfast is a great meal for add whole grains, fruit, and low-fat or fat-free milk to your day!

From L.W.Y. Cheung, H. Dart, S. Kalin, and S.L. Gortmaker, 2007, *Eat Well & Keep Moving*, 2nd ed. (Champaign, IL: Human Kinetics).

Here are three things I can do to eat more whole grains and limit sweets:

1.

2.

3.

Here are three things my family can do to eat more whole grains and limit sweets:

(Examples: Buy 100% whole wheat bread at the store; switch from soft drinks at meals to water or milk.)

1.

2.

3.

From L.W.Y. Cheung, H. Dart, S. Kalin, and S.L. Gortmaker, 2007, *Eat Well & Keep Moving*, 2nd ed. (Champaign, IL: Human Kinetics).

Keep the Fat Healthy!

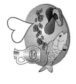

We need fat in our diets, but not all types of fat are good for us. Our bodies like the healthy fat that tends to come from plants and is liquid at room temperature. Examples are olive oil, canola oil, vegetable oil, and peanut oil. Our bodies do not like unhealthy fat, which is solid at room temperature. Examples include saturated fat (usually found in animal products such as meat and whole milk) and trans fat (found in fast-food fries and store-bought cookies). Of the unhealthy fats, trans fat is the worst and should rarely, if ever, be eaten.

Here are three things I can do to choose healthy fat and avoid unhealthy fat:

1.

2.

3.

Here are three things my family can do to choose healthy fat and avoid unhealthy fat:

(Examples: Buy healthy oils for cooking; make chicken nuggets at home in canola oil rather than buy them at fast-food restaurants.)

1.

2.

3.

From L.W.Y. Cheung, H. Dart, S. Kalin, and S.L. Gortmaker, 2007, *Eat Well & Keep Moving*, 2nd ed. (Champaign, IL: Human Kinetics)

From L.W.Y. Cheung, H. Dart, S. Kalin, and S.L. Gortmaker, 2007, *Eat Well & Keep Moving*, 2nd ed. (Champaign, IL: Human Kinetics)

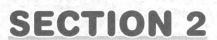

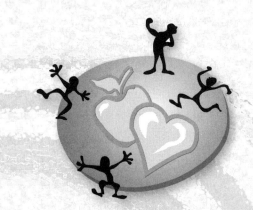

Nutrition and Physical Activity Physical Education Lessons and Microunits

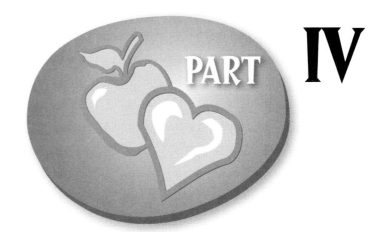

Physical Education Lessons

The physical education setting provides an ideal opportunity to teach students about the importance of both regular physical activity and good nutrition. Complementing the themes of the classroom lessons in parts I and II, the physical education lessons in part IV incorporate key nutrition concepts into physical education class. Designed to be taught by a school's physical education teacher, these lessons are based on the five components of the safe workout. Each physical activity lesson leads the students through the five steps:

1. Warm-up
2. Stretch
3. Fitness activity—an active game that involves a nutrition concept
4. Cool-down
5. Cool-down stretch

In addition to emphasizing the five parts to a safe workout as well as incorporating key nutritional concepts, these lessons focus on endurance fitness activities. Depending on the fitness levels of your students, you may want to modify these activities and slowly build up to and even beyond the target levels.

The physical education lessons offer an opportunity to reiterate one of the Principles of Healthy Living: Be physically active every day for at least an hour per day (Keep moving!). Children should get at least 60 minutes of physical activity every day. These 60 minutes should include moderate- and vigorous-intensity activities and can be accumulated throughout the day in sessions of 15 minutes or longer. (For more information on the Principles of Healthy Living, see lessons 1 and 14.)

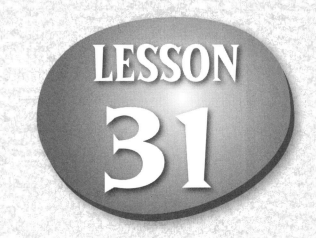

Three Kinds of Fitness Fun: Endurance, Strength, and Flexibility

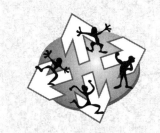

BACKGROUND

Fitness consists of three components—endurance, strength, and flexibility. Students should understand that they need to address each of these in order to become totally fit.

Each fitness component has an important job for the body. Endurance fitness helps with heart health. The key to endurance fitness is to exercise for a long duration without stopping. Choosing an appropriate pace is crucial when doing an endurance activity. Students should not exert themselves so hard that they tire after only a few minutes. Training regularly is also important in developing endurance fitness. Examples of endurance workouts are jumping rope, cycling, walking, jogging, dancing, and any other activity that is performed continuously.

To develop strength fitness, students must perform exercises that make muscles work harder than they are used to working. This is called *overloading.* The muscles must be challenged to go farther, to lift something heavier, or to go faster than they usually do. The muscle fibers that make up muscles get thicker and stronger when they are overloaded regularly. Examples of exercises that improve strength fitness include sit-ups, crunches, push-ups, weightlifting, and climbing. Sports in which strength fitness is important include basketball, baseball, tennis, and track and field.

Flexibility fitness helps prevent injuries and helps the body move more efficiently. The way you improve flexibility fitness is by stretching. Stretching regularly improves the range of motion of the joints and lengthens the fibers of muscles so they will move better with fewer chances of injury. Stretching should be done slowly and properly. Holding a stretch for 10 seconds or longer helps muscles become more flexible. Flexibility fitness is very important in all sports.

It is extremely important for students to practice what they learn in physical education class and to make fitness part of their lifestyle at home.

ESTIMATED TEACHING TIME

Estimated teaching time: 30 minutes

OBJECTIVES

1. The students will demonstrate the five parts of the safe workout.
2. The students will demonstrate different exercises that improve endurance, strength, and flexibility fitness.
3. The students will be able to identify the different parts of fitness and the different exercises that improve specific areas of fitness.

MATERIALS

1. Fitness cards (cards listing an exercise such as push-ups)
2. Fifteen containers (e.g., paper grocery bags)

3. Examples of stretches and strength fitness activities (see appendix A, pages 565-569)

SAFETY POINTS

1. Keep movements fluid and under control.
2. Perform exercises with the proper form.
3. Perform the five parts of the safe workout properly.

PROCEDURE

1. Have students form five groups. (The number of students in a group will depend on the class size; you could have more or less than five groups if needed.)
2. Place fitness cards faceup on the side of the gym opposite the students (see figure 31.1). You may have to duplicate cards more than once so that there are enough for each student to have a turn during the fitness activity.

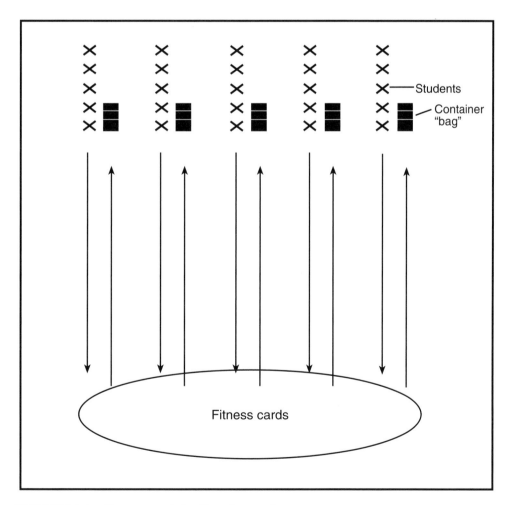

▶ FIGURE 31.1   Fitness activity line formation.

3. Place three containers next to each group—one container for each area of fitness. These will be used to collect the fitness cards chosen by each group.

4. Lead the students in a warm-up and stretch. Review with students the important points of a warm-up and stretch as well as the benefits of endurance and strength fitness activities. Remind the students they should get at least 1 hour of physical activity every day (Keep moving!) and should limit inactive TV and screen time (Freeze the screen!).

    a. Warm-up
        1. Benefits of warming up
- Helps prevent injuries
- Increases body temperature
- Gets the body ready for the rest of the workout

        2. How to warm up
- Perform a series of slow movements for 5 to 10 minutes.
- Examples include slow jogging in place and slow jumping jacks.

    b. Stretch
        1. Benefits of stretching
- Improves flexibility fitness
- Improves the ability of muscles to work
- Improves the body's ability to move
- Decreases the number of injuries

        2. How to stretch (see appendix A for diagrams, pages 565-567)
- Hold the stretch for 10 or more seconds (count out loud: 1 Mississippi, 2 Mississippi . . . 10 Mississippi).
- Don't bounce—hold the stretch gently.
- Stretch slowly.
- Use proper form to avoid injuries.
- Examples include the neck stretch, butterfly, and quadriceps burner (thigh stretch).

    c. Strength fitness (see appendix A for diagrams, pages 568-569)
        1. Benefits of strength fitness
- Improves the ability of your muscles to move or resist a force or workload
- Helps you perform your daily tasks without tiring
- Helps prevent injuries
- Improves your skills in games and sports, such as jumping rope, playing dodgeball, or shooting a basketball

        2. How to improve strength fitness
- Make your muscles work more than they are used to make them go faster, work longer, lift heavier objects, or exercise more often.
- Train, don't strain.
- Don't do too much, too soon, too often.

    d. Endurance fitness
        1. Benefits of endurance fitness
- Improves health of heart, lungs, and blood vessels (builds cardio-respiratory fitness)
- Gives you energy

    2. How to improve endurance fitness
- Do nonstop, continuous movement activities such as bike riding, walking, or rope jumping. (Students may jog or walk in place to demonstrate endurance activities in class.)
- Find a pace (speed) you can do for a long time—"Pace, don't race!"
- Find an endurance activity that you like so you will want to do it.

5. Explain to the students that they will be performing an endurance fitness activity, so they need to find a pace, or speed, that they can do for a long time without stopping. Remind students to "Pace, don't race!" Stress that the speed they pick needs to be one that works for them and that they shouldn't worry about how other students are doing.

6. Explain that at the other end of the gym there are fitness cards with exercises listed on them. Each exercise addresses a different area of fitness. Review the three different parts of fitness with the students. Talk about exercises that improve endurance fitness, strength fitness, and flexibility fitness.

7. On your signal, have the first person in each line jog or run to the fitness cards and pick one up. The first one they touch is the one they bring back to the group.

8. When they get back to the group, they should place the fitness card into the container representing the area of fitness the card addresses, and then go to the end of the line. Remember, everyone should be moving during the entire activity! When waiting in line, students should be marching or jogging in place.

9. Keep the activity going until (a) the fitness cards are gone, (b) each student has gone a designated number of times, or (c) time becomes a concern.

10. Have the groups review their choices, making sure all their cards are correctly classified.

11. Have each group share its choices with the class. Correct any misclassified fitness cards (see table 31.1).

12. Have each group demonstrate a fitness activity that they think would work well at home. Make sure that each area of fitness is covered at least once in the demonstrations.

13. Repeat the fitness activity if time allows.

14. Lead the students in a cool-down and cool-down stretch. Review the important points of each.

    a. Cool-down

        1. Benefits of cooling down
- Lets the body slow down or recover from the fitness activity
- Helps prevent injuries and muscle soreness

        2. How to cool down
- Walk slowly.
- Walk in place slowly.

    b. Cool-down stretch (see appendix A, pages 565-567)

        1. Benefits of the cool-down stretch
- Helps prevent soreness
- Improves flexibility fitness

2. How to do the cool-down stretch
- Hold stretch for 10 or more seconds (count out loud: 1 Mississippi, 2 Mississippi . . . 10 Mississippi).
- Examples include the neck stretch, butterfly, and quadriceps burner (thigh stretch).

15. Close the activity by reminding the students to get at least 1 hour of physical activity every day. It is okay to do that activity a little bit at a time—15 minutes of walking to school, 20 minutes of playing tag—just so long as it adds up to an hour each day. Mix it up to keep it fun, and try trading screen time for active time.

▶TABLE 31.1 Overview of Fitness Cards

Endurance fitness	Strength fitness	Flexibility fitness
Swimming	Push-ups	Neck stretch
Jumping rope	Sit-ups	Arm stretch
Power walking	Weightlifting	Palms to ceiling
Dancing	Pull-ups	Reach back
Basketball	Crunches	Hold up the wall
Jogging	Climbing	Shoulder stretch
In-line skating	Chin-ups	The wave
Ice hockey	Wall sits	Quad burner
Cycling	Squats	Butterfly
Running	Leg lifts	Hamstring stretch
Soccer	Curls	
Tennis		

Fitness Cards

swimming	jogging
jumping rope	in-line skating
power walking	playing ice hockey
dancing	cycling

From L.W.Y. Cheung, H. Dart, S. Kalin, and S.L. Gortmaker, 2007, *Eat Well & Keep Moving*, 2nd ed. (Champaign, IL: Human Kinetics).

(continued)

playing basketball	running
push-ups	crunches
sit-ups	climbing
weightlifting	chin-ups

(continued)

pull-ups	butterfly
neck stretch	shoulder stretch
palms to ceiling	quad burner
reach back	hamstring stretch

From L.W.Y. Cheung, H. Dart, S. Kalin, and S.L. Gortmaker, 2007, *Eat Well & Keep Moving,* 2nd ed. (Champaign, IL: Human Kinetics).

(continued)

hold up the wall	the wave
arm stretch	playing soccer
curls	playing tennis
leg lifts	wall sits
squats	

From L.W.Y. Cheung, H. Dart, S. Kalin, and S.L. Gortmaker, 2007, *Eat Well & Keep Moving*, 2nd ed. (Champaign, IL: Human Kinetics).

(continued)

hold up the wall	the wave
arm stretch	

From L.W.Y. Cheung, H. Dart, S. Kalin, and S.L. Gortmaker, 2007, *Eat Well & Keep Moving,* 2nd ed. (Champaign, IL: Human Kinetics).

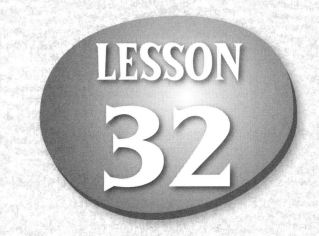

Five Foods Countdown

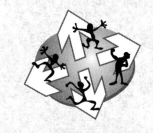

BACKGROUND

Combining a healthy diet with physical activity is important to good health. This message has been emphasized throughout the fourth- and fifth-grade classroom lessons, and this physical education lesson provides an opportunity to further reinforce this message with the students.

In this lesson, students will review nutritional concepts while simultaneously moving around the gymnasium. The lesson will reinforce the students' knowledge of nutrition and will provide an opportunity for the students to enhance their motor skills through physical activity. Furthermore, this lesson offers an opportunity to reiterate one of the Principles of Healthy Living: Be physically active every day for at least an hour per day (Keep moving!). For an overview of the Principles of Healthy Living, see teacher resource page 1 on page 467.

The gymnasium is a perfect classroom in which to learn. Students should understand that physical education is a class for learning; and they need to enter the gym knowing that although there are no desks, chairs, or pencils, they will be learning important information. Because children love to move, this lesson provides an opportunity for students not only to improve their fitness but also to have fun while learning about issues that will affect their lifelong health.

This lesson takes approximately 30 minutes to complete and leads the students through the five parts of the safe workout while also reviewing the five food groups.

ESTIMATED TEACHING TIME

Estimated teaching time: 30 minutes

OBJECTIVES

1. The students will complete an endurance workout.
2. The students will demonstrate a pace that works for them so that they can move for a long time without stopping.
3. The students will be able to list a variety of foods from the five food groups.

MATERIALS

1. Music (medium or upbeat tempo)
2. Teacher resource page 1, Principles of Healthy Living
3. Teacher resource page 2, The Balanced Plate for Health

SAFETY POINTS

1. Move with control throughout the activity.
2. Pace yourself so you have enough energy to do safe movements throughout the activity.

PROCEDURE

1. Assemble the students in an appropriate formation (circle or scattered formation) that allows them room to move, and then lead them through a warm-up and stretch while reviewing the important points of warming up and stretching.

   a. Warm-up

      1. Benefits of warming up
         - Helps prevent injuries
         - Increases body temperature
         - Gets the body ready for the rest of the workout
      2. How to warm up
         - Perform a series of slow movements for 5 to 10 minutes.
         - Examples include slow jogging in place and slow jumping jacks.

   b. Stretch

      1. Benefits of stretching
         - Improves flexibility fitness
         - Improves the ability of muscles to work
         - Improves the body's ability to move
         - Decreases the number of injuries
      2. How to stretch (see appendix A, pages 565-567)
         - Hold the stretch for 10 or more seconds (count out loud: 1 Mississippi, 2 Mississippi . . . 10 Mississippi).
         - Don't bounce—hold the stretch gently.
         - Stretch slowly.
         - Use proper form to avoid injuries.
         - Examples include the neck stretch, butterfly, and quad burner (thigh stretch).

2. As students are moving and stretching, review the important aspects of endurance and strength fitness activities.

   a. Strength fitness (see appendix A, pages 568-569)

      1. Benefits of strength fitness
         - Improves the ability of your muscles to move or resist a force or workload
         - Helps you perform your daily tasks without tiring
         - Helps prevent injuries
         - Improves your skills in games and sports, such as jumping rope, playing dodgeball, or shooting a basketball
      2. How to improve strength fitness
         - Make your muscles work more than they are used to—make them go faster, work longer, lift heavier objects, or exercise more often.
         - Train, don't strain.
         - Don't do too much, too soon, too often.

   b. Endurance fitness

      1. Benefits of endurance fitness
         - Improves health of heart, lungs, and blood vessels (builds cardiorespiratory fitness)
         - Gives you energy

2. How to improve endurance fitness
- Do nonstop, continuous movement activities such as bike riding, walking, or rope jumping (students may jog or walk in place to demonstrate endurance activities in class).
- Find a pace (speed) you can do for a long time—"Pace, don't race!"
- Find an endurance activity that you like so you will want to do it.

3. After the warm-up and stretch, have students practice jogging or walking at an endurance pace (a pace they can do for a long time) as they move in the same direction around the perimeter of the gym (see figure 32.1).

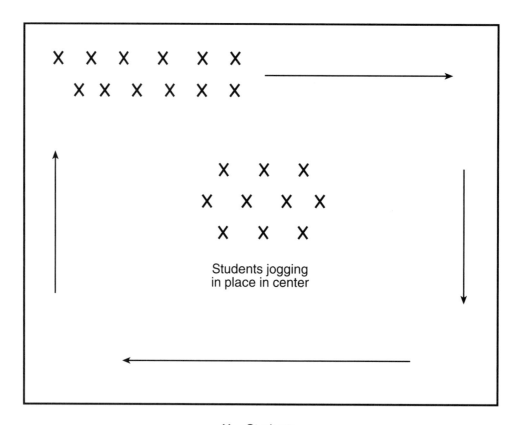

X = Students

▶ FIGURE 32.1 Fitness activity line formation.

4. Stress to the students that they should find their own pace—a speed that works for them (not a friend) that they can do without tiring. Also stress the importance of getting at least 1 hour of physical activity every day (Keep moving!) and limiting inactive TV and screen time (Freeze the screen!) to no more than 2 hours per day.

5. Pick two students to demonstrate the Five Foods Countdown activity.

6. Have the students face each other and extend one hand out in front, in a fist-at-waist level.

7. Announce a food group (e.g., fruit group). The two students take turns naming foods from the fruit group. As they announce each food, they extend a finger on their hand while making the arm motion of an umpire calling a strike. With each

food they name, they extend another finger, until all five fingers are extended. For example, one student says "apple" and makes the arm motion and extends a finger, and then the other student says "pear" and does the same. (Other counting motions may be used as well. For example, students could pat hands, shake hands, slap hands, or even do some kind of feet movement.)

8. After the demonstration of the Five Foods Countdown, have the other students practice with each other.

9. When the class is ready, start the music, and have the children start moving (walking or jogging) in the same direction around the perimeter of the gym. After each round of the Five Foods Countdown, students can reverse direction. Those students who want to jog or walk in place during the activity can do so in the center of the gym (see figure 32.1).

10. Remind the students to pace and have them use a variety of locomotive skills throughout the activity—have them walk, jog, skip, and so on. You can specify the movements or leave the choice to your students.

11. While the students move around the gym, stop the music and announce a food group. The students need to find the closest partner and start counting out five foods that come from the announced food group. The students should make sure that their partners are only naming foods that belong in the announced food group. Students must work with a different partner each time a food group is called. (See table 32.1 on teacher resource page 1, and teacher resource page 2, the Balanced Plate for Health, for a quick review of the five food groups, if needed.)

12. In addition to calling out food groups, you can also call for students to name whole-grain breakfast foods, snack foods, lunch foods, and so on.

13. When the class gets enough experience and endurance with the activity, the students can keep moving (jogging in place, for example) while they count their five foods.

14. Lead the students in a cool-down and cool-down stretch. Review the important points of each. Likewise, review the foods or food groups they had difficulty with during the activity.

   a. Cool-down
      1. Benefits of cooling down
         - Lets the body slow down or recover from the fitness activity
         - Helps prevent injuries and muscle soreness
      2. How to cool down
         - Walk slowly.
         - Walk in place slowly.
   b. Cool-down stretch
      1. Benefits of the cool-down stretch
         - Helps prevent soreness
         - Improves flexibility fitness
      2. How to do the cool-down stretch
         - Hold the stretch for 10 or more seconds (count out loud: 1 Mississippi, 2 Mississippi . . . 10 Mississippi).
         - Examples include the neck stretch, butterfly, and quad burner (thigh stretch).

15. Close the activity by reminding the students to get at least 1 hour of physical activity every day. It is okay to do that activity a little bit at a time—15 minutes of walking to school, 20 minutes of playing tag—just so long as it adds up to an hour each day. Mix it up to keep it fun, and try trading screen time for active time.

Principles of Healthy Living

- **Eat 5 or more servings of fruits and vegetables each day.**

Fruits and vegetables are packed with vitamins, minerals, antioxidants, and fiber, and they provide healthy carbohydrate that gives us energy. Choose fruits and vegetables in a rainbow of colors (choose especially dark-green and orange vegetables).

- **Choose whole-grain foods and limit foods and beverages with added sugar.**

Minimally processed whole grains make better choices than refined grains do. Whole grains contain fiber, vitamins, and minerals, and the refining process strips away many of these beneficial nutrients. Even though some refined grains are fortified with vitamins and minerals, fortification does not replace all of the lost nutrients. In addition, refined grains get absorbed very quickly, and this can cause sugar levels in the blood to spike. In response, the body quickly takes up sugar from the blood to bring the sugar levels down to normal, but the body may overshoot things a bit, making blood sugar levels a bit low. This can cause feelings of false hunger even after a big meal. Choose whole grains whenever possible, making sure that at least half of the grain servings you eat each day are made with whole grains.

In addition to selecting whole-grain foods, limit your intake of sugary beverages such as soft drinks and limit foods with added sugar. Sweetened drinks basically contain just sugar and water, and they are said to be filled with empty calories because they provide many calories but few of the nutrients the body needs to stay healthy and grow strong. A growing body of research suggests that consuming sugar-sweetened beverages is associated with excess weight gain in children and adults. For more on sugar-sweetened beverages, refer to lessons 7 and 18.

- **Choose healthy fat, limit saturated fat, and avoid trans fat.**

Plant-based foods, including plant oils (such as olive, canola, soybean, corn, sunflower, and peanut oils), nuts, and seeds, are natural sources of healthy fat, as are fish and shellfish. Healthy fat can help lower the risk of heart disease, stroke, and possibly diabetes. Unhealthy fat—namely, saturated fat and trans fat—increases the risk of heart disease, stroke, and possibly diabetes. Much of the fat that comes from animals, including dairy fat, the fat in meat or poultry skin, and lard, is saturated. Saturated fat should make up no more than 10% of your total calorie intake. Trans fat is formed when healthy vegetable oils are partially hydrogenated (a process that makes the oil solid and makes the fat more stable for use in packaged foods).

From L.W.Y. Cheung, H. Dart, S. Kalin, and S.L. Gortmaker, 2007, *Eat Well & Keep Moving*, 2nd ed. (Champaign, IL: Human Kinetics).

(continued)

This is the worst type of fat because it raises the risk of heart disease in a number of different ways, and it may possibly raise the risk of diabetes.

- **Eat a nutritious breakfast every morning.**

Breakfast is a critical meal since it gives the body the energy it needs to perform at school, work, and home. Studies have shown that breakfast can improve learning, and it helps boost overall nutrition. Many common breakfast foods are rich in whole grains; breakfast is also a great time to get started toward the daily goal of consuming 5 or more servings of fruits and vegetables.

- **Be physically active every day for at least an hour per day.**

Regular physical activity not only improves our physical health (it prevents several chronic diseases) but also benefits our emotional well-being. Children should get at least 60 minutes of physical activity every day. These 60 minutes should include moderate- and vigorous-intensity activities and can be accumulated throughout the day in sessions of 15 minutes or longer.

- **Limit TV and other screen time to no more than 2 hours per day.**

The more television you watch, the less time you have to engage in physical activity or other healthy pursuits; the same goes for surfing the Web, instant messaging (or text messaging), and playing video games. Watching more television means watching more ads for unhealthy foods, and evidence suggests that this leads to eating extra calories. Such sedentary behavior combined with poor diet can lead to excess weight gain. Children should watch no more than 2 hours of quality television or videos each day; watching less is better. Children should limit total screen time, including watching television, playing computer games, watching DVDs, and Web surfing, to no more than 2 hours each day.

From L.W.Y. Cheung, H. Dart, S. Kalin, and S.L. Gortmaker, 2007, *Eat Well & Keep Moving,* 2nd ed. (Champaign, IL: Human Kinetics).

(continued)

▶TABLE 32.1 Food Items From Each Food Group

Food group	Food items	Best choices*
Grains	Whole grains (barley, brown rice, buckwheat, bulgur, millet, quinoa, wheat), breads (whole wheat or rye bread, whole-grain rolls, stone-ground corn or whole wheat tortillas, whole wheat pitas), cereals (oatmeal, seven-grain hot cereal, ready-to-eat cereals made with whole oats, whole wheat, or other whole grains), pasta (whole wheat noodles, soba noodles), crackers (whole wheat crackers, whole rye crispbread), pancakes (whole wheat or buckwheat)	• Choose whole grains or foods made with minimally processed whole grains. • Choose foods that list a whole grain as the first ingredient.
Vegetables	Collard greens, mustard greens, spinach, kale, chard, bok choy, green cabbage, red cabbage, winter squash, summer squash, zucchini, sweet potatoes, broccoli, carrots, tomatoes, corn, turnips, string beans, lettuce, onions, okra, beets, cauliflower, brussels sprouts, dry beans and peas (kidney beans, black beans, soybeans, chickpeas, lentils, black-eyed peas)	• Choose a rainbow of colors, especially dark green and orange. • Choose dry beans and peas.**
Fruits	Peaches, nectarines, cantaloupe, watermelon, grapefruit, raisins, apples, pears, oranges, bananas, strawberries, tangerines, grapes, pineapple, mangoes, blueberries, cherries, figs, kiwi fruits, avocados	• Choose a rainbow of colors. • Choose whole fruits or sliced fruits (rather than fruit juices).
Meat, fish, and beans	Fish (salmon, trout, cod, shrimp, crab, scallops, light tuna, sardines), nuts (almonds, hazelnuts, walnuts), nut butters (peanut butter, almond butter), seeds (sunflower, pumpkin), dry beans and peas (kidney beans, black beans, soybeans, chickpeas, lentils, black-eyed peas), chicken, turkey, meat (beef, pork, ham), eggs, tofu and other high-protein vegetarian alternatives (tempeh, falafel, vegetable burgers)	• Choose dry beans and peas,** fish, poultry, nuts, and high-protein vegetarian alternatives more often than meat. • When eating meat, choose lean cuts.
Milk	Plain milk (nonfat or 1%), low-fat flavored milk, string cheese (reduced-fat mozzarella sticks), low-fat or nonfat cottage cheese, low-fat cheddar cheese, plain low-fat or nonfat yogurt, low-fat frozen yogurt	• Choose plain low-fat (1%) or nonfat milk, yogurt, and other dairy foods.***

*Best-choice foods contain the most nutrients and contribute to overall health.

**Dry beans and peas can also be considered part of the vegetable group.

***Students who cannot drink milk can choose lactose-free milk or calcium-fortified nondairy alternatives such as unflavored and unsweetened rice milk or soy milk.

From L.W.Y. Cheung, H. Dart, S. Kalin, and S.L. Gortmaker, 2007, *Eat Well & Keep Moving,* 2nd ed. (Champaign, IL: Human Kinetics).

The Balanced Plate for Health

There are five basic food groups: grains; vegetables; fruits; meat, fish, and beans (meat, poultry, fish, dry beans, eggs, nuts, and meat alternatives); and milk. Each food group provides nutritional benefits, so foods from each group should be consumed each day. The key to a balanced diet is to recognize that grains (especially whole grains), vegetables, and fruits are needed in greater proportion than are the foods from the meat, fish, and beans and milk groups. This concept is illustrated by the Balanced Plate for Health (see page 471). A healthy and balanced diet also contains a variety of foods from within each food group, since each food offers different macronutrients (the energy-providing nutrients, namely carbohydrate, protein, and fat) and micronutrients (vitamins and minerals). Eating a variety of foods also keeps our meals interesting and full of flavor. Note that the Balanced Plate for Health does not contain sweets, foods that are high in saturated or trans fats, or foods that are low in nutrients. These are "sometimes" foods, not everyday foods. "Sometimes" foods should be eaten in moderation, and they are depicted on a small side plate.

From L.W.Y. Cheung, H. Dart, S. Kalin, and S.L. Gortmaker, 2007, *Eat Well & Keep Moving,* 2nd ed. (Champaign, IL: Human Kinetics).

(continued)

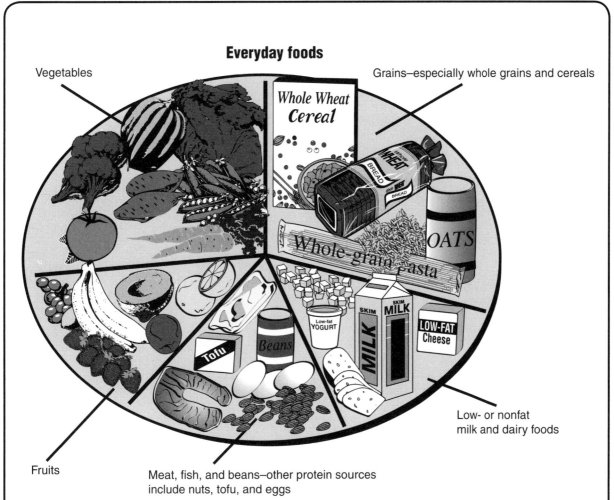

Everyday foods

Vegetables

Grains—especially whole grains and cereals

Whole Wheat Cereal

WHEAT BREAD

OATS

Whole-grain pasta

Low-fat YOGURT

SKIM MILK

LOW-FAT Cheese

Low- or nonfat milk and dairy foods

Tofu

Beans

Fruits

Meat, fish, and beans—other protein sources include nuts, tofu, and eggs

"Sometimes" foods

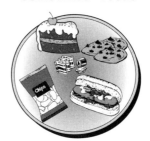

Chips

The key to a balanced diet is to recognize that grains (especially whole grains), vegetables, and fruits are needed in greater proportion than are the foods from the meat, fish, and beans and milk groups.

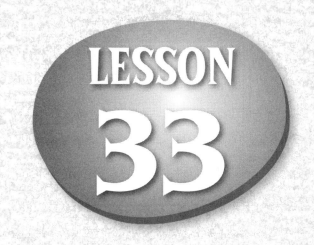

Musical Fare

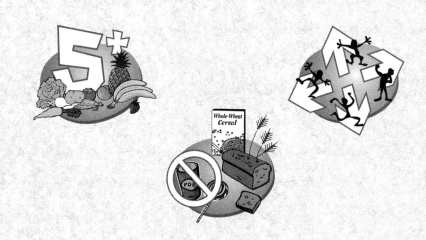

BACKGROUND

Combining a healthy diet with physical activity is important to good health. This message has been emphasized throughout the fourth- and fifth-grade classroom lessons, and this physical education lesson provides an opportunity to further reinforce this message with the students.

In this lesson, students will review nutritional concepts while simultaneously moving around the gymnasium. The lesson will reinforce the students' nutritional knowledge as well as provide an opportunity for the students to enhance their motor skills through physical activity. Furthermore, this lesson offers an opportunity to reiterate one of the Principles of Healthy Living: Be physically active every day for at least an hour per day (Keep moving!). For an overview of the Principles of Healthy Living, please see teacher resource page 1 on pages 479-480.

The gymnasium is a perfect classroom in which to learn. Students should understand that physical education is a class for learning; and they need to enter the gym knowing that although there are no desks, chairs, or pencils, they will be learning important information as they are moving. Because children love to move, this lesson provides an opportunity for students not only to improve their fitness but also to have fun while learning about issues that will affect their lifelong health.

This lesson takes approximately 30 minutes to complete and leads the students through a warm-up and stretch, a fitness activity game similar to musical chairs but involving food pictures, and finally a cool-down and cool-down stretch.

ESTIMATED TEACHING TIME

Estimated teaching time: 30 minutes

OBJECTIVES

1. Students will complete an endurance workout.
2. Students will demonstrate a pace that works for them so that they can move for a long time without stopping.
3. Students will demonstrate their knowledge of the five food groups.

MATERIALS

1. Music (medium or upbeat tempo)
2. Food pictures (cut out from magazines or food packages; the National Dairy Council produces cut-out food models of approximately 200 foods and beverages that can be ordered by calling 800-426-8271 or by contacting your local Dairy Council)
3. Teacher resource page 1, Principles of Healthy Living
4. Teacher resource page 2, The Balanced Plate for Health

SAFETY POINTS

1. Move with control throughout the exercise.

2. Pace yourself to allow safe, fluid movements throughout the lesson.

3. Move around the food pictures without stepping or slipping on them.

PROCEDURE

1. Assemble the students in an appropriate formation (circle or scattered formation) and lead them through a warm-up and stretch while reviewing the important points of the warm-up and stretch.

    a. Warm-up

        1. Benefits of warming up

- Helps prevent injuries
- Increases body temperature
- Gets the body ready for the rest of the workout

        2. How to warm up

- Perform a series of slow movements for 5 to 10 minutes.
- Examples include slow jogging in place and slow jumping jacks.

    b. Stretch

        1. Benefits of stretching

- Improves flexibility fitness
- Improves the ability of muscles to work
- Improves the body's ability to move
- Decreases the number of injuries

        2. How to stretch (see appendix A, pages 565-567)

- Hold the stretch for 10 or more seconds (count out loud: 1 Mississippi, 2 Mississippi . . . 10 Mississippi).
- Don't bounce—hold the stretch gently.
- Stretch slowly.
- Use proper form to avoid injuries.
- Examples include the neck stretch, butterfly, and quadriceps burner (thigh stretch).

2. Review with the students the important aspects of endurance and strength fitness activities.

    a. Strength fitness (see appendix A, pages 568-569)

        1. Benefits of strength fitness

- Improves the ability of your muscles to move or resist a force or workload
- Helps you perform your daily tasks without tiring
- Helps prevent injuries
- Improves your skills in games and sports, such as jumping rope, playing dodgeball, or shooting a basketball

        2. How to improve strength fitness

- Make your muscles work more than they are used to—make them go faster, work longer, lift heavier objects, or exercise more often.

- Train, don't strain.
- Don't do too much, too soon, too often.

   b. Endurance fitness

      1. Benefits of endurance fitness

- Improves health of heart, lungs, and blood vessels (builds cardio-respiratory fitness)
- Gives you energy

      2. How to improve endurance fitness

- Do nonstop, continuous movement activities such as bike riding, walking, or rope jumping (students may jog or walk in place to demonstrate endurance activities in class).
- Find a pace (speed) you can do for a long time—"Pace, don't race!"
- Find an endurance activity that you like so you will want to do it.

3. Have the students find their own space in the gym and practice moving (e.g., jogging in place) at an endurance pace (a speed they can do for a long time).

4. Stress to the students that they should find their own pace—a speed that works for them (not a friend) that they can do without tiring. Also stress the importance of getting at least 1 hour of physical activity every day (Keep moving!) and limiting inactive TV and screen time (Freeze the screen!).

5. Place food pictures from all the food groups around the perimeter of the gym and up against the wall (see figure 33.1). Make sure the pictures are not too close to one another.

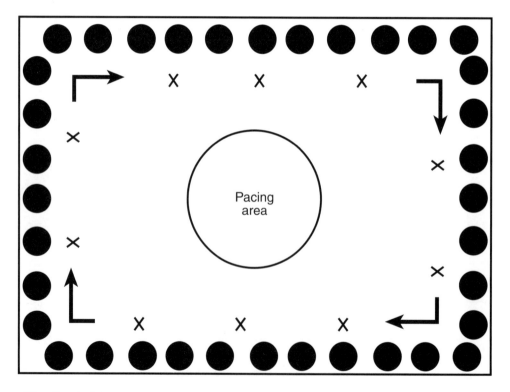

● = Food pictures

X = Students

▶ FIGURE 33.1 Fitness activity setup.

6. Explain to the students that the pictures come from the five food groups.

7. Review the different food groups (see table 33.1 on page 481) as well as the Principles of Healthy Living, and encourage the students to choose fruits and vegetables and whole grains. (While doing this, you can have the students place the food pictures around the gym.)

8. Have the music ready to go. The music should be easy to turn on and off.

9. Explain to the students that they will be playing an endurance game that is like musical chairs—but they will be using food pictures rather than chairs.

10. Stress that the students will be active throughout the workout and that they should pace themselves so that they will not get tired. They should find a speed (pace) that they can do for a long time.

11. Tell the students they may use a different locomotive skill for each round of the game. One round they can jog, the next they can walk, the next they can skip, and so on.

12. When the music begins, the students should jog around the perimeter of the room (all in the same direction and spaced out appropriately) next to the food pictures. Remind the students to be careful not to step on the pictures.

13. When the music stops, have each student stand next to the food picture he is closest to, pick it up, and hold it over his head. Then call out 1 or 2 food groups (the number of food groups you call out will depend on the class size). Those students who do not have a food that belongs to the announced food groups should put their pictures down where they found them and go to an area of the room called the *pacing area,* where they will remain (and continue walking or jogging in place) for one round.

14. Have students double-check with their neighbors to make sure they have correctly determined if their food does or does not belong to the announced food group. You can make the final determination if students are unclear on the correct answer.

> **Sample Round**
>
> When the music stops, each student picks up the food picture she is closest to and holds it above her head. Then you call out "grains group" and "milk group." Students check their foods with their neighbors, and those students who do not have a food picture belonging to the grains or milk group put their pictures down and go to the pacing area. The rest of the students then put their pictures back down on the ground, and you start the music again to begin another round. For additional game variations, see page 478.

15. Have students in the pacing area return to the main group after having missed one round.

16. Lead the students in a cool-down and cool-down stretch. Review the important points of each.
    a. Cool-down
       1. Benefits of cooling down
          • Lets the body slow down or recover from the fitness activity
          • Helps prevent injuries and muscle soreness
       2. How to cool down
          • Walk slowly.
          • Walk in place slowly.

    b. Cool-down stretch

      1. Benefits of the cool-down stretch

- Helps prevent soreness
- Improves flexibility fitness

      2. How to do the cool-down stretch

- Hold the stretch for 10 or more seconds (count out loud: 1 Mississippi, 2 Mississippi . . . 10 Mississippi).
- Examples include the neck stretch, butterfly, and quad burner (thigh stretch).

17. Close the activity by reminding the students to get at least 1 hour of physical activity every day. It is okay to do that activity a little bit at a time—15 minutes of walking to school, 20 minutes of playing tag—just so long as it adds up to an hour a day. Mix it up to keep it fun, and try trading screen time for active time.

ADDITIONAL GAME VARIATIONS

In order to keep the game exciting, you may want to modify it once in awhile. Try the following variations:

1. Have the students pair up and work as partners to play the game.

2. Change the rules so that those students who have pictures of the food groups called move into the pacing area.

Principles of Healthy Living

- **Eat 5 or more servings of fruits and vegetables each day.**

Fruits and vegetables are packed with vitamins, minerals, antioxidants, and fiber, and they provide healthy carbohydrate that gives us energy. Choose fruits and vegetables in a rainbow of colors (choose especially dark-green and orange vegetables).

- **Choose whole-grain foods and limit foods and beverages with added sugar.**

Minimally processed whole grains make better choices than refined grains do. Whole grains contain fiber, vitamins, and minerals, and the refining process strips away many of these beneficial nutrients. Even though some refined grains are forti-fied with vitamins and minerals, fortification does not replace all of the lost nutrients. In addition, refined grains get absorbed very quickly, and this can cause sugar levels in the blood to spike. In response, the body quickly takes up sugar from the blood to bring sugar levels down to normal, but the body may overshoot things a bit, making blood sugar levels a bit low, and this can cause feelings of false hunger even after a big meal. Choose whole grains whenever possible, making sure that at least half of the grain servings you eat each day are made with whole grains.

In addition to selecting whole-grain foods, limit your intake of sugary beverages such as soft drinks and limit foods with added sugar. Sweetened drinks basically contain just sugar and water, and they are said to be filled with empty calories because they provide many calories but few of the nutrients the body needs to stay healthy and grow strong. A growing body of research suggests that consuming sugar-sweetened beverages is associated with excess weight gain in children and adults. For more on sugar-sweetened beverages, refer to lessons 7 and 18.

- **Choose healthy fat, limit saturated fat, and avoid trans fat.**

Plant-based foods, including plant oils (such as olive, canola, soybean, corn, sunflower, and peanut oils), nuts, and seeds, are natural sources of healthy fat, as are fish and shellfish. Healthy fat can help lower the risk of heart disease, stroke, and possibly diabetes. Unhealthy fat—namely, saturated fat and trans fat—increases the risk of heart disease, stroke, and possibly diabetes. Much of the fat that comes from animals, including dairy fat, the fat in meat or poultry skin, and lard, is saturated. Saturated fat should make up no more than 10% of your total calorie intake. Trans fat is formed when healthy vegetable oils are partially hydrogenated (a process

From L.W.Y. Cheung, H. Dart, S. Kalin, and S.L. Gortmaker, 2007, *Eat Well & Keep Moving*, 2nd ed. (Champaign, IL: Human Kinetics).

(continued)

that makes the oil solid and makes the fat more stable for use in packaged foods). This is the worst type of fat because it raises the risk of heart disease in a number of different ways, and it may possibly raise the risk of diabetes.

- **Eat a nutritious breakfast every morning.**

Breakfast is a critical meal since it gives the body the energy it needs to perform at school, work, and home. Studies have shown that breakfast can improve learning, and it helps boost overall nutrition. Many common breakfast foods are rich in whole grains; breakfast is also a great time to get started toward the daily goal of consuming 5 or more servings of fruits and vegetables.

- **Be physically active every day for at least an hour per day.**

Regular physical activity not only improves our physical health (it prevents several chronic diseases) but also benefits our emotional well-being. Children should get at least 60 minutes of physical activity every day. These 60 minutes should include moderate- and vigorous-intensity activities and can be accumulated throughout the day in sessions of 15 minutes or longer.

- **Limit TV and other screen time to no more than 2 hours per day.**

The more television you watch, the less time you have to engage in physical activity or other healthy pursuits; the same goes for surfing the Web, instant messaging (or text messaging), and playing video games. Watching more television means watching more ads for unhealthy foods, and evidence suggests that this leads to eating extra calories. Such sedentary behavior combined with poor diet can lead to excess weight gain. Children should watch no more than 2 hours of quality television or videos each day; watching less is better. Children should limit total screen time, including watching television, playing computer games, watching DVDs, and Web surfing, to no more than 2 hours each day.

(continued)

▶ TABLE 33.1 Food Items From Each Food Group

Food group	Food items	Best choices*
Grains	Whole grains (barley, brown rice, buckwheat, bulgur, millet, quinoa, wheat), breads (whole wheat or rye bread, whole-grain rolls, stone-ground corn or whole wheat tortillas, whole wheat pitas), cereals (oatmeal, seven-grain hot cereal, ready-to-eat cereals made with whole oats, wheat, or other whole grains), pasta (whole wheat noodles, soba noodles), crackers (whole wheat crackers, whole rye crispbread), pancakes (whole wheat or buckwheat)	• Choose whole grains or foods made with minimally processed whole grains. • Choose foods that list a whole grain as the first ingredient.
Vegetables	Collard greens, mustard greens, spinach, kale, chard, bok choy, green cabbage, red cabbage, winter squash, summer squash, zucchini, sweet potatoes, broccoli, carrots, tomatoes, corn, turnips, string beans, lettuce, onions, okra, beets, cauliflower, brussels sprouts, dry beans and peas (kidney beans, black beans, soybeans, chickpeas, lentils, black-eyed peas)	• Choose a rainbow of colors, especially dark green and orange. • Choose dry beans and peas.**
Fruits	Peaches, nectarines, cantaloupe, watermelon, grapefruit, raisins, apples, pears, oranges, bananas, strawberries, tangerines, grapes, pineapple, mangoes, blueberries, cherries, figs, kiwi ftuits, avocados	• Choose a rainbow of colors. • Choose whole fruits or sliced fruits (rather than fruit juices).
Meat, fish, and beans	Fish (salmon, trout, cod, shrimp, crab, scallops, light tuna, sardines), nuts (almonds, hazelnuts, walnuts), nut butters (peanut butter, almond butter), seeds (sunflower, pumpkin), dry beans and peas (kidney beans, black beans, soybeans, chickpeas, lentils, black-eyed peas), chicken, turkey, meat (beef, pork, ham), eggs, tofu and other high-protein vegetarian alternatives (tempeh, falafel, vegetable burgers)	• Choose dry beans and peas,** fish, poultry, nuts, and high-protein vegetarian alternatives more often than meat. • When eating meat, choose lean cuts.
Milk	Plain milk (nonfat or 1%), low-fat flavored milk, string cheese (reduced-fat mozzarella sticks), low-fat or nonfat cottage cheese, low-fat cheddar cheese, plain low-fat or nonfat yogurt, low-fat frozen yogurt	• Choose plain low-fat (1%) or nonfat milk, yogurt, and other dairy foods.***

*Best-choice foods contain the most nutrients and contribute to overall health.

**Dry beans and peas can also be considered part of the vegetable group.

***Students who cannot drink milk can choose lactose-free milk or calcium-fortified nondairy alternatives such as unflavored rice milk or soy milk.

From L.W.Y. Cheung, H. Dart, S. Kalin, and S.L. Gortmaker, 2007, *Eat Well & Keep Moving,* 2nd ed. (Champaign, IL: Human Kinetics).

The Balanced Plate for Health

There are five basic food groups: grains; vegetables; fruits; meat, fish, and beans (meat, poultry, fish, dry beans, eggs, nuts, and meat alternatives); and milk. Each food group provides nutritional benefits, so foods from each group should be consumed each day. The key to a balanced diet is to recognize that grains (especially whole grains), vegetables, and fruits are needed in greater proportion than are the foods from the meat, fish, and beans and milk groups. This concept is illustrated by the Balanced Plate for Health (see page 483). A healthy and balanced diet also contains a variety of foods from within each food group, since each food offers different macronutrients (the energy-providing nutrients, namely carbohydrate, protein, and fat) and micronutrients (vitamins and minerals). Eating a variety of foods also keeps our meals interesting and full of flavor. Note that the Balanced Plate for Health does not contain sweets, foods that are high in saturated or trans fats, or foods that are low in nutrients. These are "sometimes" foods, not everyday foods. "Sometimes" foods should be eaten in moderation, and they are depicted on a small side plate.

From L.W.Y. Cheung, H. Dart, S. Kalin, and S.L. Gortmaker, 2007, *Eat Well & Keep Moving,* 2nd ed. (Champaign, IL: Human Kinetics).

(continued)

A Balanced Plate for Health

Everyday foods

Vegetables

Grains–especially whole grains and cereals

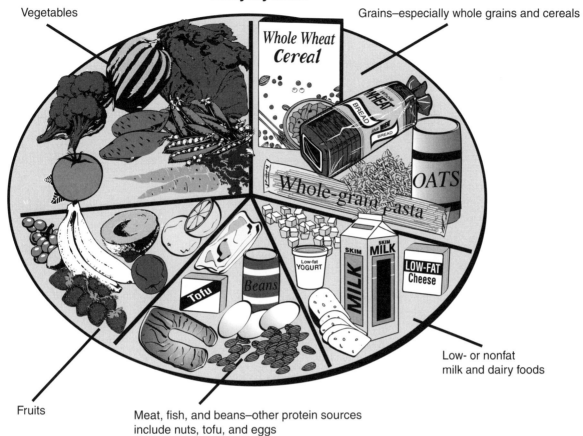

Low- or nonfat
milk and dairy foods

Fruits

Meat, fish, and beans–other protein sources
include nuts, tofu, and eggs

"Sometimes" foods

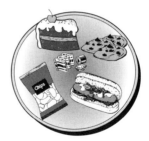

The key to a balanced diet is to recognize
that grains (especially whole grains),vege-
tables, and fruits are needed in greater
proportion than are the foods from the
meat, fish, and beans and milk groups.

From L.W.Y. Cheung, H. Dart, S. Kalin, and S.L. Gortmaker, 2007, *Eat Well & Keep Moving*, 2nd ed. (Champaign, IL: Human Kinetics).

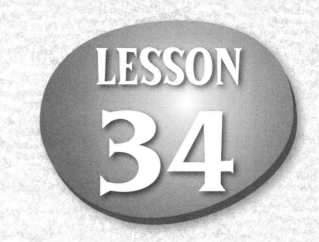

Bowling for Snacks

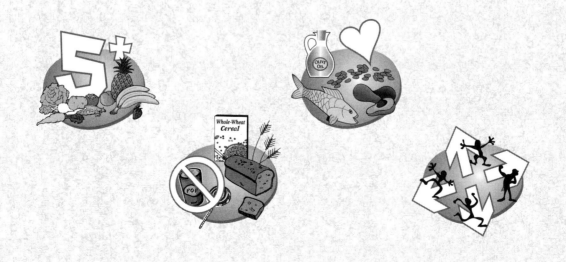

BACKGROUND

This lesson will help students understand how important physical activity and eating healthful snacks are for a healthy body.

Snacks can be an important part of a child's diet. Healthful snacks can help provide the calories and nutrients children need for growth and development. Children need guidance, however, in what they eat for snacks. They often choose snacks that are high in saturated or trans fat, sugar, salt, or calories and low in important nutrients such as vitamins and minerals. These types of snacks are said to be filled with empty calories because they provide many calories but few of the nutrients the body needs to stay healthy and grow strong.

Snacks such as fruit, low-fat plain yogurt, and whole wheat bread, on the other hand, are nutrient dense, providing both calories and nutrients. Students need to understand that they should choose nutrient-dense snacks over snacks filled with empty calories.

In this lesson, students will learn about choosing healthful, nutrient-dense snacks in a bowling activity. Cans representing healthful and less healthful snacks are set up in the gym and students attempt to knock over only those targets representing healthful, nutrient-dense snacks. The lesson also offers an opportunity to reiterate one of the Principles of Healthy Living: Be physically active every day for at least an hour per day (Keep moving!). Children should get at least 60 minutes of physical activity every day. These 60 minutes should include moderate- and vigorous-intensity activities and can be accumulated throughout the day in sessions of 15 minutes or longer.

ESTIMATED TEACHING TIME

Estimated teaching time: 30 minutes

OBJECTIVES

1. The students will complete an endurance workout.
2. The students will demonstrate a pace that they can follow for a long time without stopping.
3. The students will describe the difference between healthful, nutrient-dense snacks and empty-calorie snacks.
4. The students will be able to categorize snacks into their appropriate food groups.

MATERIALS

1. Approximately 30 to 50 pieces of equipment, such as tennis ball cans, milk cartons, plastic water bottles, plastic cups, or paper cups, that will be used as targets (pins); pictures of snacks should be attached to each target (pin)
2. Fifteen or more balls (e.g., yarn balls, Nerf balls, tennis balls, or any ball that can be safely used to roll toward and knock down the target with the attached food picture)

3. A variety of nutrient-dense snack pictures and a variety of empty-calorie snack pictures (to be attached to the targets); you may provide the pictures or have students cut them out of magazines, newspapers, or empty food packages and bring them in

4. Teacher resource page 1, Variations of Bowling for Snacks

5. Ten hula hoops (optional)

6. Two sets of food group signs (one set of originals is provided)

SAFETY POINTS

1. Choose equipment that is safe.
2. Provide enough open space for students to move freely without getting hurt.

PROCEDURE

1. Lead the students through a warm-up and stretch while reviewing the important points of each. Also review the importance of getting at least 1 hour of physical activity every day (Keep moving!) and limiting inactive TV and screen time (Freeze the screen!).

    a. Warm-up

    1. Benefits of warming up
        - Helps prevent injuries
        - Increases body temperature
        - Gets the body ready for the rest of the workout
    2. How to warm up
        - Perform a series of slow movements for 5 to 10 minutes.
        - Examples include slow jogging in place and slow jumping jacks.

    b. Stretch

    1. Benefits of stretching
        - Improves flexibility fitness
        - Improves the ability of muscles to work
        - Improves the body's ability to move
        - Decreases the number of injuries
    2. How to stretch (see appendix A, pages 565-567)
        - Hold the stretch for 10 or more seconds (count out loud: 1 Mississippi, 2 Mississippi . . . 10 Mississippi).
        - Don't bounce—hold the stretch gently.
        - Stretch slowly.
        - Use proper form to avoid injuries.
        - Examples include the neck stretch, butterfly, and quad burner (thigh stretch).

2. Review the important aspects of endurance fitness activities.

    a. Benefits of endurance fitness
        - Improves the health of the heart, lungs, and blood vessels (builds cardiorespiratory fitness)
        - Gives you energy

b. How to improve endurance fitness
- Do nonstop, continuous movement activities such as bike riding, walking, or rope jumping (students may jog or walk in place to demonstrate endurance activities in class).
- Find a pace (speed) you can do for a long time—"Pace, don't race!"
- As a goal, do endurance activities 3 to 4 days a week for 20 to 30 minutes each time.
- Find an endurance activity that you like so you will want to do it.

3. Set up half of the cans with the attached food pictures on one side of the gym and set up the other half of the cans on the other side of the gym (see figure 34.1). Make sure that healthful and less healthful snacks are distributed evenly throughout each side.

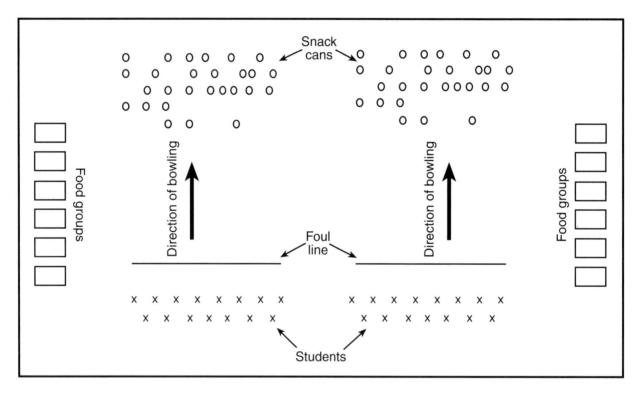

▶ FIGURE 34.1   Bowling for snacks setup.

4. If necessary, review with the students the concept of bowling—rolling a ball down a lane to knock down pins.

5. Place the food group signs parallel to each team's bowling lane (see figure 34.1). If you want, place a hula hoop next to each food group sign. During the game, the students can place their snack pictures in the proper hula hoops.

6. Review the following rules of the game with the students:

a. As in bowling, the students use balls to knock over targets (pins). Students should bowl one at a time. When a student is bowling, the objective is to knock over a target that represents a healthful snack and then place this snack in its correct food group. The first team to knock down all its healthful snacks and have them correctly categorized into the different food groups wins the game.

b. Game rules:

- Students need to move nonstop for the entire game.
- There will be two groups playing the game one group on one each side of the gym (see figure 34.1).
- Students may not cross the foul line when bowling (see figure 34.1).
- Balls should be rolled underhand on the ground toward the targets. They should not be thrown.
- If the ball hits or knocks over a target, the student may cross the foul line to see if the snack is a healthful snack or a less healthful snack.
- If it is a healthful snack, the student picks up the target and places it in the food group to which it belongs.
- If it is not a healthful snack, the student puts the target back, returns to the group, and picks an exercise to complete (such as jumping jacks, push-ups, sit-ups, or pull-ups) before getting to bowl again.
- The first group to knock down all its healthy snacks and place them in the correct food groups wins the game.
- The other team can send a person over to check to see that its opponent picked only healthy snacks and that the snacks were properly categorized.

See teacher resource page 1 for game variations.

7. After reviewing the rules, have the students play the game.

8. When the game is finished, review the choices each group made when they were bowling and discuss the differences between healthful, nutrient-dense snacks (the ones they picked and placed in the food groups) and empty-calorie snacks (the ones that remain on the bowling lane).

9. Repeat the game if time allows.

10. Lead the students in a cool-down and cool-down stretch. Review the important points of each.

   a. Cool-down

      1. Benefits of cooling down
   - Lets the body slow down or recover from the fitness activity
   - Helps prevent injuries and muscle soreness

      2. How to cool down
   - Walk slowly.
   - Walk in place slowly.

   b. Cool-down stretch

      1. Benefits of the cool-down stretch
   - Helps prevent soreness
   - Improves flexibility fitness

      2. How to do the cool-down stretch
   - Hold the stretch for 10 or more seconds (count out loud: 1 Mississippi, 2 Mississippi . . . 10 Mississippi).
   - Examples include the neck stretch, butterfly, and quad burner (thigh stretch).

11. Close the activity by reminding the students to get at least 1 hour of physical activity every day. It is okay to do that activity a little bit at a timed—15 minutes of walking to school, 20 minutes of playing tag—just so long as it adds up to an hour a day. Mix it up to keep it fun, and try trading screen time for active time.

Variations of Bowling for Snacks

You may want to change the activity to better fit your group needs or to keep the game fun and exciting. Try the following variations:

1. Have the entire class work as one team. See how many healthful snacks the class can knock over and correctly classify in 5 minutes, and then see if the students can beat their own score in the next 5-minute round.

2. Have the students switch from bowling with their dominant hand to bowling with their nondominant hand (or vice versa) with each new round.

Food Group Signs

Following is a set of food group signs. You will need to make copies of this set, as you will want two copies of each sign for the activity.

From L.W.Y. Cheung, H. Dart, S. Kalin, and S.L. Gortmaker, 2007, *Eat Well & Keep Moving*, 2nd ed. (Champaign, IL: Human Kinetics).

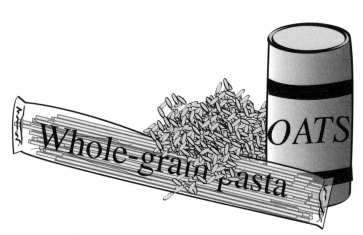

Grain

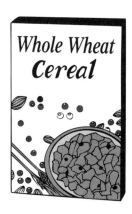

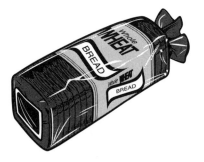

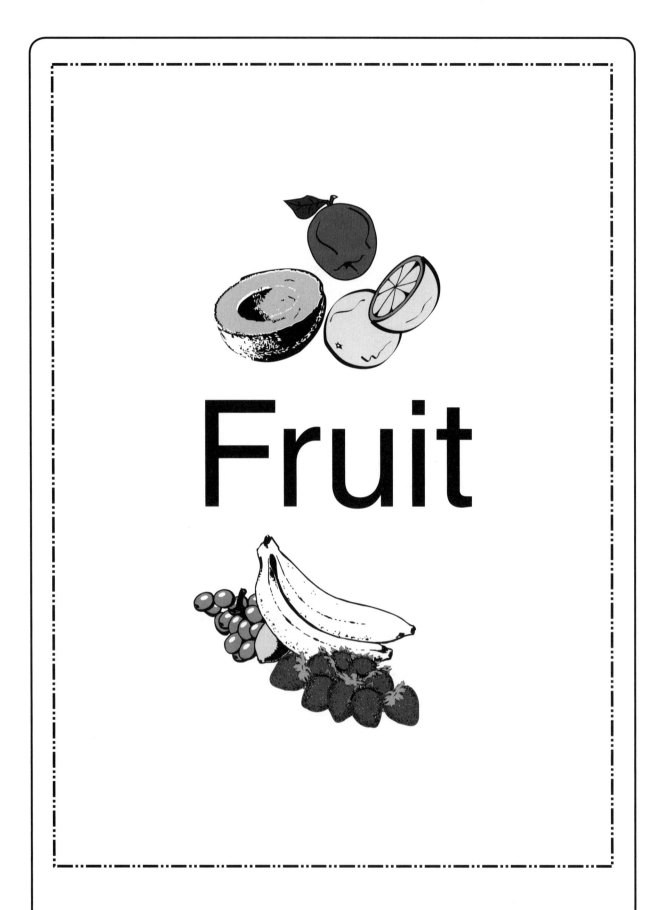

Fruit

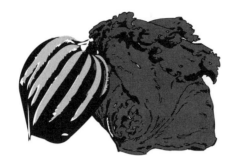

Vegetable

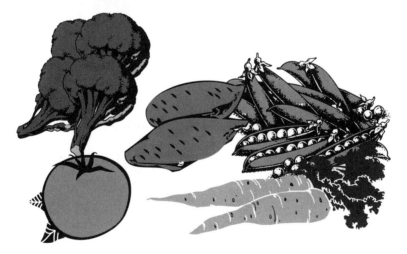

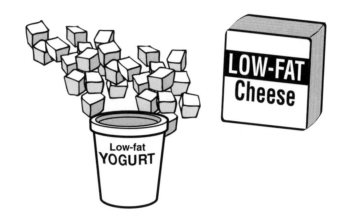

Milk, yogurt and cheese

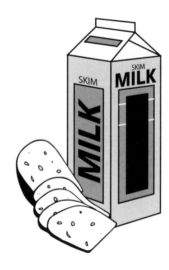

Meat, chicken, fish, and beans

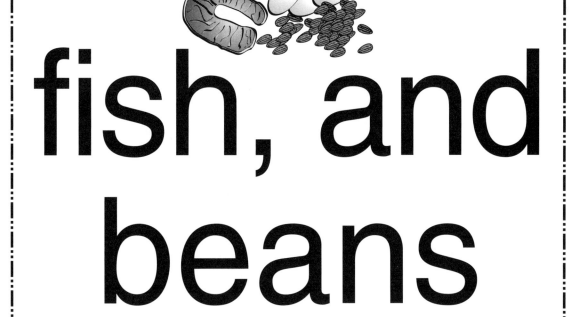

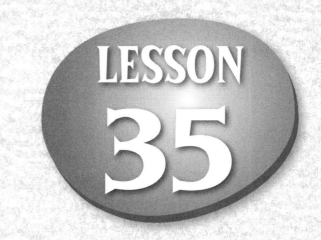

Fruits
and Vegetables

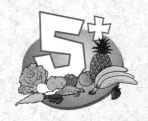 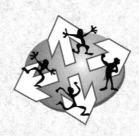

BACKGROUND

Healthy bodies are the result of combining movement with eating right. This lesson stresses doing both. Students need to understand that exercising and eating right are a winning pair.

This lesson will teach students to eat 5 or more fruits and vegetables each day. Leading health authorities recommend that both adults and children eat at least 5 daily servings of fruits and vegetables; eating more is always better. Getting at least 5 servings a day may reduce the risk of heart disease, high blood pressure, diabetes, and possibly some cancers. It is especially important to get young children excited about eating fruits and vegetables so that they establish healthy eating patterns that will last a lifetime.

This lesson takes approximately 30 minutes to complete and leads the students through the five parts of a safe workout while also reviewing the fruit and vegetable food groups. The lesson also offers an opportunity to reiterate one of the Principles of Healthy Living: Be physically active every day for at least an hour per day (Keep moving!). Children should get at least 60 minutes of physical activity every day. These 60 minutes should include moderate- and vigorous-intensity activities and can be accumulated throughout the day in sessions of 15 minutes or longer.

ESTIMATED TEACHING TIME

Estimated teaching time: 30 minutes

OBJECTIVES

1. The students will complete an endurance workout.
2. The students will demonstrate a pace that works for them so that they can move for a long time without stopping.
3. The students will learn to eat 5 or more servings of fruits and vegetables each day to help develop strong, healthy minds and bodies.

MATERIALS

1. A large variety of food pictures showing (or food words naming) at least 45 fruits and vegetables as well as other food items; food name cards are provided, you may provide the pictures or have students cut them out of magazines, newspapers, or empty food packages and bring them in.

   Examples of fruits are apple, apricot, avocado, banana, cherry, coconut, date, fig, grape, grapefruit, kiwi, lemon, lime, mango, melon, nectarine, orange, papaya, peach, pear, persimmon, pineapple, plum, prune, raisin, strawberry, and tangerine.

   Examples of vegetables are artichoke, asparagus, beet, broccoli, brussels sprouts, cabbage, carrot, cauliflower, celery, chard, corn, cucumber, eggplant, green beans, greens, kelp, lettuce, mushroom, okra, onion, parsnip, peas, pepper, pumpkin, radish, spinach, squash, sweet potato, tomato, and turnip.

Examples of other foods are barley, bread, butter, cashews, cheese, chicken, cookie, cracker, egg, tuna, tortilla, marshmallow, peanuts, pork, salmon, shrimp, soft drink, wheat, and yogurt.

2. The phrase *5⁺ A Day* written on paper, with each letter or number written on a separate page (for example, write the number *5⁺* on one sheet of paper, the letter *A* on another, and so on); each of the four teams should get one copy of the phrase (see figure 35.1)

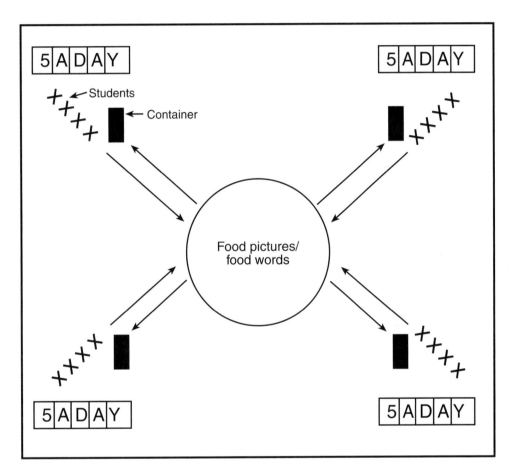

▶ FIGURE 35.1   Fitness activity setup.

3. Four containers (such as paper bags) in which each team can place the words or pictures of the foods that are not fruits and vegetables (see figure 35.1)

SAFETY POINTS

1. Move with control throughout the exercise.

2. Pace yourself to allow safe, fluid movements throughout the lesson.

PROCEDURE

1. Assemble the students in an appropriate formation (circle or scattered formation) and lead them through a warm-up and stretch while reviewing the important points of each.

    a. Warm-up

        1. Benefits of warming up

- Helps prevent injuries
- Increases body temperature
- Gets the body ready for the rest of the workout

        2. How to warm up

- Perform a series of slow movements for 5 to 10 minutes.
- Examples include slow jogging in place and slow jumping jacks.

    b. Stretch

        1. Benefits of stretching

- Improves flexibility fitness
- Improves the ability of muscles to work
- Improves the body's ability to move
- Decreases the number of injuries

        2. How to stretch (see appendix A, pages 565-567)

- Hold the stretch for 10 or more seconds (count out loud: 1 Mississippi, 2 Mississippi . . . 10 Mississippi).
- Don't bounce—hold the stretch gently.
- Stretch slowly.
- Use proper form to avoid injuries.
- Examples include the neck stretch, butterfly, and quad burner (thigh stretch).

2. Review the important points of endurance and strength fitness activities and the reasons why students should get at least 1 hour of physical activity every day (Keep moving!) and limit their inactive TV and screen time (Freeze the screen!).

    a. Strength fitness (see appendix A, pages 568-569)

        1. Benefits of strength fitness

- Improves the ability of your muscles to move or resist a force or workload
- Helps you perform your daily tasks without tiring
- Helps prevent injuries
- Improves your skills in games and sports such as jumping rope, playing dodgeball, or shooting a basketball

        2. How to improve strength fitness

- Make your muscles work more than they are used to—make them go faster, work longer, lift heavier objects, or exercise more often.
- Train, don't strain.
- Don't do too much, too soon, too often.

b. Endurance fitness

   1. Benefits of endurance fitness

- Improves the health of the heart, lungs, and blood vessels (builds cardiorespiratory fitness)
- Gives you energy

   2. How to improve endurance fitness

- Do nonstop, continuous movement activities such as bike riding, walking, or rope jumping (students may jog or walk in place to demonstrate endurance activities in class).
- Find a pace (speed) you can do for a long time—"Pace, don't race!"
- Find an endurance activity that you like so you will want to do it.

3. Divide the students into four groups.

4. Place the food pictures or food words facedown in the center of the gym (you can place the pictures before or during class) and direct each group to move to a position equidistant from the food pictures or words.

5. Place a set of 5⁺ A Day letters next to each group, and have the students lay out the letters in an area where they will not get stepped on. Have the students stand near the container or bag and line up one behind the other (see figure 35.1).

6. On your signal, the first person from each group should walk or jog (staying under control) to the food pictures, retrieve one, and then return to the group. Students picking up the picture or word card cannot peek at it until they return to their group. Stress fair play.

If the picture is a fruit or a vegetable, have the student put it on the first of the 5⁺ A Day letters—in this case, put the picture on the paper with the number 5⁺. If the food picture is not a fruit or a vegetable, the student should put it in the container or bag.

The next student in line should take a turn as soon as the first person gets back. The group is finished as soon as each sheet of paper used to spell 5 A Day is covered by a fruit or vegetable.

7. Repeat the game by returning the food pictures to the center of the gym and starting over again.

8. For each round of the game, have each group review the fruits and vegetables covering their 5⁺ A Day sign.

9. Ask the students why they should always get at least 5 servings of fruits and vegetables every day. Possible answers include that doing so will give them energy, will help them grow, and will keep them healthy.

10. Lead students in a cool-down and cool-down stretch. Review the important points of each.

   a. Cool-down

     1. Benefits of cooling down

- Lets the body slow down or recover from the fitness activity
- Helps prevent injuries and muscle soreness

> For a longer game, you can have students continue until all the food pictures are gone. In this case, simply have the students keep filling in the 5⁺ A Day letters, even if it means there is more than one picture on each letter.

> The students should be moving at a steady pace during the entire game! When they are waiting in line, they should be either marching or jogging in place.

    2. How to cool down
- Walk slowly.
- Walk in place slowly.

  b. Cool-down stretch

    1. Benefits of the cool-down stretch
- Helps prevent soreness
- Improves flexibility fitness

    2. How to do the cool-down stretch
- Hold the stretch for 10 or more seconds (count out loud: 1 Mississippi, 2 Mississippi . . . 10 Mississippi).
- Examples include the neck stretch, butterfly, and quadriceps burner (thigh stretch).

11. Close the activity by reminding the students to get at least 1 hour of physical activity every day. It is okay to do that activity a little bit at a time—15 minutes of walking to school, 20 minutes of playing tag—just so long as it adds up to an hour a day. Mix it up to keep it fun, and try trading screen time for active time.

Food Name Cards

apples	apricots
avocados	bananas
strawberries	cherries
blueberries	raspberries
blackberries	boysenberries

From L.W.Y. Cheung, H. Dart, S. Kalin, and S.L. Gortmaker, 2007, *Eat Well & Keep Moving,* 2nd ed. (Champaign, IL: Human Kinetics).

(continued)

coconuts	dates
figs	grapes
grapefruit	kiwi
kumquats	lemons
limes	mangoes

From L.W.Y. Cheung, H. Dart, S. Kalin, and S.L. Gortmaker, 2007, *Eat Well & Keep Moving,* 2nd ed. (Champaign, IL: Human Kinetics).

(continued)

melons	nectarines
oranges	papayas
peaches	pears
persimmons	pineapples
plums	prunes

From L.W.Y. Cheung, H. Dart, S. Kalin, and S.L. Gortmaker, 2007, *Eat Well & Keep Moving*, 2nd ed. (Champaign, IL: Human Kinetics).

(continued)

raisins	tangerines

From L.W.Y. Cheung, H. Dart, S. Kalin, and S.L. Gortmaker, 2007, *Eat Well & Keep Moving*, 2nd ed. (Champaign, IL: Human Kinetics).

(continued)

artichokes	asparagus
beets	broccoli
brussels sprouts	carrots
cabbage	celery
cauliflower	corn

From L.W.Y. Cheung, H. Dart, S. Kalin, and S.L. Gortmaker, 2007, *Eat Well & Keep Moving,* 2nd ed. (Champaign, IL: Human Kinetics).

(continued)

Swiss chard	eggplant
cucumbers	collard greens
green beans	iceberg lettuce
kelp	okra
mushrooms	parsnips

From L.W.Y. Cheung, H. Dart, S. Kalin, and S.L. Gortmaker, 2007, *Eat Well & Keep Moving*, 2nd ed. (Champaign, IL: Human Kinetics).

(continued)

onions	peppers
peas	radishes
pumpkin	squash
spinach	tomatoes
sweet potatoes	turnips

From L.W.Y. Cheung, H. Dart, S. Kalin, and S.L. Gortmaker, 2007, *Eat Well & Keep Moving,* 2nd ed. (Champaign, IL: Human Kinetics).

(continued)

dandelion greens	tofu
romaine lettuce	arugula
green leaf lettuce	dried beans
red leaf lettuce	legumes

From L.W.Y. Cheung, H. Dart, S. Kalin, and S.L. Gortmaker, 2007, *Eat Well & Keep Moving,* 2nd ed. (Champaign, IL: Human Kinetics).

(continued)

flour tortillas	peanuts
cashews	cookies
yogurt	butter
eggs	cheese
chicken	soft drink

From L.W.Y. Cheung, H. Dart, S. Kalin, and S.L. Gortmaker, 2007, *Eat Well & Keep Moving,* 2nd ed. (Champaign, IL: Human Kinetics).

(continued)

crackers	bread
salmon	bass
shrimp	pork
wheat	barley
marshmallows	

From L.W.Y. Cheung, H. Dart, S. Kalin, and S.L. Gortmaker, 2007, *Eat Well & Keep Moving*, 2nd ed. (Champaign, IL: Human Kinetics).

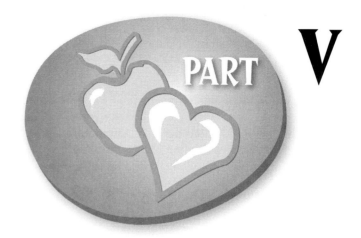

FitCheck Guide

Part V includes both the teachers' guide and the students' guide to FitCheck. These resources were adapted from the middle school curriculum *Planet Health* and are designed to teach teachers and students how to evaluate fitness progress.

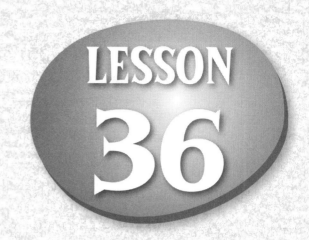

LESSON 36

Teachers' Guide to the FitCheck

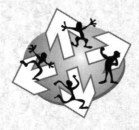
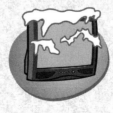

All or parts of this lesson are from J. Carter et al., 2007, *Planet Health*, 2nd ed. (Champaign, IL: Human Kinetics), microunit 11.

FITCHECK OVERVIEW

The FitCheck is a self-assessment tool that physical educators can use to help children identify, understand, and reflect on their own patterns of physical activity and inactivity. Use FitCheck if it matches your students' abilities and fits into your curriculum. This version is simplified from *Planet Health,* which targets middle school students.

FITCHECK COMPONENTS

1. *Planet Health* FitCheck journal (see pages 519-520): Students fill this journal out at home over 7 days and translate their results into FitScores and SitScores.
2. Goal Setting and Goal Evaluation sheet (see pages 521-522): Students set and evaluate goals based on their FitScores and SitScores.
3. FitScore and SitScore Progress Charts (see pages 523 and 524): Students record their scores on this chart when they complete each FitCheck at certain times you select throughout the year (select 2 or 3 times total; try to make one time close to the end of the school year).

USING THE FITCHECK JOURNAL

Lessons 37 through 41 introduce the FitCheck to students:

▶ Lesson 37, Students' Guide to the FitCheck, overviews the FitCheck.
▶ Lesson 38, Charting Your FitScore and SitScore, introduces the FitCheck journal.
▶ Lesson 39, What Could You Do Instead of Watching TV?, is the first of two lessons preparing students for goal setting (lesson 41). It presents recommendations for limiting TV use and offers alternatives to watching television and DVDs and playing computer games and video games.
▶ Lesson 40, Making Time to Stay Fit, is the second lesson preparing students for goal setting (lesson 41). Students make a group goal for class that day and evaluate their progress at the end of class. You may want to repeat this lesson several times with the students until they are comfortable with goal setting and evaluation.
▶ Lesson 41, Setting Goals for Personal Fitness, has students set goals to improve their SitScore and FitScore. At the next FitCheck, the students evaluate their progress.

USING THE FITSCORE AND SITSCORE PROGRESS CHARTS

There is no microunit accompanying the progress charts (see pages 523 and 524). After completing each FitCheck 2 or 3 times during the school year, you should have the students graph their scores so they can see their progress over time. This activity could be coordinated with a math teacher or even carried out in math class.

TIPS FOR TEACHING THE FITCHECK

1. Read through the Students' Guide to the FitCheck (lesson 37) and all the FitCheck units (lessons 38 through 41) first. These lessons are designed to be read aloud to students, and they are formatted in a way to facilitate your delivery of their messages. The bulleted lists serve as key talking points that you can discuss with your students, and they are written so that they can be read aloud to students. The text boxes provide you with additional information that you may or may not want to cover during the five minutes. The How-To sections provide you with ideas to motivate your students on how they can accomplish the goals of the unit. Finally, the questions allow you to see how well your students picked up on the concepts of the lesson.

2. Schedule FitChecks for the year. We recommend doing a check 2 to 3 times during the school year. You can spread journal assignments, charting, and goal setting and evaluation over several sessions to maximize physical activity time in your classes. If your students are not able to handle goal setting and evaluation, you can still do the journals.

3. Set up a filing system.

4. Coordinate with other teachers.
   - Because FitChecks require homework, you may want to coordinate with your students' classroom teachers ahead of time.
   - You may want to coordinate with a math teacher to do the bar graph exercise (FitScore and SitScore progress charts; see pages 523 and 524).

5. Help the students compare their FitScores and SitScores to expert recommendations for children.
   - The National Association for Sport and Physical Activity (NASPE)* recommends that "children should accumulate at least 60 minutes of activity from a variety of activities on all or most days of the week." In fact, children may accumulate up to several hours per day. The NASPE states that "this daily accumulation should include moderate and vigorous physical activity" and that most of the time should be spent in intermittent activity; the organization advises that children should accrue their physical activity in "several bouts . . . lasting 15 minutes or more each day." Because children have difficulty tracking time spent on tasks and because children's activity is intermittent by nature, we have opted to ask students to record what they did for activity rather than how long they engaged in activity.
   - The American Academy of Pediatrics recommends that children and teenagers spend no more than 1 to 2 hours per day on quality leisure-time screen media, including watching TV and movies and playing video and computer games.

6. Facilitate goal setting (if you choose to do the goal-setting unit). Help the students be realistic about their goals. Physical activity must fit in with other daily activities and family schedules and must be safe and supervised according to family rules. Students don't need to trade all their excess Sit activity time for Fit activities. Trading 1 to 2 hours per week is probably realistic.

*National Association for Sport and Physical Education. (2004). Physical Activity for Children: A Statement of Guidelines for Children Ages 5–12, 2nd Edition. Retrieved on March 17, 2007, from www.aahperd.org/naspe/template.cfm?template=ns_children.html.

FITCHECK QUESTIONS AND ANSWERS

Q. What kinds of physical activities should students choose for a goal?

A. Whatever they like. They can select an activity to get better at or they can pick an activity they are totally unfamiliar with and develop skills in that area.

Q. Do students have to choose a vigorous activity or a sport?

A. No. They can choose any physical activity to trade with their inactive time. This includes unstructured outdoor play. It could even include participating in a dance video game, such as Dance, Dance Revolution, that engages the student in moderate to vigorous physical activity.

Q. What happens if a student does not meet a goal by the next FitCheck?

A. The student can explore what prevented goal attainment. If this process is pursued in a noncritical fashion, it can help students modify their expectations and learn to set realistic goals.

Q. Is losing weight by the end of the school year a reasonable goal?

A. No. FitChecks should not be used as weight-loss tools. Many young people who think they need to lose weight really don't need to. Weight loss can be unhealthy while children are growing. Encourage children who want to lose weight to talk with their parents, the school nurse, and their physician.

FitCheck Journal*

Name _____ Date _____

Grade _____ FitCheck # _____

Start with today under column 1, Day of the week (see table 36.1). Tonight you should do the following:

1. If you did any physical activities today, list them in column 2, and mark column 3. Leave columns 2 and 3 blank if you did not do any physical activities today.

   - Include sports classes or practices, physical education class, dance, and other active classes.

   - You can also list unstructured activities like running around with friends, pickup sports, or active chores like raking or shoveling.

2. List today's TV and other screen activities in column 4. Estimate how much time these activities took in total. Mark column 5 if your total was 2 hours or less. Leave column 5 blank if your total was more than 2 hours.

   - Include watching TV shows, videos, and movies; playing computer and video games; and surfing the Internet for fun.

   - Don't include using the computer for homework.

3. Complete steps 1 and 2 for 7 nights. Then, add up the number of √s you earned.

From L.W.Y. Cheung, H. Dart, S. Kalin, and S.L. Gortmaker, 2007, *Eat Well & Keep Moving,* 2nd ed. (Champaign, IL: Human Kinetics).
*Adapted from Carter, J., J. Wiecha, K.E. Peterson, S.L. Gortmaker, and S. Nobrega, S. (2007). *Planet Health - An Interdisciplinary Curriculum for Teaching Middle School Nutrition and Physical Activity.* Champaign, IL: Human Kinetics.

(continued)

▶**TABLE 36.1 FitCheck Journal Table**

1. Day of the week	2. FitScore activities: sports, gym class, dance, games, free play, chores	3. Fit ✓s	4. SitScore activities: TV, computer and video games, Internet surfing, videos, movies	5. Sit ✓s
Total points	FitScore		SitScore	

From L.W.Y. Cheung, H. Dart, S. Kalin, and S.L. Gortmaker, 2007, *Eat Well & Keep Moving*, 2nd ed. (Champaign, IL: Human Kinetics). Adapted from Carter, J., J. Wiecha, K.E. Peterson, S.L. Gortmaker, and S. Nobrega, S. (2007). *Planet Health - An Interdisciplinary Curriculum for Teaching Middle School Nutrition and Physical Activity.* Champaign, IL: Human Kinetics.

Goal Setting

Name _____ Date _____

FitCheck # _____

What do your FitScore and SitScore mean? If your totals were 5 to 7, keep it up! If they were 0 to 4, try to increase them!

1. Your FitScore = _____.

    I need to (circle one):   Keep it up   Increase

2. Your SitScore = _____.

    I need to (circle one):   Keep it up   Increase

Make Fit and Sit goals! If you have scores you want to maintain, way to go! If you want to increase your scores, think of 1 to 3 realistic strategies you can work out with your family. For example, identify a time when you usually play computer games, and spend some or all of that time playing with friends or family instead. Or walk or bike to school instead of getting a ride.

I will try to increase my (circle one or both)   FIT   SIT   scores by doing the following:

Goal Evaluation

Date _____

Did you meet your goals?

▶ All of them

▶ Some of them

▶ None of them

Why or why not? Write how you reached your goals or why you did not reach them:

From L.W.Y. Cheung, H. Dart, S. Kalin, and S.L. Gortmaker, 2007, *Eat Well & Keep Moving,* 2nd ed. (Champaign, IL: Human Kinetics).

FitScore Progress Chart

Name _____

Find out how your FitScores changed during the school year. Draw a bar for each FitScore in the first chart. Work from left to right. How have your scores changed?

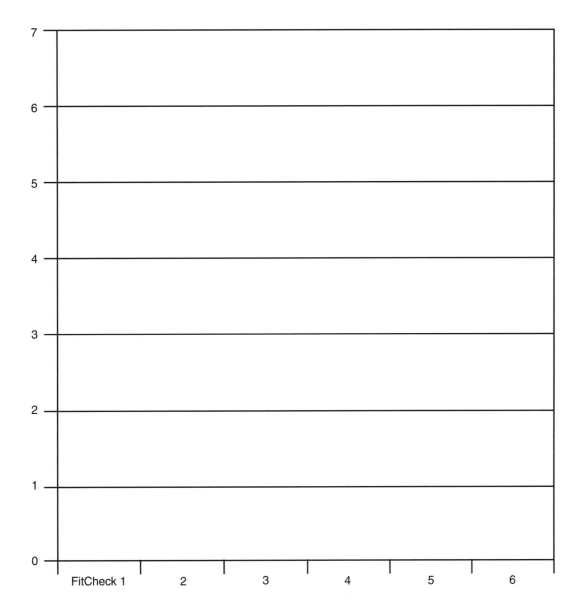

From L.W.Y. Cheung, H. Dart, S. Kalin, and S.L. Gortmaker, 2007, *Eat Well & Keep Moving,* 2nd ed. (Champaign, IL: Human Kinetics).

SitScore Progress Chart

Name _____

Find out how your SitScores changed during the school year. Draw a bar for each SitScore in the chart. Work from left to right. How have your scores changed?

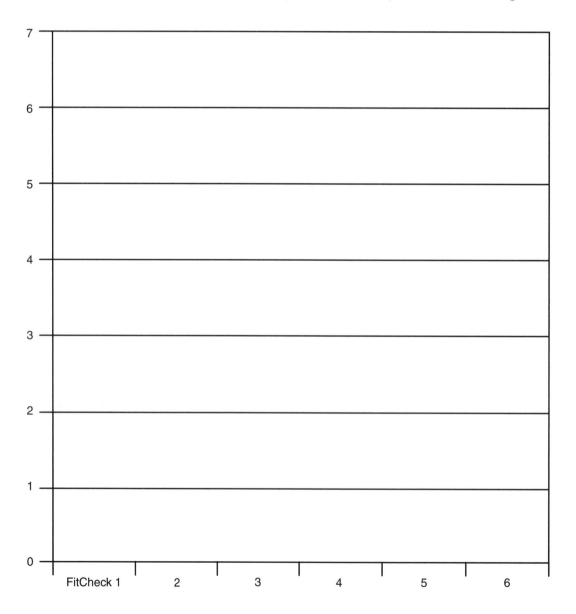

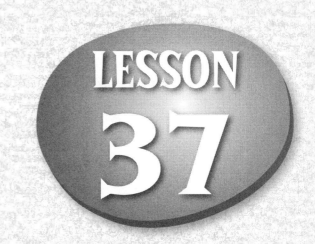

LESSON 37

Students' Guide to the FitCheck

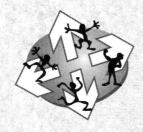 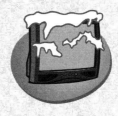

All or parts of this lesson are from J. Carter et al., 2007, *Planet Health*, 2nd ed. (Champaign, IL: Human Kinetics), microunit 11.

FITNESS TIP

FitChecks will help you choose a healthy level of activity.

FITNESS LESSON

(In this class/our next class) you will do a *Planet Health* FitCheck. The FitCheck is a way of keeping track of your physical activity (time spent in moderate activities like walking and time spent in vigorous activities like running) as well as your physical inactivity (time spent watching TV, playing video and computer games, surfing the Internet for fun, and watching movies). Based on those measurements, you can create goals to increase or maintain your current level of physical activity.

You will take your FitCheck journal (see pages 519-520) home to record your activities as a homework assignment during FitCheck weeks. After the FitCheck week comes to an end, you'll bring your FitCheck journal back to school, where I'll keep it (in/at location at school) at all times. Only you will have access to your FitCheck journal. You will use the FitCheck journal 2 or 3 times during the school year.

To chart your progress, keep track of your activities in and outside of school for 7 days. You'll figure out how often you are physically active in your physical education class, sports teams or classes, dance classes, and other activities like active play with your friends and family, helping with leaves or snow, or big cleanup projects at home. You'll also figure out how much time you spend watching TV, playing computer games, surfing the Internet for fun, and watching DVDs, videos, and movies. The time you spend doing these nonphysical activities represents time when you are not moving around.

At the end of the FitCheck week, you'll use your journal to figure out your FitScore and SitScore (see pages 523-524). You'll graph these scores for each FitCheck throughout the year so that by the end of the year you'll see how your scores have changed.

A FitCheck consists of the following (teacher note: List the FitCheck components you have chosen to use):

1. Recording physical activities
2. Recording screen time (TV, computer and video games, Internet surfing, videos, and movies)
3. Totaling your FitScore and SitScore at the end of the FitCheck week
4. Graphing your records
5. Setting goals
6. Evaluating your progress toward goals (see page 522)

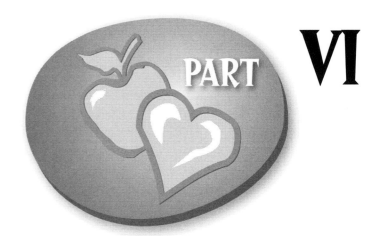

FitCheck Physical Education Microunits

Part VI includes four microunits that were developed specifically for FitCheck—5-minute lessons that cover a wide range of physical activity topics. These microunits were adapted from the middle school curriculum *Plant Health,* and they are designed to build on one another. The microunits are best taught sequentially as a set. However, the microunits can also be used intermittently—such as on days when no full-length *Eat Well & Keep Moving* physical education lesson is being taught—as long as the units are taught in the correct order.

The microunits are formatted to facilitate your delivery of their messages. The bulleted lists serve as key talking points that you can discuss with your students. The text boxes provide you with additional information that you may or may not want to cover during the 5 minutes. The How To sections provide you with ideas to motivate your students on how they can accomplish the goals of the unit. Finally, the student questions allow you to see how well your students picked up on the concepts of the lesson.

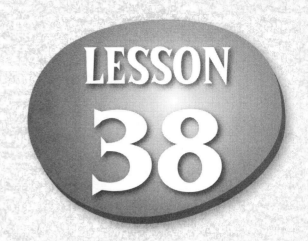

Charting Your FitScore and SitScore

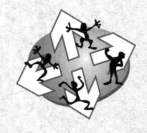 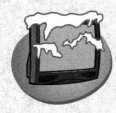

All or parts of this lesson are from J. Carter et al., 2007, *Planet Health*, 2nd ed. (Champaign, IL: Human Kinetics), microunit 4.

FITNESS TIP

You can use the FitCheck journal to find out how active you are.

FITNESS LESSON

Using the FitCheck journal, you can chart your FitScore and SitScore:

▷ Your FitScore represents the time you were physically active during the past week. It is the number of points you earn for time spent participating in moderate and vigorous physical activities.

▷ Moderate physical activities include

- walking,
- climbing on playground structures,
- easy cycling,
- easy swimming,
- easy skating,
- playing a dance video game like Dance Dance Revolution,* and
- light chores.

▷ Physical activities also include vigorous ones like

- running,
- tag games,
- basketball,
- soccer,
- rope jumping,
- in-line skating,
- fast cycling,
- fast swimming, and
- skating.

▷ Your SitScore represents the time you were not moving around during the past week. It is the total time you spent

- watching TV;
- playing computer or video games;
- surfing the Internet for fun; and
- watching DVDs, videos, and movies.

*Note: Dance video games such as Dance, Dance Revolution can also be considered vigorous physical activity.

HOW TO USE THE FITCHECK JOURNAL

Teachers, pass out a manila folder containing the FitCheck journal and a pencil to each student. Go over the instructions, making sure students understand the assignment. Show them an example (you can use yourself as the example). Have them fill out the heading of the FitCheck journal. Then, read the following to your students:

> ### Defining Moderate and Vigorous Exercise Intensities
>
> You should be able to talk easily while participating in an activity of light to moderate intensity. Vigorous activities make you breathe hard and sweat.

1. At the end of the FitCheck week, each of you will figure out your FitCheck scores.

    *   For FitScores, you will get 1 point for every day that you listed at least 1 hour of physical activity.
    *   For SitScores, you will get 1 point for every day that you spent no more than 2 hours on Sit activities.
    *   Aim for FitScores and SitScores of 5 to 7. If either score is between 0 and 4, you should set goals to improve your scores.

2. Here is how we will graph our scores.

    Go over your own graphing instructions with your students at this time.

QUESTIONS FOR STUDENTS

1. What will your scores tell you about your lifestyle?
2. How might this journal change how you spend your free time?

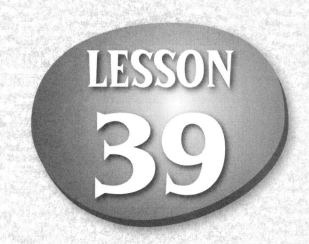

What Could You Do Instead of Watching TV?

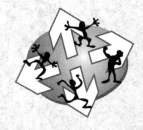
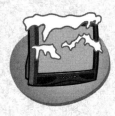

All or parts of this lesson are from J. Carter et al., 2007, *Planet Health*, 2nd ed. (Champaign, IL: Human Kinetics), microunit 5.

FITNESS TIP

Watching less than 2 hours of TV each day can help you get fit!

FITNESS LESSON

TV CUTS DOWN ON YOUR TIME TO BE ACTIVE

▶ Many children your age spend a lot of their free time doing things that require sitting down.

▶ For some kids, this includes watching TV for about 5 hours each day.

▶ Think about how this cuts into your activity time.

WATCHING TOO MUCH TV CAN MAKE YOU LESS FIT

▶ Being inactive day after day can quickly make you lose
  - flexibility,
  - muscle strength, and
  - cardiorespiratory endurance.

▶ When you sit still, you burn fewer calories than you do when you are moving around.

HOW TO CUT DOWN ON TV

1. Doctors recommend that children and teenagers watch no more than 2 hours of quality TV or videos each day. Watching less is better.

2. This means you can watch up to 4 half-hour shows every day—but you can watch less, too.

3. Watch only shows you like.

4. Take note of the times when you watch TV but you aren't really interested—when you channel surf or watch reruns—and use that time to be physically active instead.

5. Try to limit your total screen time—television, computer games, DVDs, and so on—to no more than 2 hours each day.

QUESTIONS FOR STUDENTS

1. What is the maximum amount of TV that doctors recommend children watch per day?

2. What could happen if you watch too much TV?

3. Why is being active better than watching TV and movies or playing video games?

4. What are some activities that you can do instead of watching TV?

Watching Too Much TV Can Be Harmful to Your Health

When you sit in front of the TV, you lose a chance to be active and to improve your fitness level. Also, television advertising successfully encourages kids to eat a lot of unhealthy foods. Studies show that the kids who watch the least TV are the kids who are least likely to be overweight. The combination of eating too much and moving less can cause people to gain too much weight over time. People who are overweight are more likely to develop health problems, making it harder to lead a happy, active life.

Warning!

Remember, you need plenty of healthy food for being active and growing, especially when you are growing fast. Never make a decision to cut back on the amount of food you eat without talking it over with your parents, your school nurse, or your doctor.

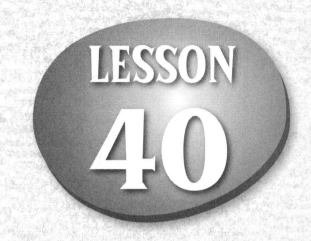
Making Time to Stay Fit

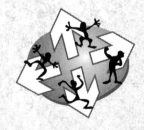
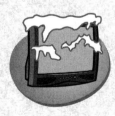

All or parts of this lesson are from J. Carter et al., 2007, *Planet Health,* 2nd ed. (Champaign, IL: Human Kinetics), microunit 6.

FITNESS TIP

It's the *regular* in regular activity that's important. Make space for fitness!

FITNESS LESSON

MAKING SPACE FOR FITNESS

▶ Find the time to be active.

▶ Set aside a specific time to exercise.

▶ Try small increases in physical activity. They can add up over time and can produce long-term health benefits.

NEVER PASS UP THE OPPORTUNITY TO BE PHYSICALLY ACTIVE

▶ Stretch when you wake up in the morning.

▶ Take the stairs instead of the escalator or elevator at the mall.

▶ If it is safe for you, walk or bike instead of getting a ride or taking the bus.

GOAL SETTING

▶ It's important to set goals for increasing your physical activity.

▶ Today we will practice setting activity goals.

▶ We'll begin by trying to write a goal that will motivate you to be more active during today's class.

QUICK IDEAS TO BECOME MORE FIT

▶ Help a younger sister or brother get started in an activity or sport.

▶ Learn how to play with young children.

▶ Try to be as active as a 2- or 3-year-old—it just might tire you out.

▶ Watch TV only if it's your favorite show.

▶ Exercise while you watch your favorite shows on TV.

▶ Borrow an exercise video from the video store or library.

▶ Take up an after-school activity or sport.

▶ Go for a walk or bike ride with a friend.

▶ After school, try to stay outside for an hour with your friends if your parents approve.

▶ Play a dance video game, such as Dance, Dance Revolution, with a friend and challenge each other to improve your scores.

HOW TO MAKE TIME FOR FITNESS

Make one goal to be completed by all the students in gym class today. For example, the goal could be, "I will warm up for 5 minutes before exercising, actively par-

Exercise With Others

Exercising with others can make doing an activity more fun. Make a plan to exercise with a friend. You can also do active things you like with your parents, brothers, or sisters. Finally, you may want to join a sports team.

Finding Active Time at School

Think about times during the day when you can trade inactive time for physical activity. Try to be more active during physical education class, and walk briskly to your classes.

Finding Active Time Away From School

In addition, you can be more active while you are away from school. Invite friends over to play active games or practice dance, aerobics, or gymnastics. Clean your room (and your house). Try vacuuming, cleaning out closets, and other tasks that require bending, stretching, and lifting. Have fun with it! Listen to music!

ticipate (break a sweat) in gym today, and spend 5 minutes cooling down at the end of class." You may want to discuss setting the goal with students and come up with one together.

1. Write the goal on the board (or in large print on sheets of paper hung on the wall) so students can see it throughout class.

2. At the end of class, leave time for students to evaluate whether they reached their goal.

3. Ask the students the following:
   - Did you reach the class goal?
   - For those of you who reached the goal, how do you know you reached your goal?
   - For those of you who didn't reach your goal, what could you have done to reach your goal?

4. You may want to repeat this lesson until students are comfortable with goal setting and evaluation.

QUESTIONS FOR STUDENTS

1. What are some ways you can make time to stay fit?

2. It's important to set realistic goals for yourself—goals that you have a reasonable chance of reaching. Which of the following goals is more realistic for a student who currently gets a ride to school from her mom? Goal 1: I will walk to and from school instead of getting a ride every day for the next month. Goal 2: I will walk to school three mornings a week for the next month.

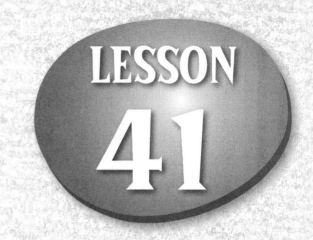

Setting Goals for Personal Fitness

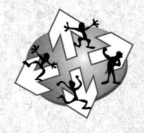 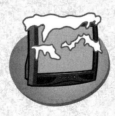

All or parts of this lesson are from J. Carter et al., 2007, *Planet Health*, 2nd ed. (Champaign, IL: Human Kinetics), microunit 7.

FITNESS TIP

Set fitness goals that fit your life. Trade some Sit time for Fit time.
If you have decided not to do goal setting, you can skip this microunit.

FITNESS LESSON

SETTING PERSONAL FITNESS GOALS

▶ Setting fitness goals is a good first step to getting fit.

▶ Today you will learn about goal setting.

▶ You will use the FitCheck sheet to set a personal fitness goal.

▶ While setting goals, keep in mind how much time you spend in front of a screen. If you have a lot of inactive time, set a goal to trade inactive time for active time.

TRADING BORED TIME FOR FUN TIME

How much of your screen time is spent

▶ channel surfing,

▶ watching shows you don't really like,

▶ watching reruns of shows you've already seen, or

▶ playing video games because you have nothing better to do?

That is the time you should trade for active time:

▶ Run around and play.

▶ Play a sport.

▶ Do an aerobics tape with a friend.

▶ Take a walk with friends.

HOW TO SET GOALS

Review the most recent FitCheck journals with your students. Make sure everyone has a pen or pencil. Read these instructions to the students:

1. Review your most recent SitScore. Is it under 5? If yes, consider trading some screen time for active time.

2. Think about when you do your screen time: before school, after school, or before bed. When could you trade some of this time for physical activity? Be specific! For example, your goal could be this: After school on Mondays and Fridays I will skate, bike, or run around for a half hour instead of playing a computer game.

3. Choose activities you like! Fill in your goal with an activity you already do well, with a new activity you would like to try, or with an activity at which you

> ### *Eat Well & Keep Moving* Fitness Goals
>
> Children should get at least 60 minutes of physical activity every day. This should include moderate- and vigorous-intensity activities. Most of this time should be spent in intermittent activities, and the 60 minutes can be accumulated throughout the day in sessions of 15 minutes or longer (NASPE, 2004). A variety of activities can contribute to children's daily total, such as team sports, free play, transportation (e.g., walking or biking to school), household chores, and school-based physical education classes (AAP, 2006). Children should spend no more than 2 hours per day watching TV, playing video or computer games, and surfing the Web.

would like to get better. Remember that making a plan with a friend could make physical activity more fun and help you do it more often.

4. Make sure your new activities are safe and supervised according to your family's rules. Make sure they fit in with your family's schedule.

Give the students time to complete their goals, and then collect the journals and goal sheets.

Goal evaluation (see the goal evaluation worksheet on p. 522 in lesson 36, Teacher's Guide to the FitCheck) will be done during every FitCheck except for the first one. If this is your first time doing the FitCheck with your class, please proceed to Questions for Students.

GOAL EVALUATION

Evaluating the previous goal will be the first thing you do in a FitCheck (beginning with the second FitCheck).

1. Put today's date in the Goal Evaluation date box.

2. Read your goal from the previous FitCheck you did.

3. To answer the question, "Did you meet your goals?" check the correct circle: all of them, some of them, or none of them.

4. In 1 or 2 sentences, explain how you reached your goal, or why you did not reach your goal.

QUESTIONS FOR STUDENTS

1. Why should you trade some of your inactive time for active time?

2. Are there times when you watch TV shows you don't like, you channel surf, or you watch reruns (shows you have already seen) simply because you are bored? Could you do some physical activity instead of being bored?

National Association for Sport and Physical Education. (2004.) Physical Activity for Children: A Statement of Guidelines for Children Ages 5 - 12, 2nd Edition. Retrieved on March 17, 2007, from www.aahperd.org/naspe/template.cfm?template=ns_children. html. American Academy of Pediatrics. (2006.) Active healthy living: prevention of childhood obesity through increased physical activity. *Pediatrics, 117*(5): 1834-1842.

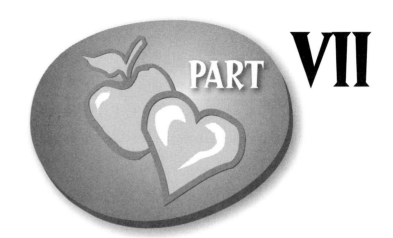

Additional Physical Education Microunits

Part VII includes five additional microunits—brief, 5-minute lessons that cover a wide range of physical activity topics. These microunits were adapted from the middle school curriculum *Planet Health,* and they are designed to build on one another. The microunits are best taught sequentially as a set. However, the microunits can also be used intermittently—such as on days when no full-length *Eat Well & Keep Moving* physical education lesson is being taught—as long as the units are taught in the correct order.

The microunits are formatted to facilitate your delivery of their messages. The bulleted lists serve as key talking points that you can discuss with your students. The text boxes provide you with additional information that you may or may not want to cover during the 5 minutes. The How To sections provide you with ideas to motivate your students on how they can accomplish the goals of the unit. Finally, the student questions allow you to see how well your students picked up on the concepts of the lesson.

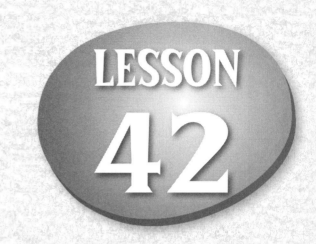

Thinking About Activity, Exercise, and Fitness

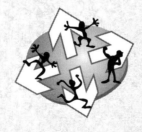
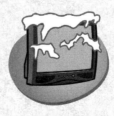

All or parts of this lesson are from J. Carter et al., 2007, *Planet Health*, 2nd ed. (Champaign, IL: Human Kinetics), microunit 1.

FITNESS TIP

Any physical activity is better than none.

FITNESS LESSON

BRIEF INTRODUCTION TO PHYSICAL FITNESS

- ▶ Being fit means you have the energy you need to
  - work,
  - exercise,
  - play, and
  - get from place to place without easily tiring.
- ▶ To get fit, you need to be physically active.

BE ACTIVE AND EAT RIGHT

- ▶ Exercise is physical activity that is planned and structured, like running a mile or playing soccer for an hour. Many people think that only exercise improves fitness.
- ▶ In fact, many kinds of movement can improve your health and fitness:
  - Dancing
  - Jumping rope
  - Walking the dog
  - Throwing a ball
  - Climbing stairs
  - Swimming
- ▶ The more active you are, the more fit you will become.
- ▶ In addition to physical activity, healthy eating will also help you stay fit.
- ▶ We'll discuss more about this aspect of fitness later.

POSITIVE EFFECTS OF PHYSICAL FITNESS

- ▶ Being physically fit
  - makes you healthier,
  - helps you build a positive self-image, and
  - helps you feel better about yourself.
- ▶ Fitness is fun, and it feels great!

HOW TO BECOME PHYSICALLY ACTIVE

1. Start thinking about the physical activities that you do as well as the activities you do that are sedentary, like
   - watching TV;
   - playing video and computer games; and
   - watching DVDs, videos, or movies.

Long-Term Health Benefits of Physical Activity

Learning to be active as a child will help you become active as an adult. If you become fit now and stay active as you get older, you'll lower your risk of having certain health problems such as obesity, heart disease, broken bones, bone loss, diabetes, and certain types of cancers. Moderate amounts of physical activity will help you prevent these health problems.

Physical Activity Recommendations for Children

Children should get at least 60 minutes of physical activity every day. These 60 minutes should include moderate- and vigorous-intensity activities. Most of the 60 minutes should be spent in intermittent activities, and the time can be accumulated throughout the day in sessions of 15 minutes or longer. A variety of activities can contribute to children's daily total, such as team sports, free play, transportation (e.g., walking or biking to school), household chores, and physical education classes. Spend no more than 2 hours per day watching TV, playing video or computer games, and surfing the Web.

2. Think about ways to increase your activity level. You can do this by replacing inactive time with active time. For instance, you can
   * ride bikes instead of watching a TV show that you don't really like, and
   * play basketball instead of playing a video game.
3. Remember, being active will help you stay healthy now and in the future as you grow up.

QUESTIONS FOR STUDENTS

1. What are some of the things that you do to be physically active?
2. What can you do to increase your physical activity?
3. What are the benefits of being fit?
4. What gets in the way of your being more physically active?

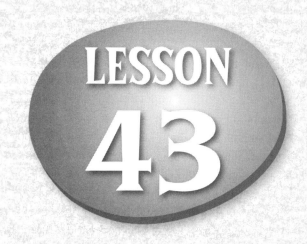

LESSON 43

Be Active Now for a Healthy Heart Later

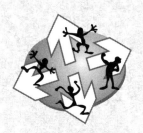

All or parts of this lesson are from J. Carter et al., 2007, *Planet Health,* 2nd ed. (Champaign, IL: Human Kinetics), microunit 19.

FITNESS TIP

Being active in your free time now can lower your risk of cardiovascular disease later in life.

FITNESS LESSON

THE NUMBER ONE KILLER

- ▶ Cardiovascular disease is a disease of the heart and blood vessels.
- ▶ It is the single largest cause of death in the United States for both men and women.

PREVENTING THE NUMBER ONE KILLER

- ▶ You can lower your risk of developing cardiovascular disease by starting a lifelong commitment to regular exercise now.
- ▶ Maintaining a healthy weight; eating a balanced diet that is low in trans fat and saturated fat (but includes a moderate amount of healthy fat from plant oils, nuts, and fish) and includes an abundance of fruits, vegetables, and whole grains; and living smoke free will also help you prevent cardiovascular disease.

HOW TO PREVENT CARDIOVASCULAR DISEASE

1. To prevent cardiovascular disease, develop good physical activity and eating habits at an early age and maintain them throughout your life.
2. Choose activities that make your heart and lungs stronger, like
   - fast walking,
   - running,
   - bicycling,
   - swimming,
   - in-line skating,
   - hiking, and
   - many more!
3. Eat at least 5 servings of fruits and vegetables a day (more is always better).
4. Eat a diet that includes healthy fat (from plant oils, nuts, and fish), limits saturated fat, and avoids trans fat.
5. Eat whole grains (e.g., whole wheat bread).
6. Finally, don't smoke!

QUESTIONS FOR STUDENTS

1. Name some physical activities that you like to do that will strengthen your heart.
2. Which of these activities do you think you will continue as an adult?

Cardiovascular Disease in the United States

Cardiovascular disease is actually a group of diseases that affect the heart and blood vessels. It includes coronary artery disease (a narrowing of the arteries in the heart that can cause a heart attack, chest pain, or both), stroke, rheumatic heart disease, and many others. According to 2004 estimates, 79 million Americans have one or more forms of cardiovascular disease. A total of 871,000 Americans died from cardiovascular disease in 2004 (36% of all deaths).

Habits That Put Adults at Risk for Cardiovascular Disease Begin in the Teenage Years

Eating diets high in saturated and trans fat and low in healthy fat (from plant oils, nuts, and fish), fruits, vegetables, and whole grains; being inactive (not moving around); and smoking are all habits that could lead to cardiovascular disease.

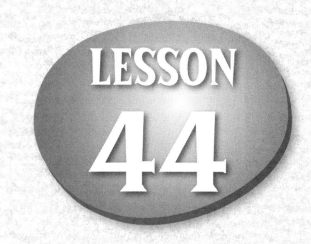

Be Active Now for Healthy Bones Later

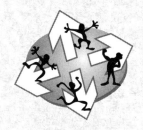

All or parts of this lesson are from J. Carter et al., 2007, *Planet Health*, 2nd ed. (Champaign, IL: Human Kinetics), microunit 20.

FITNESS TIP

Building strong bones now can help prevent fractures and bone loss later in life.

FITNESS LESSON

BUILDING STRONG BONES

- Almost 50% of your bone mass is formed during your childhood and teenage years.
- Exercising and eating a balanced diet rich in calcium and vitamin D will help you build strong bones.
- Building strong bones now is a critical part of preventing osteoporosis from developing when you are older.
- Living a healthy lifestyle with no smoking and limited alcohol consumption during adulthood will keep your bones strong.
- People with osteoporosis have weak bones that are more likely to break. For example, hip fractures are common among the elderly and are a serious injury because older peoples' bones do not heal easily.

BUILDING STRONG BONES WITH EXERCISE

- Weight-bearing exercises build strong bones.
- In weight-bearing exercises, your bones and muscles work against gravity; your feet, legs, or arms support your weight as you move. Some examples of this kind of activity are
  - walking,
  - stair-climbing,
  - hiking,
  - racket sports,
  - dancing,
  - soccer,
  - push-ups,
  - curl-ups, and
  - basketball, but
  - *not* swimming or biking.
- Weight training also builds strong bones.
- Hitting a ball or landing on your feet after jumping stimulates more calcium to be deposited in your bones. More calcium makes your bones stronger.
- Most sports and daily physical activities require weight-bearing activities. If you participate regularly in a variety of physical activities, you will build strong bones.

Osteoporosis

Osteoporosis literally means *porous bone.* While the shape of the bones looks okay, they have fewer minerals in them. The minerals calcium and phosphorus are the major building blocks of bone. Bones that are low in these minerals are brittle and break more easily than healthy bones. It is estimated that 10 million Americans have osteoporosis and 34 million have low bone density that puts them at risk for osteoporosis. Osteoporosis is more common among women than men (roughly 80% of osteoporosis cases are in women).

Preventing Osteoporosis Also Requires Consuming Enough Calcium

In order to prevent osteoporosis, you need to make sure that you consume enough calcium. Persons aged 9 to 18 require 1,300 milligrams of calcium per day, the amount found in four 8-ounce (250-milliliter) glasses of milk. Low-fat (1%) and nonfat milk and other dairy products (yogurt, cheese) offer the largest amount of calcium per serving. Other excellent sources of calcium include

- tofu,
- sardines with bones, and
- calcium-fortified foods including orange juice, cereal, soy or rice milks, and cereal bars.

Kale, broccoli, and other green leafy vegetables are good sources of calcium, but they provide a lot fewer milligrams per serving than most milk products provide. If you are unable to consume milk or milk products, you should eat other calcium-rich foods.

HOW TO BUILD STRONG BONES

1. To build strong bones and prevent osteoporosis, develop good exercise and eating habits now.
2. Choose physical activities that put some stress on your bones.
3. Eat foods rich in calcium. Have 3 servings of low-fat or nonfat dairy products like milk, cheese, and yogurt every day.

QUESTIONS FOR STUDENTS

1. How does exercise help your bones?
2. How can you help prevent osteoporosis and bone fractures?

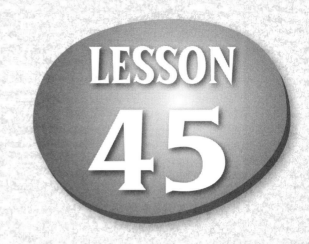

LESSON 45

Let's Get Started on Being Fit

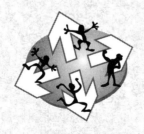

All or parts of this lesson are from J. Carter et al., 2007, *Planet Health*, 2nd ed. (Champaign, IL: Human Kinetics), microunit 8.

FITNESS TIP

For total physical fitness, work on cardiorespiratory endurance, muscle strength, and flexibility.

FITNESS LESSON

UNDERSTANDING PHYSICAL FITNESS

▶ Being physically fit means you have the energy and strength to handle the everyday demands of your life:
  - Walking to school
  - Playing soccer during gym
  - Actively listening and participating in class
  - Completing daily chores
  - Participating in after-school activities
  - Doing a good job on your homework
  - Taking the stairs when the elevator doesn't work

▶ It also means you can complete all of your daily activities without feeling overly fatigued.

OVERALL PHYSICAL FITNESS

▶ Many factors contribute to your overall physical fitness.

▶ The factors that are most important to your health are
  1. cardiorespiratory endurance (or cardiorespiratory fitness),
  2. muscle strength, and
  3. flexibility.

THREE AREAS OF PHYSICAL FITNESS

▶ Physical fitness consists of cardiorespiratory endurance, muscle strength, and flexibility. Each one of these components helps your body to be physically fit in different ways.

▶ Cardiorespiratory endurance helps you do physical work or play for a long time without getting tired. This requires your heart, blood vessels, lungs, and muscles to efficiently carry and use oxygen.

▶ Muscle strength helps you lift and move yourself and heavy objects.

▶ Flexibility helps you reach, bend, twist, and move without injury.

HOW TO GET FIT

1. To improve your cardiorespiratory endurance, do physical activities that increase your heart and breathing rate:
  - Walk briskly
  - Hike

Bone Integrity and Body Composition

Regular physical activity will help you build strong bones and maintain a healthy body composition. A fit person has strong bones and muscles and a healthy amount of body fat.

While physical activity is good for everyone, persons with disabilities may need to modify how they do activities, depending on their situation. Getting involved and staying involved is what's important.

Skill-Related Components of Physical Fitness

Success in sports and other physical activities may require you to develop some other abilities, such as

- agility,
- balance,
- power, and
- speed,
- coordination,
- reaction time.

- Swim
- Play dodgeball
- Play basketball
- Jump rope
- Play soccer
- Dance
- Ride your bike
- Do in-line skating

2. To improve your strength and muscular endurance, do work, play, or exercise that makes you repeatedly lift or move a load (an object, your body, a weight) that is heavier than what you are used to lifting or moving.

- Do push-ups, pull-ups, and sit-ups.
- Pedal your bike up an incline.
- Shovel snow.

3. Performing strength activities in sets of repetitions will improve your muscle strength and endurance.

4. To improve your flexibility, stretch regularly. Activities like gymnastics, yoga, dance, and figure skating require good flexibility.

5. To best improve your overall physical fitness, participate in a variety of physical activities.

6. Be sure to do activities that work and stretch your upper and lower body.

QUESTIONS FOR STUDENTS

1. Can you name some activities that will improve each component of physical fitness?

2. Which area of fitness do you think you need to improve the most?

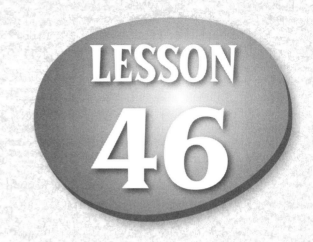

More on the Three Areas of Physical Fitness

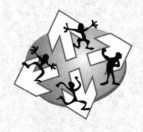

All or parts of this lesson are from J. Carter et al., 2007, *Planet Health*, 2nd ed. (Champaign, IL: Human Kinetics), microunit 9.

FITNESS TIP

To get fit, choose a mixture of activities that you can do regularly to build your cardiorespiratory endurance, muscle strength, and flexibility.

FITNESS LESSON

PHYSICAL FITNESS

▶ We learned that, in order to be physically fit and to meet the daily demands of work and play, we must possess an adequate level of
  - cardiorespiratory endurance,
  - muscular strength, and
  - flexibility.

▶ To be fit, we need to work in all three areas of fitness because each area has a different effect on our bodies.

WORKING THE DIFFERENT AREAS

▶ To be fit, you need to participate in a variety of physical activities.

▶ You need to be able to identify which activities belong to different fitness areas.

▶ Then you need to identify activities in each area that you can enjoy and do.

HOW TO WORK THE THREE AREAS OF FITNESS

1. Think about some daily activities and exercises you do, and figure out what areas of physical fitness they address. For example, what area of physical fitness do you work on when you
   - carry heavy boxes or grocery bags (improves upper-body strength),
   - bike to your friend's house (increases your cardiorespiratory endurance), and
   - shovel snow (improves muscle strength and endurance and cardiorespiratory endurance)?

2. Share your activities and exercises with your class and work together to identify the components of physical fitness that they address.

Different Activities for Different Areas

Aerobic activities generally improve cardio-respiratory and muscle endurance but not strength and flexibility. Similarly, many activities that build muscular strength and flexibility don't do much for endurance. These activities only improve the body part being worked. In addition to performing general aerobic and strength activities, you must perform strength and flexibility exercises by each muscle group and at each joint.

QUESTIONS FOR STUDENTS

1. Name three components of physical fitness.
2. Which component do you need to work on the most?
3. What activity will you do today during gym class? What components of fitness will you work on during this activity?

Stretch and Strength Fitness Diagrams

STRETCH FITNESS DIAGRAMS

Stretching positions are the same for all people. However, the extent of the stretch depends on the flexibility of the individual. Safety is important, so stretches should not be taken beyond comfortable levels. The recommended time to hold each stretch is 10 to 15 seconds.

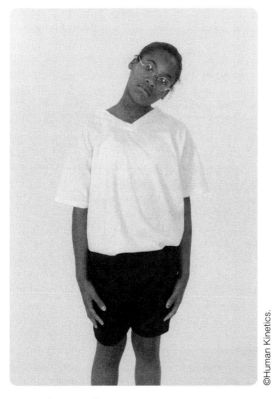

▶ Neck stretch.

▶ Arm and shoulder stretch.

From L.W.Y. Cheung, H. Dart, S. Kalin, and S.L. Gortmaker, 2007, *Eat Well & Keep Moving,* 2nd ed. (Champaign, IL: Human Kinetics).

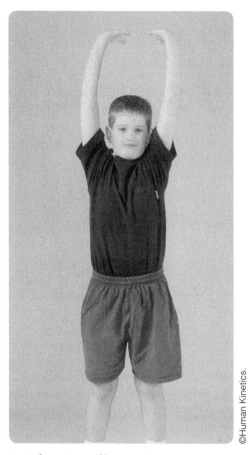

▶ Palms to ceiling.

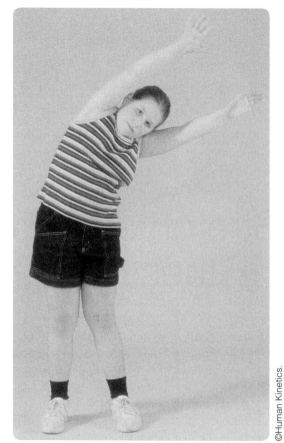

▶ The wave.

©Human Kinetics.

©Human Kinetics.

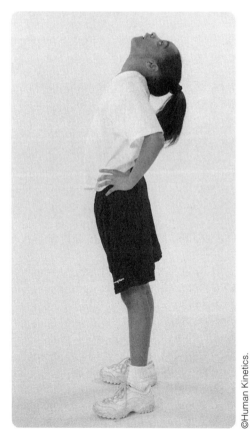

▶ Reach back.

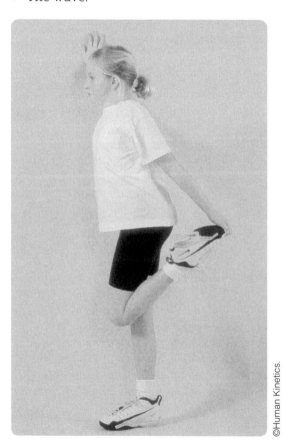

▶ Quad burner.

©Human Kinetics.

©Human Kinetics.

From L.W.Y. Cheung, H. Dart, S. Kalin, and S.L. Gortmaker, 2007, *Eat Well & Keep Moving*, 2nd ed. (Champaign, IL: Human Kinetics).

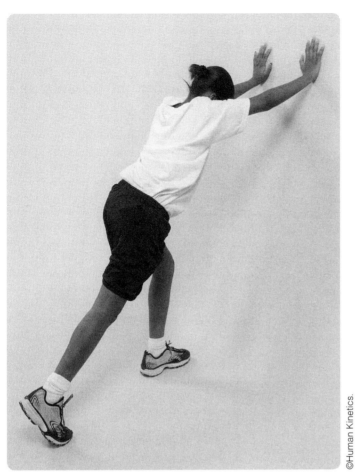

©Human Kinetics.

▶ Hold-up-the-wall hamstring stretch.

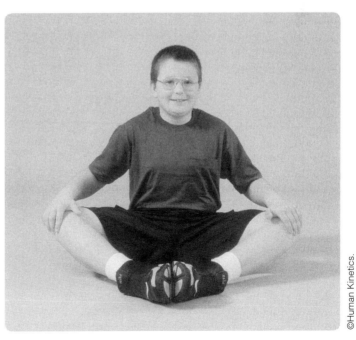

©Human Kinetics.

▶ Butterfly.

From L.W.Y. Cheung, H. Dart, S. Kalin, and S.L. Gortmaker, 2007, *Eat Well & Keep Moving*, 2nd ed. (Champaign, IL: Human Kinetics).

STRENGTH FITNESS DIAGRAMS

UPPER-BODY STRENGTH

Regular Push-Ups

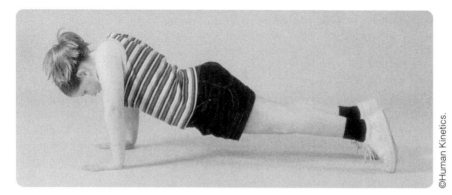

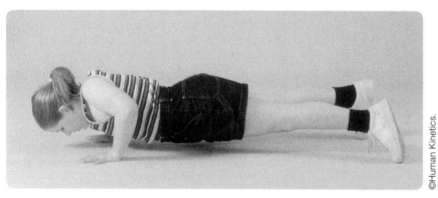

Modified Push-Ups

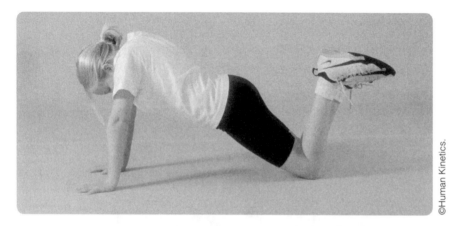

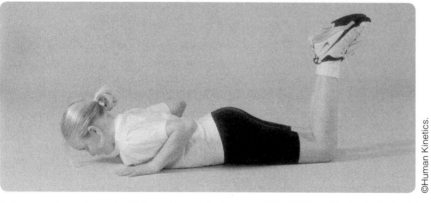

From L.W.Y. Cheung, H. Dart, S. Kalin, and S.L. Gortmaker, 2007, *Eat Well & Keep Moving*, 2nd ed. (Champaign, IL: Human Kinetics).

STOMACH STRENGTH

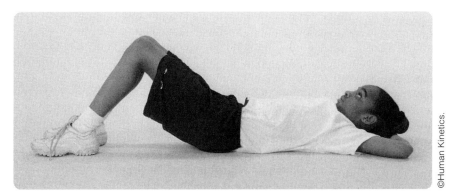

Abdominal Crunches

©Human Kinetics.

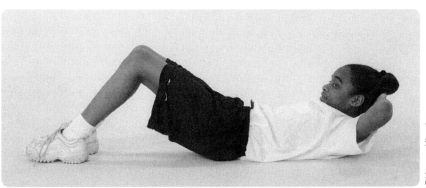

©Human Kinetics.

From L.W.Y. Cheung, H. Dart, S. Kalin, and S.L. Gortmaker, 2007, *Eat Well & Keep Moving,* 2nd ed. (Champaign, IL: Human Kinetics).

Appendix B

Eat Well Cards and Keep Moving Cards

Eat Well cards and Keep Moving cards reinforce key messages and link the classroom and the food service and physical education components of the program. The cards, which contain a mix of text and graphics, present intriguing information to pique the interest of students and can be reviewed with students in as little as 3 minutes. The cards can also be reprinted in the school's parent newsletter, providing a valuable link between home and school.

Stir-Fry With Healthy Fat!

Stir-fry means to cook over high heat while briskly stirring the ingredients so that they cook evenly. Because the vegetables are cut into small pieces, they cook quickly, stay crisp and delicious, and retain most of their nutrients and fresh flavor.

Unlike foods fried in butter, which is high in saturated (unhealthy) fat, stir-fry dishes often have healthy fat, because they are often cooked in vegetable oil and sometimes with another liquids like chicken broth.

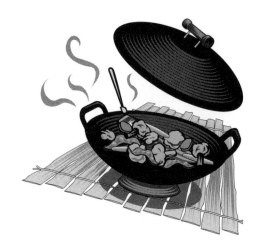

From L.W.Y. Cheung, H. Dart, S. Kalin, and S.L. Gortmaker, 2007, *Eat Well & Keep Moving,* 2nd ed. (Champaign, IL: Human Kinetics).

From L.W.Y. Cheung, H. Dart, S. Kalin, and S.L. Gortmaker, 2007, *Eat Well & Keep Moving,* 2nd ed. (Champaign, IL: Human Kinetics).

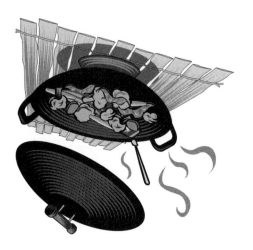

chicken broth.
and sometimes with another liquids like
they are often cooked in vegetable oil
dishes often have healthy fat, because
high in saturated (unhealthy) fat, stir-fry
Unlike foods fried in butter, which is

nutrients and fresh flavor.
and delicious, and retain most of their
pieces, they cook quickly, stay crisp
the vegetables are cut into small
so that they cook evenly. Because
while briskly stirring the ingredients
Stir-fry means to cook over high heat

Stir-Fry With Healthy Fat!

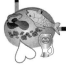

What's the New Food?
It's Chunky Vegetable Stew

What's in chunky vegetable stew?

Tomatoes

Tomatoes have lots of vitamin C to help you heal cuts and scrapes. Vitamin C can also help you fight infections.

Carrots

Carrots have a lot of vitamin A, which helps keep your eyesight good.

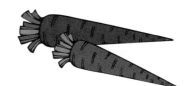

Sweet Potatoes

Sweet potatoes are packed with energy to help you run, dance, and think. They are also rich in several vitamins and minerals such as potassium, which is very important for working muscles.

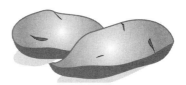

From L.W.Y. Cheung, H. Dart, S. Kalin, and S.L. Gortmaker, 2007, *Eat Well & Keep Moving,* 2nd ed. (Champaign, IL: Human Kinetics).

From L.W.Y. Cheung, H. Dart, S. Kalin, and S.L. Gortmaker, 2007, *Eat Well & Keep Moving,* 2nd ed. (Champaign, IL: Human Kinetics).

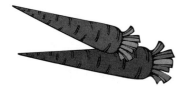

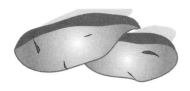

Sweet Potatoes

Sweet potatoes are packed with energy to help you run, dance, and think. They are also rich in several vitamins and minerals such as potassium, which is very important for working muscles.

Carrots

Carrots have a lot of vitamin A, which helps keep your eyesight good.

Tomatoes

Tomatoes have lots of vitamin C to help you heal cuts and scrapes. Vitamin C can also help you fight infections.

What's in chunky vegetable stew?

It's Chunky Vegetable Stew
What's the New Food?

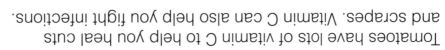
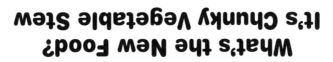

To Nourish Your Body as Well as Your Soul . . .
At Least 5 A Day Should Be Your Goal!

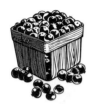

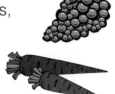

Fruits and vegetables not only are colorful and naturally beautiful but also are packed with vitamins, minerals, and fiber. Research has even shown that they can help keep our hearts healthy.

Eat a rainbow of colors, especially dark-green vegetables like romaine lettuce or spinach and bright orange vegetables like carrots or sweet potatoes. Blueberries, grapefruit, strawberries, pumpkin, and broccoli are a few of the many colorful and nutrient-rich fruits and vegetables you can eat.

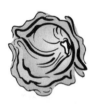

So, if you do not already eat at least 5 servings of fruits and vegetables each day, give it a try. If you already eat 5, go for more—more is always better. It will do wonders for your health!

From L.W.Y. Cheung, H. Dart, S. Kalin, and S.L. Gortmaker, 2007, *Eat Well & Keep Moving*, 2nd ed. (Champaign, IL: Human Kinetics).

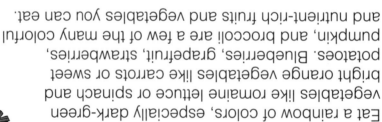

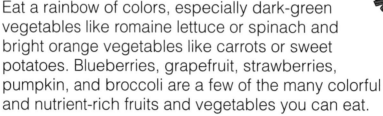

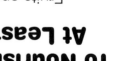

From L.W.Y. Cheung, H. Dart, S. Kalin, and S.L. Gortmaker, 2007, *Eat Well & Keep Moving*, 2nd ed. (Champaign, IL: Human Kinetics).

It will do wonders for your health!

already eat 5, go for more—more is always better. If you fruits and vegetables each day, give it a try. If you So, if you do not already eat at least 5 servings of

and nutrient-rich fruits and vegetables you can eat. pumpkin, and broccoli are a few of the many colorful potatoes. Blueberries, grapefruit, strawberries, bright orange vegetables like carrots or sweet vegetables like romaine lettuce or spinach and Eat a rainbow of colors, especially dark-green

they can help keep our hearts healthy. minerals, and fiber. Research has even shown that naturally beautiful but also are packed with vitamins, Fruits and vegetables not only are colorful and

At Least 5 A Day Should Be Your Goal!
To Nourish Your Body as Well as Your Soul . . .

Calcium Is Right for Pearly Whites!

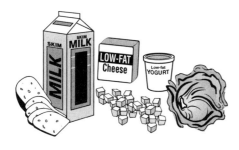

Calcium is crucial for all the growing bones in your body. Low-fat or nonfat dairy products are high in calcium, and there are many other calcium-rich foods to choose from. Leafy greens like kale and bok choy, baked beans, and black-eyed peas have calcium as well as other vitamins and minerals and fiber. Soy products like tofu and canned fish (like salmon and sardines) have calcium, protein, and healthy fat! Some 100% orange juice has calcium added to it.

Smile!

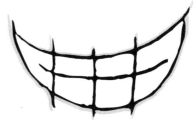

Did you know that calcium is great for helping to keep your teeth healthy and strong?

So eat calcium-rich foods, smile, and show off those pearly whites!

From L.W.Y. Cheung, H. Dart, S. Kalin, and S.L. Gortmaker, 2007, *Eat Well & Keep Moving*, 2nd ed. (Champaign, IL: Human Kinetics).

From L.W.Y. Cheung, H. Dart, S. Kalin, and S.L. Gortmaker, 2007, *Eat Well & Keep Moving*, 2nd ed. (Champaign, IL: Human Kinetics).

those pearly whites!
So eat calcium-rich foods, smile, and show off

to keep your teeth healthy and strong?
Did you know that calcium is great for helping

Smile!

has calcium added to it.
sardines) have calcium, protein, and healthy fat! Some 100% orange juice
minerals and fiber. Soy products like tofu and canned fish (like salmon and
calcium as well as other vitamins and
baked beans, and black-eyed peas have
from. Leafy greens like kale and bok choy,
many other calcium-rich foods to choose
products are high in calcium, and there are
bones in your body. Low-fat or nonfat dairy
Calcium is crucial for all the growing

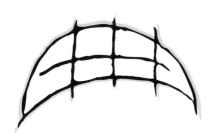

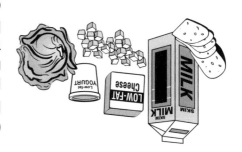

Calcium Is Right for Pearly Whites!

Oranges for Each Day's Journey

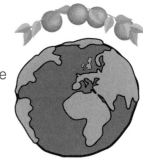

Originally, oranges grew in Asia and the East Indies—do you know where these areas are on the map? Oranges were brought to Europe and then to the New World (North America) by explorers. Orange trees were first planted in the San Gabriel Mission in San Gabriel, California, in 1804. In 1841, William Wolfskill planted a commercial orange grove in Los Angeles. By 1849, this entrepreneur sold oranges to gold rushers to prevent scurvy, a disease marked by overall weakness, spots on the skin, and, in the worst cases, bleeding gums.

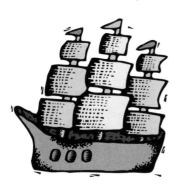

The vitamin C in oranges and other citrus fruits (like lemons, limes, and grapefruit) helped keep the gold rushers and the early explorers, like Columbus, Magellan, and Marco Polo, healthy during their long journeys. Just like the explorers, you can keep healthy and strong on your daily journeys (to school, to home, and to the store) by eating oranges and other citrus fruit. It's as easy as pouring a small glass of 100% orange juice or eating the orange wedges served in the cafeteria. You'll have energy for playing, and the vitamin C will help you grow strong, heal cuts and bruises, and fight off infections.

From L.W.Y. Cheung, H. Dart, S. Kalin, and S.L. Gortmaker, 2007, *Eat Well & Keep Moving*, 2nd ed. (Champaign, IL: Human Kinetics).

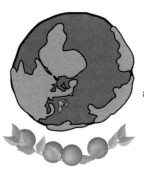

From L.W.Y. Cheung, H. Dart, S. Kalin, and S.L. Gortmaker, 2007, *Eat Well & Keep Moving*, 2nd ed. (Champaign, IL: Human Kinetics).

grow strong, heal cuts and bruises, and fight off infections. You'll have energy for playing, and the vitamin C will help you juice or eating the orange wedges served in the cafeteria. fruit. It's as easy as pouring a small glass of 100% orange to home, and to the store) by eating oranges and other citrus can keep healthy and strong on your daily journeys (to school, healthy during their long journeys. Just like the explorers, you early explorers, like Columbus, Magellan, and Marco Polo, limes, and grapefruit) helped keep the gold rushers and the The vitamin C in oranges and other citrus fruits (like lemons,

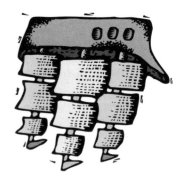

overall weakness, spots on the skin, and, in the worst cases, bleeding gums. oranges to gold rushers to prevent scurvy, a disease marked by orange grove in Los Angeles. By 1849, this entrepreneur sold California, in 1804. In 1841, William Wolfskill planted a commercial trees were first planted in the San Gabriel Mission in San Gabriel, and then to the New World (North America) by explorers. Orange where these areas are on the map? Oranges were brought to Europe Originally, oranges grew in Asia and the East Indies—do you know

Oranges for Each Day's Journey

Punch Out Fruit Punch—Pick Whole Fruit

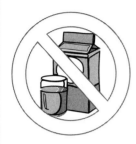

It's easy to tell the difference between fruit punch and 100% fruit juice. Only the pure juice will say "100% juice" right on the label—this goes for orange juice, grapefruit juice, or any kind of juice. It is even better to eat whole fruit instead of juice. While 100% juice is packed with vitamins and minerals, whole fruit has that and more! Whole fruit can have up to three times the fiber that juice has, and it is easy to grab on the go.

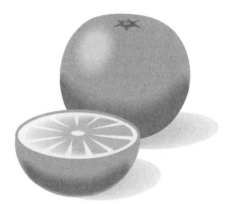

Other fruit drinks and colored punches that don't say "100% juice" on the label may look like pure juice, but they usually contain very little juice (often none at all) and a lot of sugar. When in doubt, grab a whole piece of fruit instead of juice!

From L.W.Y. Cheung, H. Dart, S. Kalin, and S.L. Gortmaker, 2007, *Eat Well & Keep Moving*, 2nd ed. (Champaign, IL: Human Kinetics).

From L.W.Y. Cheung, H. Dart, S. Kalin, and S.L. Gortmaker, 2007, *Eat Well & Keep Moving*, 2nd ed. (Champaign, IL: Human Kinetics).

fruit instead of juice!

Other fruit drinks and colored punches that don't say "100% juice" on the label may look like pure juice, but they usually contain very little juice (often none at all) and a lot of sugar. When in doubt, grab a whole piece of fruit instead of juice!

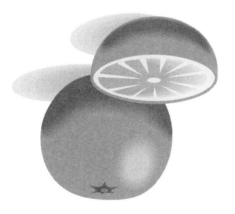

Whole fruit can have up to three times the fiber that juice has, and it is easy to grab on the go.

vitamins and minerals, whole fruit has that and more! fruit instead of juice. While 100% juice is packed with juice, or any kind of juice. It is even better to eat whole right on the label—this goes for orange juice, grapefruit 100% fruit juice. Only the pure juice will say "100% juice" It's easy to tell the difference between fruit punch and

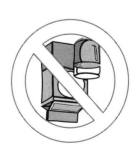

Punch Out Fruit Punch—Pick Whole Fruit

Have a Little Slice of Spring

Pri-ma-ver-a *adjective*

1. Made with different kinds of sliced or diced vegetables
2. From Latin, meaning *early spring* (*primus = first* + *ver = spring*)

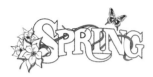

The word *primavera* can be traced back to the Latin roots *primus,* meaning *first,* and *ver,* meaning *spring.* Some of the spring vegetables you might find in a primavera dish (whole wheat pasta primavera or pizza primavera, for example) are peas, green beans, tomatoes, asparagus, and mushrooms. But don't be surprised if you find other kinds of vegetables in your primavera, like broccoli, onions, or carrots. Great chefs like to be creative!

This winter, when you're dreaming of warmer days, have some whole wheat pizza primavera for lunch. It's like having a little slice of spring.

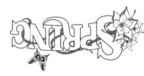

From L.W.Y. Cheung, H. Dart, S. Kalin, and S.L. Gortmaker, 2007, *Eat Well & Keep Moving*, 2nd ed. (Champaign, IL: Human Kinetics).

From L.W.Y. Cheung, H. Dart, S. Kalin, and S.L. Gortmaker, 2007, *Eat Well & Keep Moving*, 2nd ed. (Champaign, IL: Human Kinetics).

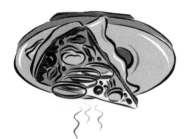

This winter, when you're dreaming of warmer days, have some whole wheat pizza primavera for lunch. It's like having a little slice of spring.

Great chefs like to be creative!
your primavera, like broccoli, onions, or carrots. But don't be surprised if you find other kinds of vegetables in mushrooms. primavera, for example) are peas, green beans, tomatoes, asparagus, and primavera dish (whole wheat pasta primavera or pizza Some of the spring vegetables you might find in a roots *primus,* meaning *first,* and *ver,* meaning *spring.* The word *primavera* can be traced back to the Latin

2. From Latin, meaning *early spring* (*primus = first* + *ver = spring*)
1. Made with different kinds of sliced or diced vegetables

Pri-ma-ver-a *adjective*

Have a Little Slice of Spring

What a Treat to Eat a Sweet Peach!

Peaches are rich in vitamins and minerals, especially vitamin A and potassium. They also contain iron, niacin, and vitamin C.

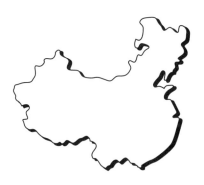

The peach originated in China around 2000 BC and was regarded as a symbol of life. Peaches are still used to help celebrate birthdays in China. A special peach dessert is often served at Chinese birthday parties.

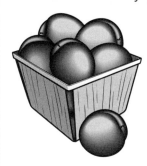

Fresh peaches are best tasting and most available in the summer, but you can eat canned or frozen peaches year-round! They are delicious for breakfast, as a snack, or for dessert. Eat them by themselves, sliced with other fruit on whole-grain cereal, mixed in with oatmeal, baked with cinnamon and rolled oats, or even made into peach salsa.

From L.W.Y. Cheung, H. Dart, S. Kalin, and S.L. Gortmaker, 2007, *Eat Well & Keep Moving*, 2nd ed. (Champaign, IL: Human Kinetics).

From L.W.Y. Cheung, H. Dart, S. Kalin, and S.L. Gortmaker, 2007, *Eat Well & Keep Moving*, 2nd ed. (Champaign, IL: Human Kinetics).

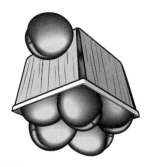

peach salsa.
baked with cinnamon and rolled oats, or even made into
other fruit on whole-grain cereal, mixed in with oatmeal,
or for dessert. Eat them by themselves, sliced with
year-round! They are delicious for breakfast, as a snack,
the summer, but you can eat canned or frozen peaches
Fresh peaches are best tasting and most available in

Chinese birthday parties.
China. A special peach dessert is often served at
are still used to help celebrate birthdays in
and was regarded as a symbol of life. Peaches
The peach originated in China around 2000 BC

contain iron, niacin, and vitamin C.
especially vitamin A and potassium. They also
Peaches are rich in vitamins and minerals,

What a Treat to Eat a Sweet Peach!

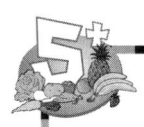

Pick Peppers

Peppers come in many different shapes, colors, and sizes, but they all are packed with vitamins and minerals. Green, red, orange, and yellow bell peppers have a mild, sweet taste and are good sources of vitamin C and fiber. Other crisp, sweet peppers include pimientos, which are red and heart shaped, and banana peppers, which are yellow and shaped like the fruit. Jalapeño and green hot chili peppers pack in flavor and nutrients. They are good for you and taste great!

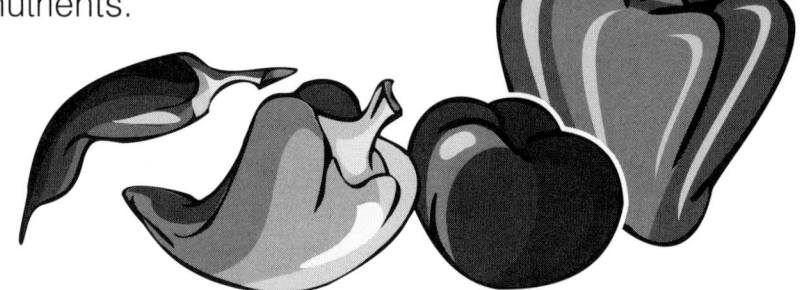

From L.W.Y. Cheung, H. Dart, S. Kalin, and S.L. Gortmaker, 2007, *Eat Well & Keep Moving,* 2nd ed. (Champaign, IL: Human Kinetics).

From L.W.Y. Cheung, H. Dart, S. Kalin, and S.L. Gortmaker, 2007, *Eat Well & Keep Moving,* 2nd ed. (Champaign, IL: Human Kinetics).

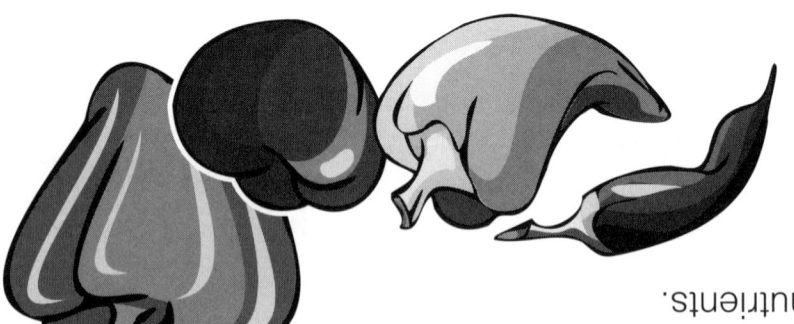

taste great!
for you and
They are good
pack in flavor and nutrients.
the fruit. Jalapeño and green hot chili peppers
peppers, which are yellow and shaped like
which are red and heart shaped, and banana
of vitamin C and fiber. Other crisp, sweet peppers include pimientos,
yellow bell peppers have a mild, sweet taste and are good sources
all are packed with vitamins and minerals. Green, red, orange, and
Peppers come in many different shapes, colors, and sizes, but they

Pick Peppers

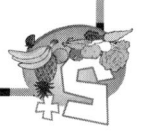

A Message From Bobby Broccoli

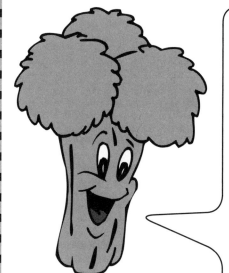

Hi, kids! My name is Bobby Broccoli and I would like to fill you in on (and up with) some tasty tidbits of news. . . .

▶ Broccoli is now more popular than ever! Did you know that the average person in the United States eats 6 pounds (3 kilograms) of broccoli a year?

▶ Broccoli is loaded with vitamin C and fiber, is very low in unhealthy fat, and is rich in beta-carotene—nutrients that keep our hearts healthy!

▶ Broccoli is also a terrific vegetable source of calcium. It's good for your teeth and bones!

I know we're going to like each other!

From L.W.Y. Cheung, H. Dart, S. Kalin, and S.L. Gortmaker, 2007, *Eat Well & Keep Moving,* 2nd ed. (Champaign, IL: Human Kinetics).

I know we're going to like each other!

▶ Broccoli is also a terrific vegetable source of calcium. It's good for your teeth and bones!

▶ Broccoli is loaded with vitamin C and fiber, is very low in unhealthy fat, and is rich in beta-carotene—nutrients that keep our hearts healthy!

▶ Broccoli is now more popular than ever! Did you know that the average person in the United States eats 6 pounds (3 kilograms) of broccoli a year?

Hi, kids! My name is Bobby Broccoli and I would like to fill you in on (and up with) some tasty tidbits of news. . . .

A Message From Bobby Broccoli

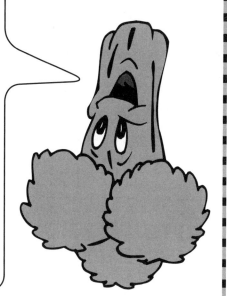

What's the New Food?
It's Sweet Potatoes and Orange Juice

Sweet potatoes contain a lot of vitamin A, which is needed for strong bones and good eyesight. They also give you energy for playing and learning.

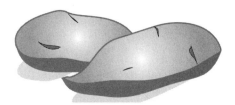

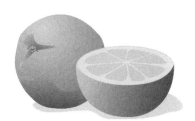

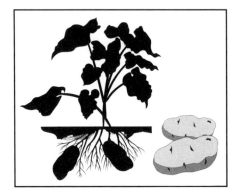

From L.W.Y. Cheung, H. Dart, S. Kalin, and S.L. Gortmaker, 2007, *Eat Well & Keep Moving,* 2nd ed. (Champaign, IL: Human Kinetics). From the Grolier Multimedia Encyclopedia, 1999 Edition. Copyright 1999 by Grolier Incorporated. Reprinted by permission.

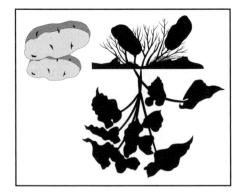

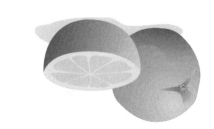

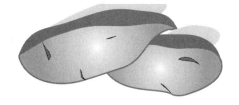

energy for playing and learning. They also give you and good eyesight. A, which is needed for strong bones Sweet potatoes contain a lot of vitamin

It's Sweet Potatoes and Orange Juice
What's the New Food?

That's One Sweet Potato!

Sweet potatoes contain a lot of vitamin A, which is needed for strong bones, fighting infections, and good eyesight. In general, fruits and vegetables that are orange (like sweet potatoes and carrots) are a great source of vitamin A.

The sweet potato is very hardy and grows underground. It grows especially well in southern states, where the climate is warm.

Sweet potatoes are a sweet, delicious, and nutritious addition to many meals. Try some today!

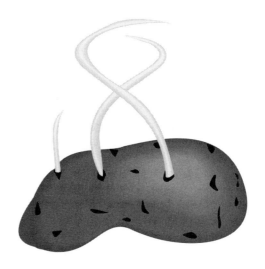

From L.W.Y. Cheung, H. Dart, S. Kalin, and S.L. Gortmaker, 2007, *Eat Well & Keep Moving,* 2nd ed. (Champaign, IL: Human Kinetics).

From L.W.Y. Cheung, H. Dart, S. Kalin, and S.L. Gortmaker, 2007, *Eat Well & Keep Moving,* 2nd ed. (Champaign, IL: Human Kinetics).

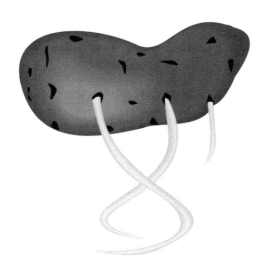

That's One Sweet Potato!

Sweet potatoes contain a lot of vitamin A, which is needed for strong bones, fighting infections, and good eyesight. In general, fruits and vegetables that are orange (like sweet potatoes and carrots) are a great source of vitamin A.

The sweet potato is very hardy and grows underground. It grows especially well in southern states, where the climate is warm.

Sweet potatoes are a sweet, delicious, and nutritious addition to many meals. Try some today!

The Power of Whole Grains

What in the world are whole grains?

They are grains like wheat, oats, and rice that have not been changed much from their natural state.

Whole grains still have their natural outer shell (the bran) and inner core (the germ). The bran and germ are packed with vitamins, minerals, and fiber. Most grains eaten in the United States are "refined" grains, meaning that the nutritious bran and germ are removed.

Why are whole grains powerfully good?

Whole grains taste great! They have more vitamins, more minerals, and more fiber than refined grains. They give you energy that lasts.

Where can I find whole grains?

Whole grains are everywhere! Choose plain oatmeal for breakfast. At lunch, ask for a sandwich on whole wheat bread, or pick brown rice pilaf or tabbouleh as a side dish. For great whole-grain snacks, try popcorn or a bowl of whole-grain cereal. Feeling adventurous? Try barley, buckwheat, millet, or quinoa (pronounced "KEEN-wah").

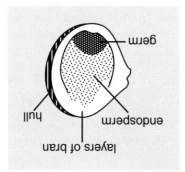

▶ A whole wheat kernel.

From L.W.Y. Cheung, H. Dart, S. Kalin, and S.L. Gortmaker, 2007, *Eat Well & Keep Moving*, 2nd ed. (Champaign, IL: Human Kinetics).

From L.W.Y. Cheung, H. Dart, S. Kalin, and S.L. Gortmaker, 2007, *Eat Well & Keep Moving*, 2nd ed. (Champaign, IL: Human Kinetics).

Where can I find whole grains?

Whole grains are everywhere! Choose plain oatmeal for breakfast. At lunch, ask for a sandwich on whole wheat bread, or pick brown rice pilaf or tabbouleh as a side dish. For great whole-grain snacks, try popcorn or a bowl of whole-grain cereal. Feeling adventurous? Try barley, buckwheat, millet, or quinoa (pronounced "KEEN-wah").

Why are whole grains powerfully good?

Whole grains taste great! They have more vitamins, more minerals, and more fiber than refined grains. They give you energy that lasts.

◀ A whole wheat kernel.

Whole grains still have their natural outer shell (the bran) and inner core (the germ). The bran and germ are packed with vitamins, minerals, and fiber. Most grains eaten in the United States are "refined" grains, meaning that the nutritious bran and germ are removed.

What in the world are whole grains?

They are grains like wheat, oats, and rice that have not been changed much from their natural state.

The Power of Whole Grains
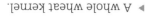

What's the New Food? Tabbouleh

Tabbouleh (pronounced "tah-BOO-lee") is a traditional dish from the Middle Eastern region of the world. It has become popular dish in the United States because of its delicious mix of flavors.

The main ingredient in tabbouleh is bulgur, a form of whole wheat. Tabbouleh is also made with lots of tasty vegetables—tomatoes, cucumbers, onions, parsley—and healthy vegetable oil. Lemon juice and mint add flavor.

Here's why you should try tabbouleh:

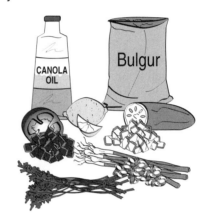

- ▶ It tastes great!

- ▶ It is a healthy, whole-grain food.

- ▶ It can work toward your five or more servings of fruits and vegetables a day. (Remember—when it comes to vegetables, more is always better.)

- ▶ It tastes great!

From L.W.Y. Cheung, H. Dart, S. Kalin, and S.L. Gortmaker, 2007, *Eat Well & Keep Moving*, 2nd ed. (Champaign, IL: Human Kinetics).

- ▶ It tastes great!

- ▶ It can work toward your five or more servings of fruits and vegetables a day. (Remember—when it comes to vegetables, more is always better.)

- ▶ It is a healthy, whole-grain food.

- ▶ It tastes great!

Here's why you should try tabbouleh:

The main ingredient in tabbouleh is bulgur, a form of whole wheat. Tabbouleh is also made with lots of tasty vegetables—tomatoes, cucumbers, onions, parsley—and healthy vegetable oil. Lemon juice and mint add flavor.

Tabbouleh (pronounced "tah-BOO-lee") is a traditional dish from the Middle Eastern region of the world. It has become popular dish in the United States because of its delicious mix of flavors.

What's the New Food? Tabbouleh

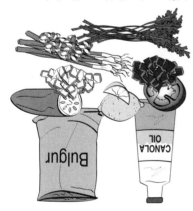

Bulgur Facts

▶ Bulgur (pronounced "BUHL-gur") is whole wheat that has been cooked in water, dried, and ground. It has a nutty taste. It's fast and easy to prepare! Put the bulgur in a bowl. Pour hot water over it. Cover it, and wait ten minutes.

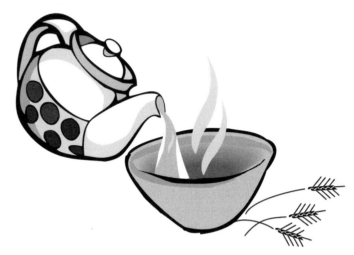

▶ One cup of bulgur has 8 grams of fiber. That's 8 times more fiber than a slice of white bread or a cup of white rice! Bulgur's also packed with B vitamins, iron, and magnesium.

From L.W.Y. Cheung, H. Dart, S. Kalin, and S.L. Gortmaker, 2007, *Eat Well & Keep Moving,* 2nd ed. (Champaign, IL: Human Kinetics).

From L.W.Y. Cheung, H. Dart, S. Kalin, and S.L. Gortmaker, 2007, *Eat Well & Keep Moving,* 2nd ed. (Champaign, IL: Human Kinetics).

magnesium.
vitamins, iron, and
also packed with B
of white rice! Bulgur's
white bread or a cup
fiber than a slice of
That's 8 times more
has 8 grams of fiber.
▶ One cup of bulgur
ten minutes.
it. Cover it, and wait
and easy to prepare! Put the bulgur in a bowl. Pour hot water over
cooked in water, dried, and ground. It has a nutty taste. It's fast
▶ Bulgur (pronounced "BUHL-gur") is whole wheat that has been

Bulgur Facts

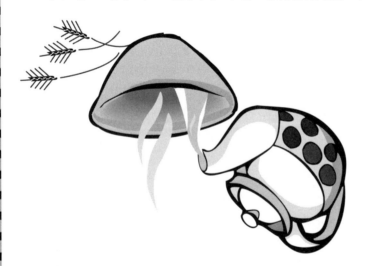

Cool Beans

Here is a riddle for you: What do a chick and a pigeon have in common?

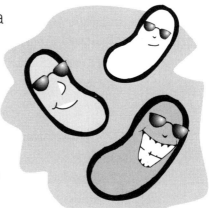

"They are both birds," you say?
Guess again.
They are both types of beans. Yes, beans.

Humans have grown beans and their close relatives, peas, for thousands of years. Chickpeas, also called garbanzo beans, have been found in ancient ruins more than 10,000 years old. Pigeon peas, also called *gandules* or red gram, have been found in Egyptian tombs!

Dry beans and peas come in many colors—red, white, black, brown, tan, yellow, and green. Some are solid-colored, and some are speckled. Some are large, and some are small. The five most popular types of dry beans in the United States are pinto, navy, kidney, black, and Great Northern.

From L.W.Y. Cheung, H. Dart, S. Kalin, and S.L. Gortmaker, 2007, *Eat Well & Keep Moving,* 2nd ed. (Champaign, IL: Human Kinetics).

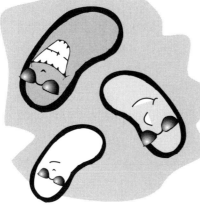

Cool Beans

Here is a riddle for you: What do a chick and a pigeon have in common?

"They are both birds," you say?
Guess again.
They are both types of beans. Yes, beans.

Humans have grown beans and their close relatives, peas, for thousands of years. Chickpeas, also called garbanzo beans, have been found in ancient ruins more than 10,000 years old. Pigeon peas, also called *gandules* or red gram, have been found in Egyptian tombs!

Dry beans and peas come in many colors—red, white, black, brown, tan, yellow, and green. Some are solid-colored, and some are speckled. Some are large, and some are small. The five most popular types of dry beans in the United States are pinto, navy, kidney, black, and Great Northern.

From L.W.Y. Cheung, H. Dart, S. Kalin, and S.L. Gortmaker, 2007, *Eat Well & Keep Moving,* 2nd ed. (Champaign, IL: Human Kinetics).

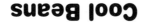

Great Ways to Eat Beans

Beans taste great by themselves or mixed with other foods:

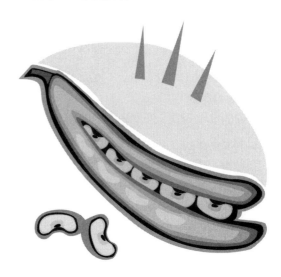

- ▶ Vegetable chili is made of red kidney beans, tomatoes, and green peppers.

- ▶ Hummus is made of chickpeas, lemon juice, garlic, and sesame paste. It makes a great dip for vegetables or whole wheat crackers.

- ▶ Rice and beans is a traditional side dish in many cultures.

- ▶ Did you know that dry beans and peas are actually the seeds of plants? That's why they are power-packed with vitamins, minerals, protein, and carbohydrate. So try some cool beans today!

From L.W.Y. Cheung, H. Dart, S. Kalin, and S.L. Gortmaker, 2007, *Eat Well & Keep Moving,* 2nd ed. (Champaign, IL: Human Kinetics).

From L.W.Y. Cheung, H. Dart, S. Kalin, and S.L. Gortmaker, 2007, *Eat Well & Keep Moving,* 2nd ed. (Champaign, IL: Human Kinetics).

- ▶ Did you know that dry beans and peas are actually the seeds of plants? That's why they are power-packed with vitamins, minerals, protein, and carbohydrate. So try some cool beans today!

- ▶ Rice and beans is a traditional side dish in many cultures.

- ▶ Hummus is made of chickpeas, lemon juice, garlic, and sesame paste. It makes a great dip for vegetables or whole wheat crackers.

- ▶ Vegetable chili is made of red kidney beans, tomatoes, and green peppers.

mixed with other foods:

Beans taste great by themselves or

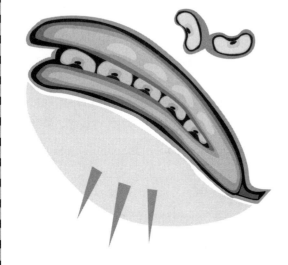

Great Ways to Eat Beans

Have You Ever Heard of Pineapple Oranges?
(How About Valencia, Temple, Navel, or Blood Oranges?)

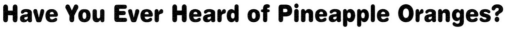

The oranges you usually see in the cafeteria are called *pineapple oranges.* Pineapple oranges are popular because they have few seeds and have the familiar bright orange skin.

All types of oranges are sweet and juicy, but each type has a different name and looks a little bit different from the others. Some are light orange on the inside, some are bright orange on the inside, and some are even bright red on the inside (these oranges are called *blood oranges).*

Some oranges have thin skin, like Valencia oranges, which also have few seeds and so are great for juicing, and some have thick, easily peeled skin, like navel oranges. Oranges also come in different sizes, ranging from the smaller temple to the larger navel.

Because oranges are so delicious, they make a great snack and a sweet dessert! You can eat them peeled or cut into wedges, or you can drink them as a small glass of 100% orange juice. Eating oranges in any of these ways lets you enjoy them and gives you a boost of vitamin C that helps you grow, play, and learn.

From L.W.Y. Cheung, H. Dart, S. Kalin, and S.L. Gortmaker, 2007, *Eat Well & Keep Moving,* 2nd ed. (Champaign, IL: Human Kinetics).

Have You Ever Heard of Pineapple Oranges?
(How About Valencia, Temple, Navel, or Blood Oranges?)

The oranges you usually see in the cafeteria are called *pineapple oranges.* Pineapple oranges are popular because they have few seeds and have the familiar bright orange skin.

All types of oranges are sweet and juicy, but each type has a different name and looks a little bit different from the others. Some are light orange on the inside, some are bright orange on the inside, and some are even bright red on the inside (these oranges are called *blood oranges).*

Some oranges have thin skin, like Valencia oranges, which also have few seeds and so are great for juicing, and some have thick, easily peeled skin, like navel oranges. Oranges also come in different sizes, ranging from the smaller temple to the larger navel.

Because oranges are so delicious, they make a great snack and a sweet dessert! You can eat them peeled or cut into wedges, or you can drink them as a small glass of 100% orange juice. Eating oranges in any of these ways lets you enjoy them and gives you a boost of vitamin C that helps you grow, play, and learn.

From L.W.Y. Cheung, H. Dart, S. Kalin, and S.L. Gortmaker, 2007, *Eat Well & Keep Moving,* 2nd ed. (Champaign, IL: Human Kinetics).

Whole Wheat Bread Versus White Bread

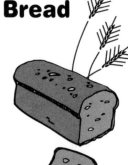

Try the wonderful world of whole wheat bread! It may look a little different, but whole wheat bread tastes good and is good for you. The more you eat it, the more you'll like it!

And it's more nutritious than white bread. White bread is made from wheat flour that has had the bran and wheat germ removed from the grain.

vs.

Even when the white flour is enriched by adding back nutrients, only 5 nutrients are added back. Compared to whole wheat flour, the enriched white flour lacks much of the fiber and 18 other vitamins and minerals found in whole wheat flour.

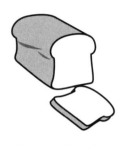

From L.W.Y. Cheung, H. Dart, S. Kalin, and S.L. Gortmaker, 2007, *Eat Well & Keep Moving*, 2nd ed. (Champaign, IL: Human Kinetics).

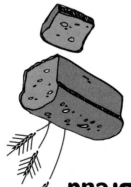

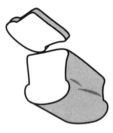

vs.

From L.W.Y. Cheung, H. Dart, S. Kalin, and S.L. Gortmaker, 2007, *Eat Well & Keep Moving*, 2nd ed. (Champaign, IL: Human Kinetics).

and minerals found in whole wheat flour.
flour lacks much of the fiber and 18 other vitamins
Compared to whole wheat flour, the enriched white
back nutrients, only 5 nutrients are added back.
Even when the white flour is enriched by adding

wheat germ removed from the grain.
is made from wheat flour that has had the bran and
And it's more nutritious than white bread. White bread

more you'll like it!
good and is good for you. The more you eat it, the
look a little different, but whole wheat bread tastes
Try the wonderful world of whole wheat bread! It may

Whole Wheat Bread Versus White Bread

Amber Waves of Grain

Although wild wheat was not native to America, wheat seeds were brought here by Columbus and European immigrants, who planted them across the country. Are you familiar with the phrase *amber waves of grain* from our national hymn, "America the Beautiful"? It refers to wheat fields that spread far and wide and look as large and impressive as an ocean.

Today, the United States is the world's largest producer of wheat, growing 600 million bushels a year that are ground into 20 billion pounds (9 billion kilograms) of flour. Because more than 60% of the wheat grown here is exported, wheat is very important to our economy. American wheat provides people around the world with an excellent source of nutrition. Pick whole wheat and whole-grain foods, such as 100% whole wheat bread, barley, whole wheat pasta, and brown rice, which are packed with vitamins, minerals, and fiber.

From L.W.Y. Cheung, H. Dart, S. Kalin, and S.L. Gortmaker, 2007, *Eat Well & Keep Moving*, 2nd ed. (Champaign, IL: Human Kinetics).

Amber Waves of Grain

Although wild wheat was not native to America, wheat seeds were brought here by Columbus and European immigrants, who planted them across the country. Are you familiar with the phrase *amber waves of grain* from our national hymn, "America the Beautiful"? It refers to wheat fields that spread far and wide and look as large and impressive as an ocean.

Today, the United States is the world's largest producer of wheat, growing 600 million bushels a year that are ground into 20 billion pounds (9 billion kilograms) of flour. Because more than 60% of the wheat grown here is exported, wheat is very important to our economy. American wheat provides people around the world with an excellent source of nutrition. Pick whole wheat and whole-grain foods, such as 100% whole wheat bread, barley, whole wheat pasta, and brown rice, which are packed with vitamins, minerals, and fiber.

From L.W.Y. Cheung, H. Dart, S. Kalin, and S.L. Gortmaker, 2007, *Eat Well & Keep Moving*, 2nd ed. (Champaign, IL: Human Kinetics).

A Piece of the Pie?

Our days can be divided into many different parts. We sleep. We sit. We are active. The following pie chart shows how a lot of students, like you, spend their days.

How would your own pie chart look?

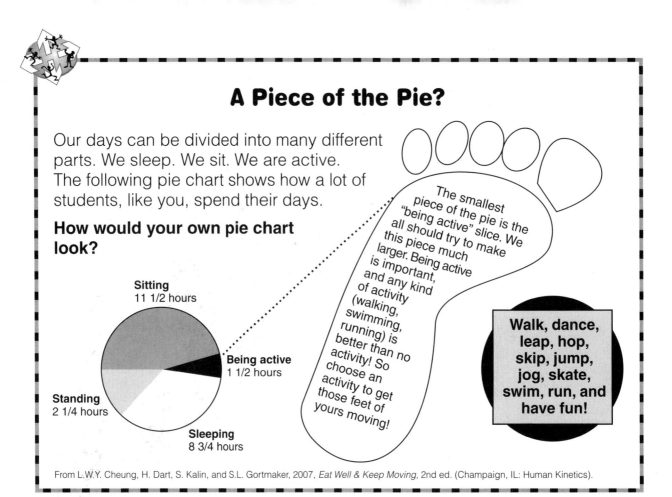

Sitting
11 1/2 hours

Being active
1 1/2 hours

Standing
2 1/4 hours

Sleeping
8 3/4 hours

The smallest piece of the pie is the "being active" slice. We all should try to make this piece much larger. Being active is important, and any kind of activity (walking, swimming, running) is better than no activity! So choose an activity to get those feet of yours moving!

Walk, dance, leap, hop, skip, jump, jog, skate, swim, run, and have fun!

From L.W.Y. Cheung, H. Dart, S. Kalin, and S.L. Gortmaker, 2007, *Eat Well & Keep Moving*, 2nd ed. (Champaign, IL: Human Kinetics).

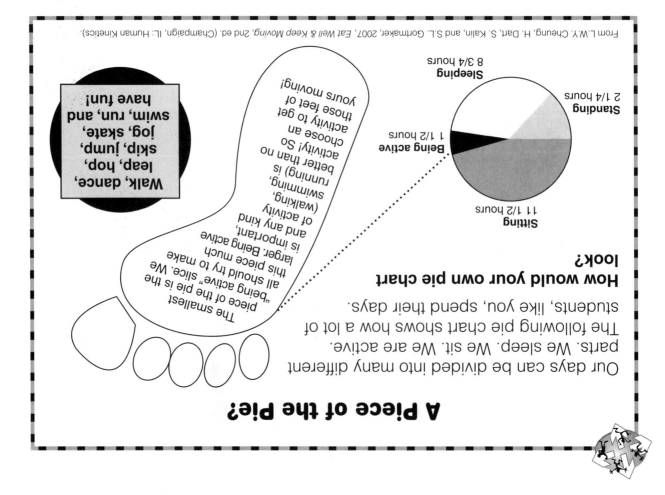

A Piece of the Pie?

Our days can be divided into many different parts. We sleep. We sit. We are active. The following pie chart shows how a lot of students, like you, spend their days.

How would your own pie chart look?

Sitting
11 1/2 hours

Being active
1 1/2 hours

Standing
2 1/4 hours

Sleeping
8 3/4 hours

The smallest piece of the pie is the "being active" slice. We all should try to make this piece much larger. Being active is important, and any kind of activity (walking, swimming, running) is better than no activity! So choose an activity to get those feet of yours moving!

Walk, dance, leap, hop, skip, jump, jog, skate, swim, run, and have fun!

From L.W.Y. Cheung, H. Dart, S. Kalin, and S.L. Gortmaker, 2007, *Eat Well & Keep Moving*, 2nd ed. (Champaign, IL: Human Kinetics).

Be Wise . . . Warm Up for 5 Before You Exercise

Before you get your feet moving, warm up your body!

QUESTION: What is the very first thing you should do before you exercise?
Answer: Warm up for 5 minutes!

5 minutes = 1/12 of an hour = 300 seconds = 1/288 of a day

Why Warm Up?

Just like warming up a car gets it ready to drive, warming up your body gets it ready for activity. Warming up also keeps you from getting hurt, which can happen if your muscles and joints haven't been loosened up.

How Do You Warm Up?

Do slow movements—like jogging in place or slow jumping jacks. Anything that keeps you moving slowly for 5 minutes will work!

From L.W.Y. Cheung, H. Dart, S. Kalin, and S.L. Gortmaker, 2007, *Eat Well & Keep Moving*, 2nd ed. (Champaign, IL: Human Kinetics).

From L.W.Y. Cheung, H. Dart, S. Kalin, and S.L. Gortmaker, 2007, *Eat Well & Keep Moving*, 2nd ed. (Champaign, IL: Human Kinetics).

How Do You Warm Up?

Do slow movements—like jogging in place or slow jumping jacks. Anything that keeps you moving slowly for 5 minutes will work!

Why Warm Up?

Just like warming up a car gets it ready to drive, warming up your body gets it ready for activity. Warming up also keeps you from getting hurt, which can happen if your muscles and joints haven't been loosened up.

5 minutes = 1/12 of an hour = 300 seconds = 1/288 of a day

Answer: Warm up for 5 minutes!

QUESTION: What is the very first thing you should do before you exercise?

Before you get your feet moving, warm up your body!

Be Wise . . . Warm Up for 5 Before You Exercise

About the Authors

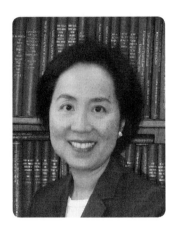

Lillian W.Y. Cheung, DSc, is a lecturer and director of health promotion and communication in the department of nutrition at the Harvard School of Public Health. She was the coprincipal investigator for the original *Eat Well & Keep Moving* controlled trial in Baltimore Public Schools, the curriculum of which became the foundation for the first edition of this book. She was the principal investigator for the *Qualitative Study of the School Health Index*, funded by the Centers for Disease Control and Prevention. As a registered dietitian and a DSc in nutrition, she has more than 20 years of experience promoting healthy eating and physical activity to the public, with a special emphasis on children.

Dr. Cheung is editorial director of the Nutrition Source Web site at the Harvard School of Public Health and is coauthor of *Be Healthy! It's a Girl Thing: Food, Fitness, and Feeling Great*, a book for girls aged 9 to 13 that promotes a healthy lifestyle. She was also coeditor of *Child Health, Nutrition, and Physical Activity* (1995). In her leisure time, she enjoys gardening, yoga, cooking, meditation, and chi gong.

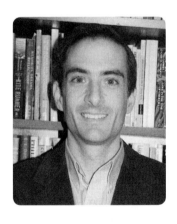

Hank Dart, MS, is a health communications consultant who works in prevention and control for the Siteman Cancer Center at Washington University School of Medicine. He has worked for nearly 20 years in health communication and health education, both on the federal level and in academia. He managed the education component of the *Eat Well & Keep Moving* study, and he developed all the educational materials for the program. He also managed the development of the popular health risk assessment Web site *Your Disease Risk*, and he coauthored a book titled *Healthy Women, Healthy Lives*. In his spare time, he enjoys trail running, Nordic skiing, and "writing mediocre poetry."

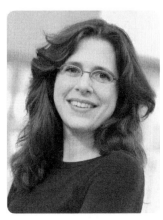

Sari Kalin, MS, is a program coordinator in the department of nutrition at Harvard School of Public Health, where she manages the Nutrition Source, a Web site that explores the latest science on healthy eating. A professional writer and editor for more than 15 years, she recently contributed to a forthcoming textbook for graduate students, *Nutrition in the Lifecycle: An Evidence-Based Approach*. She was the 2006 recipient of a Schweitzer fellowship to work with Operation Frontline in Boston, where she taught nutrition and cooking classes to adults and youth in underserved communities. She enjoys gardening, fitness walking, cooking healthy foods, and playing jazz piano.

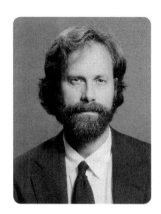

Steven L. Gortmaker, PhD, is a professor of the practice of health sociology at the Harvard School of Public Health, where he has been a faculty member for 30 years. He directs the Harvard School of Public Health Prevention Research Center, whose mission is to design, implement, and evaluate programs that improve physical activity and nutrition, reduce overweight, and decrease chronic disease risk among children. He was the coprincipal investigator for the original *Eat Well & Keep Moving* controlled trial in Baltimore Public Schools, and he has more than 120 research publications to his credit. He helped develop the first school curriculum that proved, through a randomized controlled trial, to reduce obesity prevalence among girls. This middle school curriculum—*Planet Health*—focuses on improving diet, increasing physical activity, and reducing television viewing. He enjoys playing sports with his family, golfing, playing tennis, hiking, and reading.

CD-ROM Contents

▶ *EAT WELL & KEEP MOVING, SECOND EDITION* TEXTBOOK (PDF VERSION)

▶ MANUALS

Acknowledgments
Contributors
Manual 1:   Program Overview
Manual 2:   Education Guide
Manual 3:   Parent and Community Involvement Guide
Manual 4:   Food Service Guide
Writers

To see how the *Eat Well & Keep Moving* classroom lessons match up to educational frameworks in your state, visit the *Eat Well & Keep Moving* Web site, www.eatwellandkeepmoving.org

▶ TRAINING SESSIONS

Training 1	Introduction—Nutrition Education and Wellness Training for Food Service Staff
Training 1	Module 1 PowerPoint—Let's *Eat Well & Keep Moving:* An Introduction to the Program
Training 1	Module 1 PDF of Slides—Let's *Eat Well & Keep Moving:* An Introduction to the Program*
Training 1	Module 1 PDF of Talking Points—Let's *Eat Well & Keep Moving:* An Introduction to the Program
Training 1	Module 2 PowerPoint—The Good Life—Wellness
Training 1	Module 2 PDF of Slides—The Good Life—Wellness*
Training 1	Module 2 PDF of Talking Points—The Good Life—Wellness
Training 1	Module 3 PowerPoint—*Eat Well & Keep Moving* Principles of Healthy Living
Training 1	Module 3 PDF of Slides—*Eat Well & Keep Moving* Principles of Healthy Living*
Training 1	Module 3 PDF of Talking Points—*Eat Well & Keep Moving* Principles of Healthy Living
Training 1	Module 4 PowerPoint—Tour de Health and Nutrition Facts
Training 1	Module 4 PDF of Slides—Tour de Health and Nutrition Facts*
Training 1	Module 4 PDF of Talking Points—Tour de Health and Nutrition Facts
Training 1	Lunch Break PowerPoint—*Eat Well & Keep Moving* Lunch Break
Training 1	Lunch Break PDF of Slides—*Eat Well & Keep Moving* Lunch Break*
Training 1	Lunch Break PDF of Talking Points—*Eat Well & Keep Moving* Lunch Break

*Print and copy these Slides on transparencies if a computer with a projector is not available.

▶ WEB SITES FOR HEALTHY EATING AND ACTIVE LIVING

*Print and copy these Slides on transparencies if a computer with a projector is not available.

▶ PARENT NEWSLETTER ARTICLES

Fat in Foods

Fruits and Veggies

Keep Moving!

Parent Newsletter Articles

Stay Cool

Be Sugar Smart

Super Snacks

Tune Out the TV

Whole Grains

▶ FACT SHEETS

Activate Your Family!

Dietary Fats

Eat More Whole Grains…

Fruits and Vegetables

Healthy Snacks

Take Control of TV

Activate Your Family (Spanish)

Dietary Fats (Spanish)

Fruits and Vegetable (Spanish)

Take Control of TV (Spanish)

Whole Grains (Spanish)

▶ ADDITIONAL RESOURCES

Background

The Balanced Plate for Health

Basic Cuts

Breakout

Brochure

Cycle Menu

Food Facts

Food Group Examples

Food Ovals

Food Waste

Getting Acquainted

Lifestyle Change Card

Menu Boards

Menu Cards

Needs Assessment

Numbers

Principles of Healthy Living

Recipes

Stress Test

Student Survey

Tips

Transparency Presentation PowerPoint

Transparency Presentation PDF of Slides

Transparency Presentation PDF of Talking Points

Vendor Letter

Weights and Measures

Wellness Bell

Wellness Session Introduction

Wellness Session PowerPoint

Wellness Session PDF of Slides

Wellness Session PDF of Talking Points

▶ ART

Menu Board

Stir Fry With Healthy Fat!

What's the New Food? It's Chunky Vegetable Stew

To Nourish Your Body as Well as Your Soul . . . At Least
    5 A Day Should Be Your Goal!

Calcium Is Right for Pearly Whites!

Oranges for Each Day's Journey

Punch Out Fruit Punch—Pick Whole Fruit

Have You Ever Heard of Pineapple Oranges?

Have a Little Slice of Spring

What a Treat to Eat a Sweet Peach!

Pick Peppers

A Message From Bobby Broccoli

What's the New Food? It's Sweet Potatoes and Orange Juice

That's One Sweet Potato!

Cool Beans

Great Ways to Eat Beans

Bulgur Facts

What's the New Food? Tabbouleh
The Power of Whole Grains
Whole Wheat Bread Versus White Bread
Amber Waves of Grain
A Piece of the Pie?
Be Wise . . . Warm Up for 5 Before You Exercise
Brown Rice Pilaf
Caribbean Chicken on Brown Rice
Chicken Stir-Fry With Vegetables on Brown Rice
Pizza Primavera
Vegetable Chili
Chicken Gyro With Cucumber Sauce on Whole Wheat Pita
Tarragon Tuna Whole Wheat Pita Pocket
Turkey and Cheese Roll-Up
Herbed Broccoli and Cauliflower Polonaise
Chunky Vegetable Stew
Sweet Potatoes and Orange Juice
Seasoned Collards
Marinated Black Bean Salad
Hummus
Peach Salsa
Tabbouleh

▶ RECIPES

Recipe List
Caribbean Chicken on Brown Rice
Chicken Stir-Fry With Vegetables on Brown Rice
Pizza Primavera
Vegetable Chili
Chicken Gyro With Cucumber Sauce on Whole Wheat Pita
Tarragon Tuna Pita Pocket
Turkey and Cheese Roll-Up
Herbed Broccoli and Cauliflower Polonaise
Brown Rice Pilaf
Chunky Vegetable Stew
Peach Salsa
Sweet Potatoes and Orange Juice
Seasoned Collards
Hummus
Marinated Black Bean Salad
Tabbouleh
Chunky Typhoon Dip

CD-ROM User Instructions

System Requirements

You can use this CD-ROM on either a Windows®-based PC or a Macintosh computer.

Windows

- IBM PC compatible with Pentium® processor
- Windows® 98/2000/XP/Vista
- Adobe Reader® 8.0
- Microsoft® PowerPoint® Viewer 97
- 4x CD-ROM drive

Macintosh

- Power Mac® recommended
- System 9.x or higher
- Adobe Reader® 8.0
- Microsoft® PowerPoint® Viewer OS9 or OS10
- 4x CD-ROM drive

User Instructions

Windows

1. Insert the *Eat Well & Keep Moving CD-ROM.* (Note: The CD-ROM must be present in the drive at all times.)
2. Select the "My Computer" icon from the desktop.
3. Select the CD-ROM drive.
4. Open the file you wish to view. See the "start.pdf" file for a list of the contents.

Macintosh

1. Insert the *Eat Well & Keep Moving CD-ROM.* (Note: The CD-ROM must be present in the drive at all times.)
2. Double-click the CD icon located on the desktop.
3. Open the file you wish to view. See the "start.pdf" file for a list of the contents.

For customer support, contact Technical Support:

Phone: 217-351-5076 Monday through Friday (excluding holidays) between 7:00 a.m. and 7:00 p.m. (CST).
Fax: 217-351-2674
E-mail: support@hkusa.com

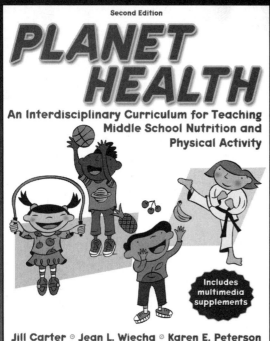